THE ILLUSTRATED HORSE'S FOOT

A COMPREHENSIVE GUIDE

CHRISTOPHER C. POLLITT, BVSC, PHD

Honorary Professor of Equine Medicine
School of Veterinary Science
The University of Queensland
Brisbane, Australia

ELSEVIER

ELSEVIER

3251 Riverport Lane
St. Louis, Missouri 63043

THE ILLUSTRATED HORSE'S FOOT: A COMPREHENSIVE GUIDE   ISBN: 978-0-7020-4655-1

Notices

Knowledge and best practice in this field are constantly changing. As new research and experience broaden our understanding, changes in research methods, professional practices, or medical treatment may become necessary.

Practitioners and researchers must always rely on their own experience and knowledge in evaluating and using any information, methods, compounds, or experiments described herein. In using such information or methods they should be mindful of their own safety and the safety of others, including parties for whom they have a professional responsibility.

With respect to any drug or pharmaceutical products identified, readers are advised to check the most current information provided (i) on procedures featured or (ii) by the manufacturer of each product to be administered, to verify the recommended dose or formula, the method and duration of administration, and contraindications. It is the responsibility of practitioners, relying on their own experience and knowledge of their patients, to make diagnoses, to determine dosages and the best treatment for each individual patient, and to take all appropriate safety precautions.

To the fullest extent of the law, neither the Publisher nor the authors, contributors, or editors, assume any liability for any injury and/or damage to persons or property as a matter of products liability, negligence or otherwise, or from any use or operation of any methods, products, instructions, or ideas contained in the material herein.

International Standard Book Number: 978-0-7020-4655-1

Content Strategy Director: Penny Rudolph
Content Development Manager: Jolynn Gower
Publishing Services Manager: Julie Eddy
Project Manager: Abigail Bradberry
Designer: Amy Buxton

To Sandra, my soulmate and mother of my children, Benjamin and Jane, my love and gratitude for running our home while writing this book made me an absentee husband, parent, and now grandparent. As a fellow scientist and writer, Sandra also proofread all the drafts and improved my grammar, syntax, and punctuation with meticulous skill.

When I was 14, my father, Cal, bought me my first camera, and from my mother, Mabel, I scrounged up the money to buy ever-increasing quantities of film, processing chemicals, and printing paper. To them I am grateful for nurturing my love of photography and for being the caring parents who made it possible for me to become a veterinarian.

To Keith Swan, my first farrier colleague, who transformed so many horses' feet with his skill and showed me the meaning of balance. We, and the farriers he taught, have learned much from each other.

My friend and veterinary colleague, Dr. Don Walsh, Director of the Animal Health Foundation, Missouri, USA, shares my quest to understand the horse's foot and laminitis, and he is thanked for allocating precious, donated funds for many postgraduate students and me to pursue years of productive scientific research.

Finally, Dr. Simon Collins introduced me to Mimics software and shared his passion and superior skill to create virtual 3-D anatomic models of horsefoot anatomy and pathology. The images he created advanced understanding for a new generation and will be his legacy; many are presented for the first time in this book. Simon passed away in 2014 and is deeply missed. May his busy, brilliant, eccentric mind now be at peace.

Preface

In an earlier version of this book, entitled *Color Atlas of the Horse's Foot*, the photography required film to produce color slides, and the text was either handwritten or dictated and subsequently typed. This was before digital photography and word processing. Now, my Nikon D200 and various Nikkor lenses are used to create high-resolution digital photographs processed using Adobe Photoshop CS6. Using a well-lit tabletop studio to photograph specimens enhanced sharpness, and depth of field was achieved using focus stacking software (www.heliconsoft.com). Uniform color balance was maintained by incorporating a grayscale in each composition for later Photoshop processing. An Olympus BX50 microscope, coupled with a Tucsen digital camera and ISCapture V3.6 software (www.tucsen.com), was used to create the photomicrographs, again with Helicon 6 focus stacking software. A big step forward, and a major incentive to illustrate the horse's foot again, was being able create three-dimensional models from computed tomography (CT) and magnetic resonance (MR) data using Mimics software (www.materialise.com). Simon Collins's infectious enthusiasm for the value of the Mimics horse foot models inspired their use throughout this book.

This book is intended to supplement, not replace, the major textbooks on equine lameness, anatomy, and surgery, which often dedicate little space for figures. The major texts should be studied in tandem with *The Illustrated Horse's Foot* with the expectation that conditions and problems are better understood when clearly and comprehensively illustrated.

Thus, this illustrated text will provide the student of the horse's foot (whether veterinarian, farrier, trimmer, or the informed horse owner) with the means to more fully appreciate and understand equine foot anatomy and the problems associated with it. Much folklore and fallacy surround mankind's association with the horse, but nowhere more so than with the foot. Much confabulated nonsense has become entrenched dogma and, having entered the literature, is now difficult to counter with logic.

> *It isn't until late in life—if ever—that most of us learn not to argue with the Unconvincibles. In Grandma's famous phrase, we might as well save our breath to cool our porridge.*
> **SYDNEY J. HARRIS**

The spirit of taking a fresh look at the horse's foot and sifting fact from fiction is embodied in the philosophy of this book. Facts and evidence are presented from which readers can draw their own conclusions, just as Darwin's theory of evolution by natural selection never needed proof because the evidence was overwhelmingly convincing.

The resolution of horse foot problems will often depend on collaboration among veterinarian, farrier, trimmer, and the horse's owner. This book should provide information for all the foot-care professions and thus promote greater mutual understanding and cooperation. This should benefit not only the horse but also its owner. It is envisaged that the illustrations in this book will be used to communicate information among all concerned. With better communication should come greater understanding and better relations between the professions and their clients.

A particular effort has been made to illustrate foot problems using case histories to enable readers to see for themselves what actually happened—for better or for worse. Brief details of the treatments are supplied to put the case history in its context.

The major blood vessels of the foot have been injected with contrast medium, colored latex, polyurethane, or acrylic and then dissected (virtually or in reality) so that their relationships with other structures are clearly depicted. My research into the microcirculation of the foot dermis using the technique of corrosion casting and scanning electron microscopy is again shown, but this time enhanced with digital colorization.

This book has sprung from my compulsion as a university lecturer in equine medicine to gather material with which to teach and communicate. My photographic record of the horse's foot, over the past 35 years of my teaching career, is the cornerstone of this book. I am grateful to Elsevier for their patience in persevering with me during the gestation of this book—perhaps its welcome birth will see the concept grow to be authored by others following in our footsteps. With the current ubiquity and ease of digital photography, this should not be too difficult.

A journalist once wrote to ask what made a good investigator of the horse's foot. I wrote this in reply:

People who care about horses and especially their feet come from all walks of life. They need to be well educated, but can be self-taught through reading and learning from others. An ability to think in pictures (like Einstein) rather than in the abstract is vital—understanding the three-dimensional foot in the mind's eye is difficult but essential—few really get it. An empathy with horse behavior is a must. Working with relaxed horses gets you far—with the horse and its owner. Perhaps most important is to be rational—absorb information from all sources, analyze it, and draw your own common (horse)-sense conclusions. Don't be an irrational acolyte to anyone—treat self-proclaimed gurus with analytical suspicion—make your own trail but look back and make corrections when necessary. The one scientific principle that really needs to be acquired is the understanding of "evidence." Believe nobody until you are persuaded by the results of controlled trials.

People have a great aversion to intellectual labor; but even supposing knowledge to be easily attainable, more people would be content to be ignorant than would take even a little trouble to acquire it.

ENRICO FERMI (1901–1954)

Christopher C. Pollitt, BVSc, PhD

No hour of life is wasted that is spent in the saddle.

WINSTON CHURCHILL

Acknowledgments

Over the years, many horse owners have generously donated the feet of their euthanized horses so that they could be photographed, scanned, dissected, and analyzed; some of this material is presented here. This is not always easy to do when the horse is a treasured companion, so I and the readers of this book are grateful for such foresight. The expectation is that others will learn from the case histories presented herein with better outcomes for horses in the future. One particular horse owner, Ms. Talea Bongers (encouraged by her friend, Stephanie Rutherford), shared the details of Case History 4 in Chapter 14, and she is especially thanked. In addition, the veterinarians, farriers, and hoof trimmers who shared case material and gave access to records, photographs, and radiographs are sincerely thanked; without them, this would have been a lesser book.

Introduction

The modern horse foot is an impressive example of evolutionary bioengineering.[1-3] A detailed fossil record tracing 52 million years of evolution shows numerous extinct branches to the Equid evolutionary lineage with the modern equids (horses, donkeys, zebras, onagers, kiangs, and Przewalski's horse) the only ones to survive.[5] Their specialized feet, along with other anatomic and physiologic adaptions, enabled this survival by playing an important part in fitting the horse to the ever-changing environment of planet Earth.

The horse foot makes contact with the ground via hooves (ungulae) that encase only the third finger or toe bone, on the end of each of their four limbs. Locomotion on hooves makes horses unguligrade, like other ungulates such as cattle, camels, and rhinoceroses. This is quite different from plantigrade humans, walking on the padded bones of their tarsal, metatarsal, and phalangeal bones—the human ankle is the anatomic equivalent of the horse hock. The horse's terminal finger bone (or toe bone in the rear limbs) is called the *distal phalanx* and is encased in a tough, horny capsule, the equivalent of our fingernail. It is more precise to say that the horse makes four-legged contact with the ground on just four modified finger (or toe) nails. Horses belong to the order Perissodactyla (odd-toed ungulates,) and having just one uncloven hoof means they are solipeds (unlike the other Perissodactyla, rhinoceroses and tapirs, which have three), making the Equidae unique in the animal kingdom. The tough hoof capsule protects the softer, more sensitive structures within, allowing the horse to gallop over dry, abrasive rocky terrain, usually with impunity. Modern equids, despite being relatively large animals (an adult Thoroughbred weighs around 450 kg), move with great speed and agility. Having single digits, encased in tough hooves, on the end of relatively lightweight limbs, endows speed and versatility to the unguligrade horse.

However, this comes at a price. Exploiting an evolutionary niche, which is successful most of the time, horses are extremely dependent on the health of a complex suspensory apparatus between the distal phalanx and their hooves. Failure of attachment between skeleton and hoof and subsequent descent of the distal phalanx (as occurs with the foot disease laminitis or founder) cripples the horse, and this is evidence that a suspensory apparatus of the distal phalanx (SADP) exists.

Considerable selection pressure for a reliable SADP (and thus against laminitis) must have existed among ancestral Equidae, as a foundered animal would quickly attract the attention of predators. In fact, it can be argued that laminitis results from the association of horses with humans, as it is commonly the artificial environment and inappropriate diet that results in the development of the disease. This applies not only to the starch-laden grains[4] but also to carbohydrate-rich pastures, selected to maximize sheep and cattle production, that our horses consume.[6] Equids are normally mobile and athletic, but when they develop laminitis and become crippled, we realize, belatedly, how dependent they are on an intact, functional, pain-free foot.

References

1. Pollitt, C.C. (1992). Clinical anatomy and physiology of the normal equine foot. *Equine Vet, 4,* 219–224.
2. Pollitt, C.C. (1998). The anatomy and physiology of the hoof wall. *Equine Vet Education, 10,* 318–325.
3. Pollitt, C.C. (2004). Anatomy and physiology of the hoof wall. *Clinical Techniques in Equine Practice, 4,* 3–21.
4. Pollitt, C.C., Visser, M.B. (2010). Carbohydrate alimentary overload laminitis. Veterinary clinics of North America. *Equine Practice, 26,* 65–78.
5. Simpson, G.G. (1951). *Horses: the story of the horse family in the modern world and through sixty million years of history.* New York: Oxford University Press.
6. Watts, K. (2010). Pasture Management to Minimize the Risk of Equine Laminitis. *Veterinary Clinics of North America-Equine Practice, 26,* 361–369.

Contents

Foot Structure and Function

The *hoof,* or *ungula,* is a term sometimes used to describe the whole foot,[1] but in this text the International Committee on Veterinary Gross Anatomical Nomenclature (1994)[1,2] will be followed, and *hoof* will mean the cornified epidermis, the dermis, and the tela subcutanea (subcutaneous tissue) of the foot.[2,5,16]

The hoof is shaped like a truncated cone (a cone without an apex) and encapsulates the inner structures of the foot. The equine hoof is one of the most complex and specialized integumentary structures in the animal kingdom.[3] The distal rim of the hoof wall is the load-bearing border. The wall can be divided into three sections: the *stratum externum* (periople), the *stratum medium* (the tubular bulk of the hoof wall), and the *stratum internum* (the primary and secondary epidermal lamellae [SELs]). The term *stratum lamellatum* is sometimes used interchangeably with *stratum internum,* but used correctly *lamellatum* refers to both dermal and epidermal lamellae. An alternate nomenclature notates the hoof wall according to the tissues from which it is proliferated. Thus coronary horn (the *stratum medium*) derives from the coronary segment, periople (*stratum externum*) from the perioplic segment, terminal horn (the white line) from terminal papillae, and the epidermal lamellae (*stratum internum*) from the wall segment.[11]

THE HOOF WALL

The wall of the hoof is topographically divided into a frontal region (the toe), the lateral or medial sides (the quarters), and palmar (plantar) to the heels (see Figures 2-1, 2-2, 2-3, 2-4, 2-5 and 2-6). The proximal heels are called the *heel bulbs.* In front feet the toe is three times taller than the heels; in hind feet the ratio is 2:1.[11] A line drawn from the proximal border of the toe to the heel (the coronary band angle) slopes at an angle of approximately 20 degrees relative to the ground surface.[10]

The *Stratum Externum* (Periople)

The *stratum externum* or periople (also, limbus = edge or border between two parts) consists of a narrow band of soft, flexible horn, yellowish-white in color, which joins the hairy skin to the hard horn of the *stratum medium* (Figure 1-1). At the toe it

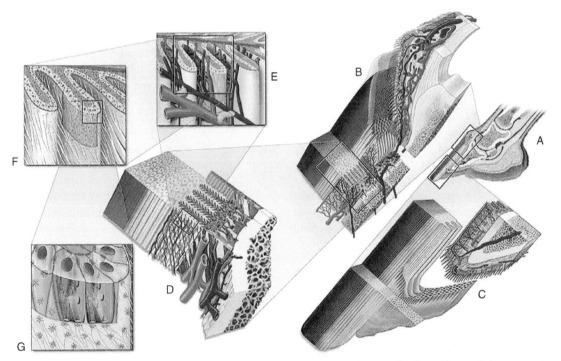

● **Figure 1.1** Hierarchical chart of the structures illustrated in the following chapters. Starting with an artistic representation of the classic sagittal section (A and Figure 5.4) the coronary band region is then detailed in a three dimensional format (B and Figure 3-4). Moving distally is a diagram of the terminal papillae at the epidermal sole-wall junction and how they form the white line (C and Figure 7-30). At higher magnification the lamellar circulation and its relationship to the parietal surface of the distal phalanx, the sublamellar connective tissue and the epidermal lamellae are illustrated (D and Figure 7-26). The lamellar microcirculation is illustrated next in a figure showing the arteriovenous anastomoses between axial arteries and veins and the lamellar capillaries within the secondary dermal lamellae (E and Figure 7-44). At higher magnification still the epidermal basal cells of secondary epidermal lamellae, the lamellar basement membrane and the collagen filaments of suspensory apparatus of the distal phalanx attached to the basement membrane are shown (F and Figure 2-13). Finally, the most important cell of the entire hoof system, the epidermal basal cell, is illustrated to show the ultrastructure of its attachments to the basement membrane and to the cells around it (G and Figure 8-21).

bulges forward (dorsally) and projects downward (distally) over the hard *stratum medium* for a few millimeters. The periople becomes white and obvious when the foot has been soaked in water. The hard edge of the proximal *stratum medium* can be palpated through the soft periople. This landmark is important clinically because it forms the proximal limit of the *stratum medium* and, identified with a radiopaque marker on lateral-medial radiographs, is used to estimate the vertical distance between proximal hoof wall and the dorsal limit of the extensor process of the distal phalanx—the so-called founder distance.[9]

The periople is narrow in horses living in natural conditions; the distal parts get abraded away as the hoof makes contact with sticks, stones, and sandy substrates in its environment. Horses kept in stables or on soft bedding, such as straw and wood shavings, may have a very long periople, covering up to half of the hoof wall.

The *Stratum Medium* (Coronary Horn)

The *stratum medium* is the thickest of the three layers and is characterized by its tubular and intertubular horn structure (Figure 1-1). It is the main load-transmission platform of the equine limb and serves to transfer ground reaction forces to the bony skeleton.

Examination of the hoof capsule, with its contents removed, shows thousands of small, circular holes pocking the surface of the concave, coronary groove. A sagittal section of the proximal hoof wall shows that the holes continue distally into the body of the wall a distance of 4 to 5 mm, tapering to a point, thus forming a socket. A layer of confluent epidermal basal cells covers the surface of the sockets and the surface of the coronary groove between the sockets. Coronary basal cells undergo mitosis throughout the life of the horse, producing *stratum medium* daughter cells that mature and cornify, undertaking a journey, up to eight months in duration, in the direction of the ground surface. Cornifying keratinocytes, arising from basal cells lining the sockets, become organized into thin, elongated cylinders or tubules approximately 0.2 mm in diameter. The basal cells between the sockets also proliferate to produce intertubular horn that embeds the tubules. The surfaces of the periople, terminal wall horn, sole, and frog also have sockets and a tubular architecture.

The *Stratum Internum* (Epidermal Lamellae)

Projecting from the inner surface of the hoof wall and bars in proximodistal parallel rows are 550 to 600 epidermal lamellae.[6] In common with all epidermal hair and hornlike structures, the lamellae of the inner hoof wall are avascular and depend on the microcirculation in the adjacent lamellar dermis (lamellar corium) to supply nutrients. The epidermal cells adjacent to the dermis (the lamellar epidermal basal cells, or LEBCs) are especially important because it is these cells that maintain a vital attachment, via collagenous connective tissue, to the parietal (outer) surface of the distal phalanx. The attachment between LEBCs and the distal phalanx is known as the suspensory apparatus of the distal phalanx. As their anatomic name suggests, the lamellar epidermal basal cells are expected to be germinative or proliferative cell layer, but interestingly, this is not the case with the basal cells of the lamellae. They do not proliferate to any great extent, in sharp contrast to the epidermal basal cells of the coronet and sole, which proliferate continuously to form the tough, but flexible, hoof wall and sole, respectively. The primary function of the lamellar basal cells therefore is to suspend the distal phalanx within the hoof capsule.[14a] A proportion of the lamellar basal cells comprises p63-expressing stem cells,[4] ready to proliferate should the hoof wall be injured and healing is required.

Secondary Epidermal Lamellae

Microscopic examination of the inner hoof wall shows that the surface area of the lamellae is further expanded by the addition of secondary lamellae upon each primary lamella. At the toe there are about 125 to 150 secondary lamellae along the length of each primary lamella. Fewer SELs are present at the heels and bars, approximately 95 and 82, respectively. The axial tips of the lamellae (both primary and secondary) point toward the distal phalanx, indicating the direction of the tension to which the lamellar suspensory apparatus is subject. The surface area of the equine inner hoof wall has been calculated to average just under 1 square meter,[6] which is a considerable increase over the bovine hoof that lacks secondary lamellae.

The Basement Membrane

At the interface of the lamellar epidermis and dermis is a tough, unbroken sheet of connective tissue called the *basement membrane*. This key structure is the bridge attaching the basal cells of the lamellar hoof epidermis on one side and the tough connective tissue (tendonlike collagen) on the parietal surface of the distal phalanx on the other. The basement membrane is constructed of a unique, fibrillar collagen called *type IV collagen*. Woven into the matlike type IV collagen framework is laminin, one of several basement membrane glycoproteins. It forms receptor sites and ligands for a complex array of growth factors, cytokines, adhesion molecules, and integrins that together direct the functional behavior of the epidermis. Without an intact, functional basement membrane, the epidermis, to which it is normally firmly attached, falls into disarray.

Hemidesmosomes

The lamellar basement membrane is attached to the feet or base of the epidermal basal cells at discrete sites called hemidesmosomes. Hemidesmosomes resemble "spot-welds" on sheet metal and are attachment discs that serve to keep the sheet of basement membrane firmly adhered to all the basal cells of the lamellar hoof. Each hemidesmosome is constructed of several proteins that stain darkly when viewed with the transmission electron microscope. Bridging the gap between the dense plaque of the hemidesmosome and the basement membrane proper (the *lamina densa*) are numerous submicroscopic anchoring filaments. Each filament consists of a single glycoprotein molecule called laminin-332, which is unique to hemidesmosomes. If either the anchoring filaments or the hemidesmosomes are damaged and made to disintegrate, the basement membrane separates from the basal cell.

Basal Cell Cytoskeleton

Within the cytoplasm of each basal cell is a criss-crossing network of fine keratin filaments that make up part of the internal skeleton (cytoskeleton) of the cell. The cytoskeleton bestows rigidity and the correct shape to the cell. All of the cellular organelles (mitochondria, Golgi apparatus, endoplasmic reticulum), as well as the all-important nucleus, are suspended and fixed to the three-dimensional lattice of the keratin cytoskeleton. Where the keratin cytoskeleton approaches the basal wall of the cell adjacent to the basement membrane, it is woven into the disc of the hemidesmosome. Where the cytoskeleton approaches the inner side and top walls of the cell, adjacent to the neighboring basal cells and parabasal cells, it is woven into the discs of the desmosomes. Thus the keratin cytoskeleton forms a direct line of communication between neighboring cells, the basement membrane, and the exterior. Actin is also part of the cytoskeleton and joins the side walls of the basal cells together via an attachment plaque called the *adherens junction.*

If damage should occur to the hemidesmosomes, desmosomes, adherens junctions, or the basement membrane, the basal cell cytoskeleton collapses and the basal cell is cut off from the information that controls its normal shape and proper function. Under these circumstances the basal cell may also separate from its basement membrane and from its neighbors, stretch, and deform, leading to collapse of the suspensory apparatus of the distal phalanx: the hallmark lesion of laminitis.

HOOF WALL GROWTH

The hoof wall grows throughout the life of the horse to replace hoof lost to wear and tear at the ground surface. Continual regeneration of the hoof wall occurs at the coronet where germinal cells (epidermal basal cells) produce populations of daughter cells (keratinocytes or keratin-producing cells), which mature and keratinize, continually adding to the proximal hoof wall. Similarly, mitosis in the proximal hoof primary epidermal lamellae (PELs) also occurs.[12] Although mitotic figures (MFs) among the basal cells of the proximal lamellar zone are easily observed, there is no convincing evidence that the more distal lamellae proliferate to the same extent. The fundamental question is: how do the inner hoof wall lamellae remain attached to the connective tissue embedded on the surface of the stationary distal phalanx, while one moves over the other? Is it by continuous proliferation of the lamellar epidermis (laminar flow) or by some other remodeling process that may somehow be involved in laminitis pathogenesis?

Cells in mitosis are infrequent in normal lamellae below the proximal, proliferative zone. To determine precisely where in the hoof wall epidermal cell proliferation occurs, a proliferative index (PI) for basal cells of the coronet, lamellae,

and toe of the dorsal hoof wall of ponies was calculated.[7] The thymidine analog (5-bromo-2-deoxyuridine, or BRdU), injected intravenously into living ponies, was incorporated into all cells undergoing mitosis, during a 1-hour study period. Histologic sections of hoof tissue were stained immunohistochemically, using monoclonal antibodies against BRdU. As expected, the highest proliferative rates (mean $\pm$ standard error) were in the coronet: 12.04% $\pm$ 1.59 and proximal lamellae (7.13% $\pm$ 1.92). These are the growth zones of the proximal hoof wall.

Distal to this, proliferative rates in more distal lamellae were very much lower. They ranged from 0.11% $\pm$ 0.04 to 0.97% $\pm$ 0.29, significantly lower ($P < 0.05$) than the proximal lamellar growth zone. Evidence for a constant supply of new cells in the lamellar region, generating a downward laminar flow, was not provided by this study. A twentyfold proliferative rate decrease between proximal and more distal lamellae suggests that the majority of the normal lamellae are nonproliferative and their main function is to suspend the distal phalanx within the hoof capsule. More recently, in laminitis validation studies, a similar low rate of proliferation in normal lamellae was documented using immunohistochemistry, specifically, the proliferative marker TPX2.[8]

Similar proliferation and keratinization occur in the tubular horn production of the white line, frog, and sole. The epidermal basal cells of the distal lamellae proliferate rapidly to form the tubular and intertubular horn of the white line. This new horn surrounds and incorporates the keratinized axis of the primary epidermal lamellae, bestowing a characteristic appearance to the white zone.

Remodeling within the hoof wall epidermal lamellae, which must occur as the hoof wall moves past the stationary distal phalanx, appears to be a process not requiring mitosis.

The molecular components of desmosomes, hemidesmosomes, and basement membranes are substrates for matrix metalloproteinase activity, so the mechanistic concept[13] of "formation and destruction of desmosomes in a staggered ratchet-like manner" now has a well-referenced, biological explanation.

Lamellar epidermal cells and their adjacent basement membrane are constantly responding to the stresses and strains of growth and locomotion by releasing proteases and intrinsic inhibitors to accomplish whatever cellular reorganization is required. Because this involves enzymes capable of destroying key components of the attachment apparatus between distal phalanx and inner hoof wall, it is clear that triggering this "loaded gun" will have dire consequences for the future health of the foot. Inadvertent or uncontrolled lamellar protease activation makes unguligrade horses, with their generic reliance on a single digit per limb, uniquely susceptible to the destructive effects of laminitis. Interestingly, laminitis can be stopped in its tracks if global enzyme activity in the foot is inhibited by cooling the distal limb to around 5° C.[17]

THE DERMIS

The highly vascular dermis (corium) underlies the hoof wall and consists of a dense matrix of tough connective tissue containing a network of arteries, veins, and capillaries, and sensory and vasomotor nerves. All parts of the dermis, except for the lamellar dermis, have papillae that fit tightly into the sockets in the adjacent hoof. The lamellar dermis has dermal lamellae that interlock with the epidermal lamellae of the inner hoof wall and bars. The vascular system within the dermis provides the hoof with nourishment. The dense matrix of dermal connective tissue connects the basement membrane of the dermal–epidermal junction to the parietal surface of the distal phalanx and thus suspends the distal phalanx from the inner wall of the hoof capsule (the suspensory apparatus of the distal phalanx).

The Coronary Dermis

The coronary dermis fills the coronary groove and blends distally with the lamellar dermis. Its inner surface is attached to the extensor tendon and the ungual cartilages of the distal phalanx by the subcutaneous tissue of the coronary cushion. Collectively the coronary dermis and the germinal epidermal cells that rest on its basement membrane are known as the coronet or coronary band. A feature of the coronary dermis is the large number of hairlike papillae projecting from its surface. Each tapering papilla fits into one of the sockets on the surface of the epidermal coronary groove and, in life, is responsible for nurturing an individual hoof wall tubule.

To explore the microanatomy of the basement membrane its surface was examined with the scanning electron microscope after treatment of hoof tissue blocks with a detergent enzyme mixture.[14] A clean separation could be made between dermal and epidermal tissues, enabling the surface of the dermal basement membrane to be examined in detail. The basement membrane of the coronary and terminal papillae was folded into numerous ridges parallel with the long axis of the papilla.

These longitudinal ridges on the surface of the papillae are analogous to the secondary dermal lamellae and probably share the similar role of increasing the surface area of attachment between the epidermal hoof and the connective tissue on the parietal surface of the distal phalanx. They may also act as guides or channels directing columns of maturing keratinocytes in a correctly oriented proximodistal direction. The density of coronary papillae is greatest at the periphery and least adjacent to the lamellae. This mirrors the arrangement of the hoof wall tubules of the *stratum medium* in zones based on tubule size and density.[15]

The Sole Dermis

As in the coronet, each dermal papilla of the sole dermis fits into a socket in the epidermal (horn) sole. At the distal end of each dermal lamella is a set of papillae known as the *terminal papillae*. The epidermis surrounding the terminal papillae is nonpigmented and forms the inner part of the white zone (white line). The white zone is relatively soft and flexible and effectively "seals" the sole to the hoof wall. It is sometimes subject to degeneration and infection, usually described as "seedy toe" or "white line disease."

References

1. Anon. (2015). *Nomina Anatomica Veterinaria.* Hannover, International Committee on Veterinary Gross Anatomical Nomenclature.
2. Anon. (2012). *Nomina Anatomica Veterinaria.* Hannover: International Committee on Veterinary Gross Anatomical Nomenclature.
3. Bragulla, H., & Hirschberg, R. M. (2003). Horse hooves and bird feathers: Two model systems for studying the structure and development of highly adapted integumentary accessory organs—The role of the dermo-epidermal interface for the micro-architecture of complex epidermal structures. *Journal of Experimental Zoology, 298B,* 140–151.
4. Carter, R. A., Engiles, J. B., Megee, S. O., Senoo, M., & Galantino-Homer, H. L. (2011). Decreased expression of p63, a regulator of epidermal stem cells, in the chronic laminitic equine hoof. *Equine Veterinary Journal, 43,* 543–551.
5. Constantinescu, G. M., & Constantinescu, I. A. (2004). *Clinical dissection guide for large animals: Horse and large ruminants.* St Louis, MO: Mosby-Year Book Inc.
6. Daradka, M. (2000). The Equine Hoof Wall: Growth, Repair and Dimensions. In, *School of Veterinary Science.* Australia: The University of Queensland.
7. Daradka, M., & Pollitt, C. C. (2004). Epidermal cell proliferation in the equine hoof wall. *Equine Veterinary Journal, 36,* 236–241.
8. de Laat, M. A., Patterson-Kane, J. C., Pollitt, C. C., Sillence, M. N., & McGowan, C. M. (2012). Histological and morphometric lesions in the pre-clinical, developmental phase of insulin-induced laminitis in Standardbred horses. *Veterinary Journal, 195,* 305–312.
9. Eustace, R. A., Emery, S. L., & Cripps, P. J. (2012). A retrospective study of 23 cases of coronary band separation longer than 8 cm as a sequel to severe laminitis. *Journal of Equine Veterinary Science, 32,* 235–244.
10. Hampson, B. A., de Laat, M. A., Mills, P. C., & Pollitt, C. C. (2013). The feral horse foot. Part A: Observational study of the effect of environment on the morphometrics of the feet of 100 Australian feral horses. *Australian Veterinary Journal, 91,* 14–22.
11. König, H. E., & Liebich, H.-G. (Eds.), (2009). *Veterinary anatomy of domestic animals.* Stuttgart: Scattauer.
12. Leach, D. H. (1980). *The structure and function of the equine hoof wall.* PhD thesis, University of Saskatchewan—Saskatoon.
13. Leach, D. H., & Oliphant, L. W. (1983). Ultrastructure of the equine hoof wall secondary epidermal lamellae. *American Journal of Veterinary Research, 44,* 1561–1570.
14. Pollitt, C. C. (1994). The basement membrane at the equine hoof dermal epidermal junction. *Equine Veterinary Journal, 26,* 399–407.
14a. Pollitt, C. C. & S. N. Collins (2015). The suspensory apparatus of the distal phalanx in normal horses. *Equine Veterinary Journal.* DOI: 10.1111/evj.12459.
15. Reilly, J. D., Collins, S. N., Cope, B. C., Hopegood, L., & Latham, R. J. (1998). Tubule density of the stratum medium of horse hoof. *Equine Veterinary Journal Supplement, 26,* 4–9.
16. Sack, W. O. (1992). Integumentum commune, Common integument. *Illustrated Veterinary Anatomical Nomenclature.* O. Schaller. Stuttgart, Enke Verlag: 542-561.
17. van Eps, A. W., Leise, B. S., Watts, M., Pollitt, C. C., & Belknap, J. K. (2012). Digital hypothermia inhibits early lamellar inflammatory signalling in the oligofructose laminitis model. *Equine Veterinary Journal, 44,* 230–237.

2 The Hoof Capsule

THE TUBULAR HOOF WALL

At the proximal *stratum medium*, maturing keratinocytes become organized into thin, elongated cylinders (tubules). In cross-section the keratinocytes of individual hoof wall tubules are arranged around a central hollow medulla in nonpigmented concentric layers. Each hairlike tubule is continuous, from its origin at the proximal coronary groove, all the way to the ground surface (a distance of 5 to 15 cm, depending on the breed). The keratinocytes between the hoof wall tubules mature into intertubular hoof, thus forming a keratinized cellular matrix in which tubules are embedded. The intertubular horn is formed at right angles to the tubular horn and bestows on the hoof wall the unique property of a mechanically stable, multidirectional, fiber-reinforced composite.[3]

Interestingly, hoof wall is stiffer and stronger at right angles to the direction of the tubules, a finding at odds with the usual assumption that the ground reaction force is transmitted proximally up the hoof wall parallel to the tubules. The hoof wall appears to be reinforced by the tubules, but it is the intertubular material that accounts for most of its mechanical strength, stiffness, and fracture toughness. The tubules are three times more likely to fracture than intertubular horn.[2,10] The *stratum medium* is considered to have an anatomic design that confers strength in all directions. Unlike bone, which is a living tissue and remodels to become stronger along lines of stress, the *stratum medium* is nonliving tissue, but is anatomically constructed to resist stress in every direction and to never require remodeling. During normal locomotion, the *stratum medium* only experiences one tenth of the compressive force required to cause its structural failure.[12] The basal cell daughters, whether destined to be tubular or intertubular hoof, do not keratinize immediately. As the distance between basal cells and their daughters increases (each generation is pushed further away from the basal cell layer by the production of successive generations), the intracellular skeleton of the maturing cells becomes denser by the manufacture of more intermediate filaments composed of various keratin molecules. Then, by increasing the number of desmosomes, stronger attachment zones are formed between the cell membranes of adjoining keratinocytes. Desmosomes are points of intercellular contact, which function like spot-welds between adjacent cells. Within the cell, keratin intermediate filaments also attach to the desmosomes to form the three-dimensional internal skeleton (the cytoskeleton) of the cell. Thus the keratinocytes transform, becoming sturdier and more durable to stress and strain. The final stage of keratinocyte maturation is abrupt. The cell nucleus fragments and disappears, and the cell is declared officially dead. Granular, densely staining material (membrane-coating granules) migrates through the cytoplasm to be deposited on the outside of the cell as an intercellular cement substance. At this late stage of keratinocyte maturation, the cell loses its nucleus (becomes anuclear), and the cytoplasm is densely packed with tough keratin filaments that interconnect with each other and to the desmosomes. Thus the cell membrane of each cell becomes firmly cemented to its neighbor. Finally, the keratin filaments are embedded in a dense, amorphous matrix, rich in sulfur-containing amino acids (but not keratin), to form the mature corneocyte. The fully keratinized cells (anuclear corneocytes) of the tubular and intertubular hoof, cemented firmly to each other, form a continuum—the tough yet flexible *stratum medium* of the hoof wall. Mature corneocytes, firmly cemented together, form a tough, protective barrier, preventing the passage of water and water-soluble substances inwards, and the loss of body fluids, imparted by the highly vascular dermis, outwards. In addition to acting as a permeability barrier, hoof wall corneocytes, arranged in their specialized tubular and intertubular configuration, have the crucial job of ultimately supporting the entire weight of the horse.

The tubules of the equine hoof wall are not arranged randomly. The tubules of the *stratum medium* are arranged in three distinct zones based on the density of tubules in the intertubular horn.[4] The zone of highest tubule density is the outermost layer, and the density declines stepwise toward the internal lamellar layer. The tubule density gradient across the wall appears to be a mechanism for smooth energy transfer, from the rigid (high tubule density) outer wall to the more plastic (low tubule density) inner wall, and ultimately to the distal phalanx. The gradient in tubule density mirrors the gradient in water content across the hoof wall, and together these factors represent an optimum design for equine hoof wall. Tubule zonation is also a crack-stopping mechanism.[11] The zones confer on the hoof wall the design properties of a laminated composite; the interface between zones absorbs energy and prevents the propagation of cracks toward sensitive inner structures. In addition, the anisotropy (the condition of having greater strength in one direction) of the *stratum medium* ensures that cracks, when they occur, propagate from the bearing surface upward, parallel with the tubules, that is, along the weakest plane. They do not extend to the innermost layers of the hoof wall because in this region the relatively high water content confers high crack resistance.[12] The hoof wall also has a powerful dampening function on vibrations generated when the hoof wall makes contact with the ground during locomotion. It is able to reduce both the frequency and maximal amplitude of the vibrations.[8] By the time the shock of impact with the ground reaches the first phalanx, around 90% of the energy has been dissipated, mainly at the lamellar interface.

The Dermis

The highly vascular corium, or dermis (often referred to as the "quick"), underlies the hoof wall and consists of a dense matrix of tough, connective tissue (tendonlike collagen) containing a network of arteries, veins, and capillaries, and sensory and vasomotor nerves. All parts of the corium, except for the lamellar corium, have papillae that fit tightly into the holes in the adjacent hoof. The lamellar corium has dermal lamellae that interlock with the epidermal lamellae of the inner hoof wall and bars. The corium provides the hoof with nourishment, and its dense matrix of connective tissue connects the basement membrane of the dermal-epidermal junction to the periosteal surface of the distal phalanx and thus suspends the distal phalanx from the inner wall of the hoof capsule—the suspensory apparatus of the distal phalanx.

The Coronary Dermis

The coronary dermis fills the coronary groove and blends with the lamellar dermis of the inner hoof wall. Its inner surface is firmly attached to the extensor tendon and the cartilages of the distal phalanx. Thus, wherever the distal phalanx goes, the coronary band goes with it. This fact becomes important when laminitis precipitates a downward displacement of the distal phalanx. Collectively, the coronary dermis and the germinal epidermal cells that rest upon its basement membrane are known as the coronary band. A feature of the coronary corium is the large number of hairlike papillae projecting from its surface. In life each tapering papilla fits snugly into a hole on the surface of the epidermal coronary groove. Each papilla is responsible for nurturing an individual hoof wall tubule.

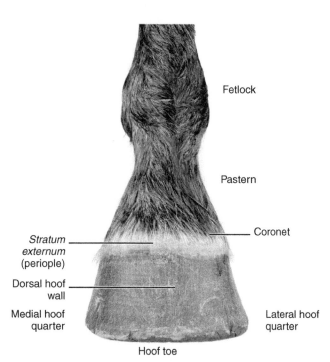

• **Figure 2.1** Surface anatomy of the dorsal aspect of a normal distal forelimb. The horse was an unbroken, three-year-old Australian Stock Horse with a body weight of 420 kg. The horse was running in rocky, mountainous terrain, and the hooves had never been trimmed. The attributes of the hoof are the result of interaction with the environment and an active lifestyle. Typically the medial and lateral hoof wall angles differ as the medial being steeper than the lateral. Here the medial is 74° and the lateral 69°, both angle less acute than the medial and lateral hoof wall angles of the Australian feral horses studied by Hampson et al.[9]

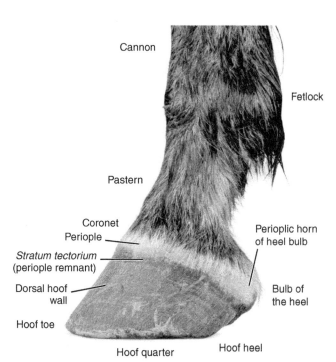

• **Figure 2.2** Surface anatomy of the lateral aspect of a normal distal forelimb from the same horse as in figure 2.1. The dorsal hoof wall angle is 53° similar to the dorsal hoof wall angles (mean 52.4 ± 2.4) of Australian feral horses from similar country.[9] The foot had been soaked in water so the periople is opaque. Distal to the periople and extending a few millimeters down the hoof wall is the shiny remnant of the periople, the *stratum tectorium.*

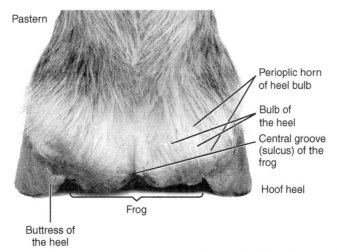

Pastern

Perioplic horn
of heel bulb

Bulb of
the heel

Central groove
(sulcus) of the
frog

Hoof heel

Frog

Buttress of
the heel

• **Figure 2.3** Surface anatomy of the palmar aspect of a normal distal forelimb from the same horse as in figure 2.1. The heel buttresses are well developed with straight tubules and are platform for the palmar ground contact. The frog is broad and does not make contact with the ground. The mean distance between the frog and the ground surface in feral horses from similar country was 2.30 ± 1.6 cm.[9]

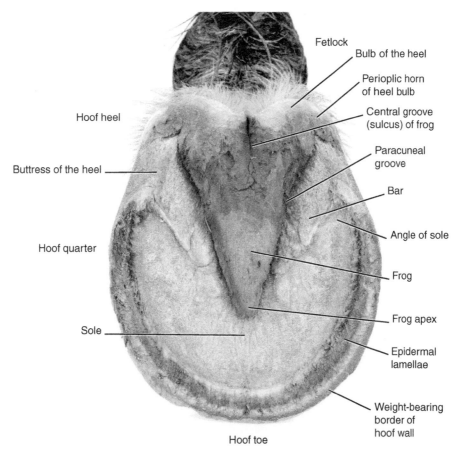

Fetlock

Bulb of the heel

Perioplic horn
of heel bulb

Central groove
(sulcus) of frog

Paracuneal
groove

Bar

Angle of sole

Frog

Frog apex

Epidermal
lamellae

Weight-bearing
border of
hoof wall

Hoof heel

Buttress of the heel

Hoof quarter

Sole

Hoof toe

• **Figure 2.4** Surface anatomy of the solear aspect of a normal distal front foot from the same horse as in figure 2.1. The sole is circular in shape, and the heel buttresses, bars, and frog are well developed. The border of the hoof wall from toe to buttress is making contact with the ground and is bearing weight. The distal hoof wall extends past the sole and there are remnants of primary epidermal lamellae on the axial (inner) surface of the wall. Extension of the wall past the sole suggests that the horse spent at least some of its time on sandy, nonabrasive country. Feral horses inhabiting sandy country had similar extended wall growth.[9]

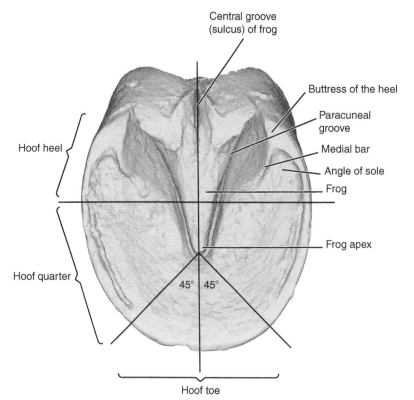

Central groove
(sulcus) of frog

Buttress of the heel

Paracuneal
groove

Medial bar

Angle of sole

Frog

Frog apex

Hoof heel

Hoof quarter

45° 45°

Hoof toe

• **Figure 2.5** Divisions of the hoof. Normal left front foot in a Standardbred.

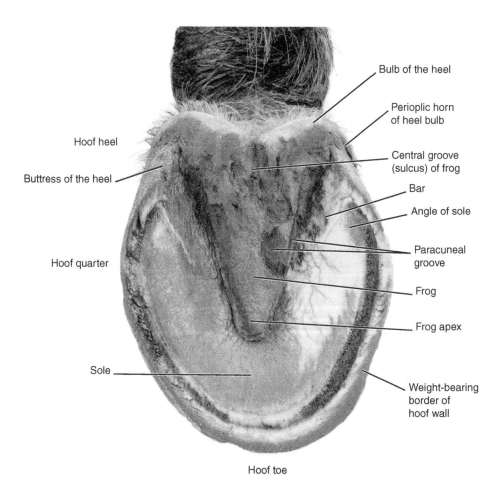

Bulb of the heel

Perioplic horn
of heel bulb

Central groove
(sulcus) of frog

Bar

Angle of sole

Paracuneal
groove

Frog

Frog apex

Weight-bearing
border of
hoof wall

Hoof heel

Buttress of the heel

Hoof quarter

Sole

Hoof toe

• **Figure 2.6** Surface anatomy of the solear aspect of a normal distal hind from the same horse as in figure 2.1. The shape of the solear aspect differs between front and hind feet. In this hind foot the shape is oval compared with round in the front foot (Figure 2.4).

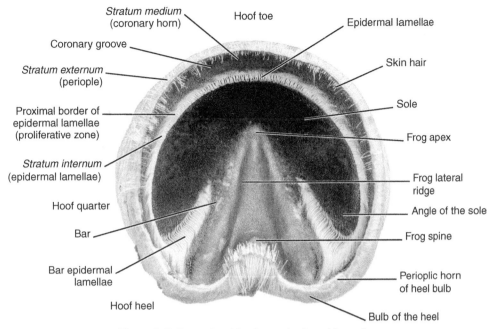

Stratum medium (coronary horn)
Hoof toe
Epidermal lamellae
Coronary groove
Stratum externum (periople)
Skin hair
Sole
Proximal border of epidermal lamellae (proliferative zone)
Frog apex
Stratum internum (epidermal lamellae)
Frog lateral ridge
Hoof quarter
Angle of the sole
Bar
Frog spine
Bar epidermal lamellae
Perioplic horn of heel bulb
Hoof heel
Bulb of the heel

• **Figure 2.7** Exungulated hoof capsule viewed from above.

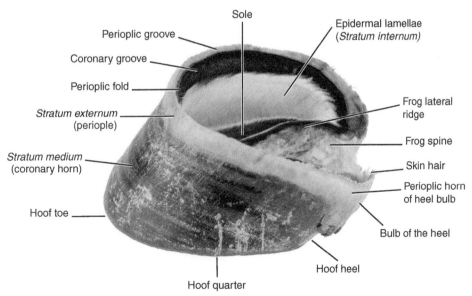

Sole
Perioplic groove
Epidermal lamellae (Stratum internum)
Coronary groove
Perioplic fold
Stratum externum (periople)
Frog lateral ridge
Stratum medium (coronary horn)
Frog spine
Skin hair
Perioplic horn of heel bulb
Hoof toe
Bulb of the heel
Hoof quarter
Hoof heel

• **Figure 2.8** A hoof capsule exungulated from a foot that has been soaked in water. Perioplic horn absorbs water, swells, and becomes opaque, thus making the periople prominent. The palmar periople expands over the bulbs of the heel.

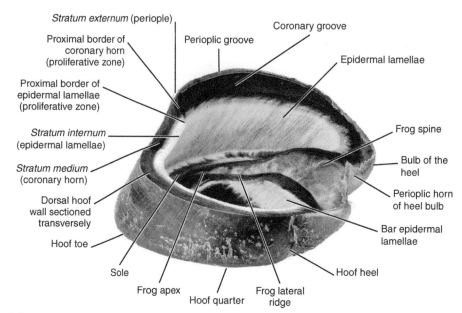

• Figure 2.9 A pigmented hoof capsule exungulated from its dermis and the rest of the foot. Half the hoof wall is cut away to show the inner surfaces of the perioplic and coronary grooves, lamellae, sole bars, and frog. There are approximately 560 nonpigmented, epidermal lamellae in parallel rows lining the internal surface of the wall and bars. The toe lamellae are taller than the heel lamellae. The surface of the concave perioplic and coronary grooves and the entire sole and frog are dotted with numerous holes, which, in life, contain the papillae of the perioplic, coronary, sole, and frog dermis (corium) respectively. The longitudinal section of the hoof at the toe shows the curve of the coronary groove, the pigmented *stratum medium* of the tubular hoof wall, and the nonpigmented inner hoof wall (*stratum internum*), which bear the epidermal lamellae. The hoof wall cut in transverse section shows the cut edges of the lamellae lining the nonpigmented inner hoof wall. At the proximal border of the coronary groove is the soft, nonpigmented, flexible periople, which expands at the heels to form the bulbs of the heel. The periople, or limbus (junction between two anatomic regions), joins the hoof wall *stratum medium* to the skin of the coronet. In the center of the frog is a spine to which is attached the digital cushion. Note the thickness and height of the wall is greater at the toe than at the heels.

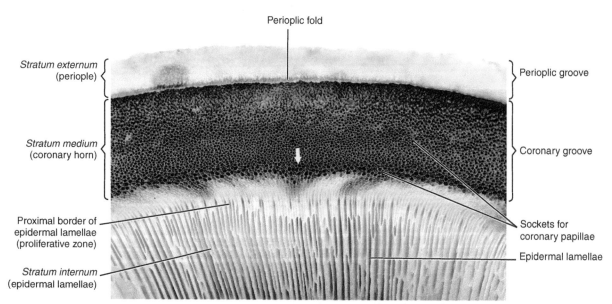

• Figure 2.10 The proximal dorsal hoof wall exungulated from a normal, adult horse foot, viewed from the inner, lamellar surface. The most proximal structure, the white, hydrated periople of the *stratum externum,* has separated cleanly from the skin and merges distally into the pigmented *stratum medium* (coronary horn). Stripped of their dermis, both the periople and the *stratum medium* remain as concentric, concave grooves in the proximal border of the hoof wall. Both are constructed of tubular and intertubular horn and have sockets to accept complementary dermal components, notably papillae. The sockets and papillae of the *stratum externum* are much smaller than those of the *stratum medium.* The sockets of the *stratum medium* vary in size commensurate with the size of the tubules they generate. Thus the outer, middle, and inner sockets get progressively larger, as do the diameters of the three zones of tubules in the more distal hoof wall. The basal cells lining the surface of the intertubular and tubular epidermis proliferate constantly, adding new horn to the ever-growing hoof wall. The largest sockets adjoin the nonpigmented, proximal epidermal lamellae, which arise in this zone also by constant proliferation of epidermal basal cells. Interestingly, only the sockets and lamellae in the dead center of the hoof (*arrow*) are aligned in straight lines; the remainder radiate from the center.

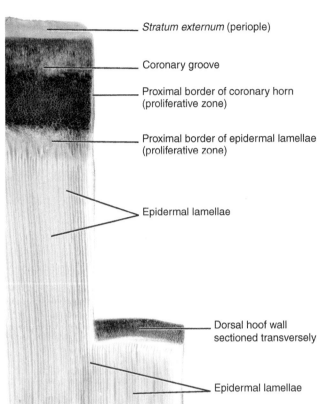

Stratum externum (periople)

Coronary groove

Proximal border of coronary horn
(proliferative zone)

Proximal border of epidermal lamellae
(proliferative zone)

Epidermal lamellae

Dorsal hoof wall
sectioned transversely

Epidermal lamellae

• **Figure 2.11** A section of exungulated dorsal hoof wall cut longitudinally and transversely and viewed from the inner, lamellar surface. Parallel rows of nonpigmented epidermal lamellae line the entire inner surface of the hoof wall. Normal epidermal lamellae are remarkably symmetric, equidistant from each other and similar in length and thickness depending on their location. The longest lamellae (measured proximal to distal) are at the toe and the shortest at the heels and bars. Constant basal cell proliferation at proximal lamellar border creates keratinized primary epidermal lamellae that migrate distally, attached to the inner hoof wall, itself migrating distally at approximately the same rate. In life dermal lamellae of matching dimensions fit between their epidermal counterparts and attach firmly to the basement membrane at the dermal-epidermal interface.

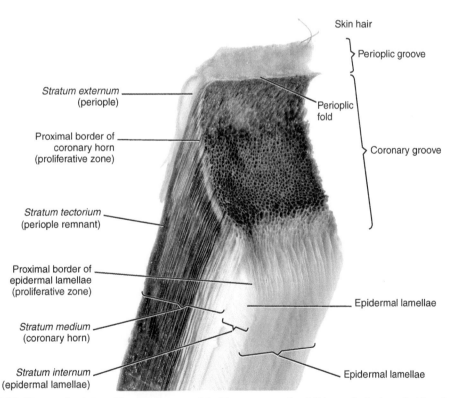

Skin hair

Perioplic groove

Stratum externum
(periople)

Perioplic
fold

Proximal border of
coronary horn
(proliferative zone)

Coronary groove

Stratum tectorium
(periople remnant)

Proximal border of
epidermal lamellae
(proliferative zone)

Epidermal lamellae

Stratum medium
(coronary horn)

Stratum internum
(epidermal lamellae)

Epidermal lamellae

• **Figure 2.12** The proximal dorsal hoof wall exungulated from a normal, adult horse foot, viewed obliquely from the lateral and inner surfaces. The most proximal structure, the white, hydrated periople of the *stratum externum,* has separated cleanly from the skin and merges distally into the pigmented *stratum medium* (coronary horn). The perioplic fold forms a clear boundary between periople and the pigmented *stratum medium.* Stripped of their dermis, both the periople and the *stratum medium* are concave grooves in the proximal border of the hoof wall. Both are constructed of tubular and intertubular horn and have sockets to accept complementary dermal components, notably papillae. The sockets and papillae of the *stratum externum* are much smaller than those of the *stratum medium.* The nonpigmented epidermal lamellae arise in this zone by constant proliferation of epidermal basal cells. The lamellae adjoining the most proximal *stratum medium* are short (in the transverse plane) but increase in length distally, forming a rounded or curved shoulder to each proximal lamella. From this point distally they remain the same length (3 to 4 mm).

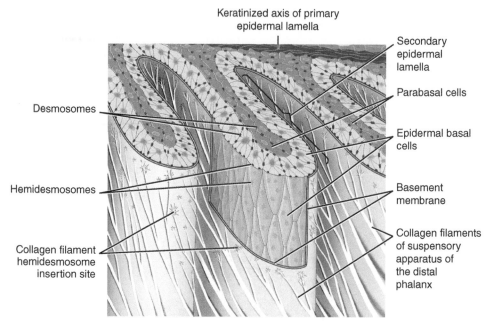

Keratinized axis of primary
epidermal lamella

Secondary
epidermal
lamella

Parabasal cells

Epidermal basal
cells

Basement
membrane

Collagen filaments
of suspensory
apparatus of
the distal
phalanx

Desmosomes

Hemidesmosomes

Collagen filament
hemidesmosome
insertion site

• Figure 2.13 Diagram of secondary epidermal lamellae (SELs) and the suspensory apparatus of the distal phalanx (SADP). The collagen filaments of the SADP insert on the lamellar basement membrane at hemidesmosome attachment sites. Note the oblique angle of the SADP collagen bundles as they insert on the basement membrane covered surface of the secondary epidermal lamellae. The lamellar epidermal basal cells (LEBCs) are fusiform, and the long axes of the LEBCs are aligned proximodistally, similar to the load-bearing collagen bundles of the SADP. Desmosomes link adjoining LEBCs to each other and to the more keratinized parabasal cells forming the central backbone of the SEL. Figure designed by the author.

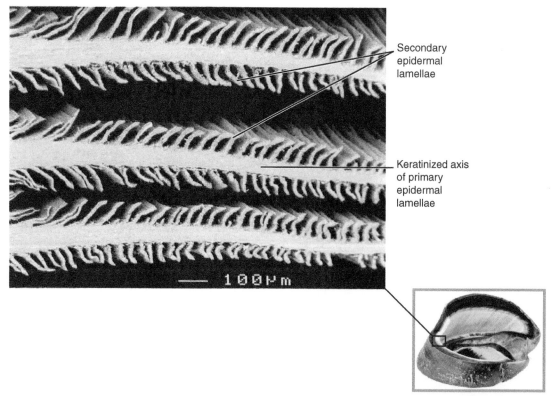

Secondary
epidermal
lamellae

Keratinized axis
of primary
epidermal
lamellae

100µm

• Figure 2.14 Scanning electron microscopic (SEM) image of three epidermal lamellae cut in transverse section. The dermal lamellae have been removed by treatment with detergent and enzyme. The surface area of each primary epidermal lamella is expanded by subdivisions into microscopically visible secondary epidermal lamellae. The number of SELs per primary lamella is approximately 135.

Keratinized axis of primary
epidermal lamellae

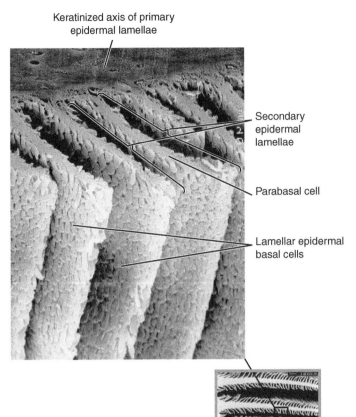

Secondary
epidermal
lamellae

Parabasal cell

Lamellar epidermal
basal cells

• Figure 2.15 Scanning electron microscopic (SEM) image of secondary epidermal lamellae cut in transverse section. The dermal lamellae and basement membrane have been removed by treatment with detergent and enzyme exposing the lamellar epidermal basal cells (LEBCs). The long axis of each LEBC is arranged proximodistally, aligning with the orientation of the SADP collagen filaments in this region.

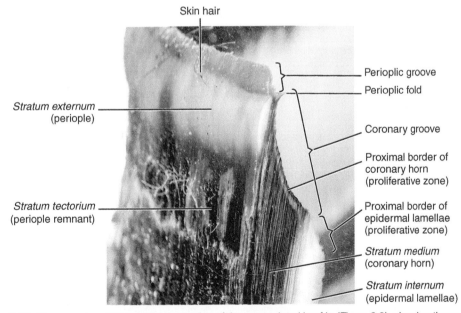

Skin hair

Perioplic groove

Perioplic fold

Coronary groove

Proximal border of
coronary horn
(proliferative zone)

Proximal border of
epidermal lamellae
(proliferative zone)

Stratum medium
(coronary horn)

Stratum internum
(epidermal lamellae)

Stratum externum
(periople)

Stratum tectorium
(periople remnant)

• Figure 2.16 Close-up view of the proximal cut edge of the exungulated hoof in (Figure 2.9), showing the curved perioplic and coronary grooves, the pigmented *stratum medium* and its nonpigmented inner zone and the *stratum internum* (epidermal lamellae). The soft, rubbery periople, or limbus (junction between two anatomic regions), joins the skin of the coronet to the hoof wall *stratum medium*. Some skin hairs remain at the proximal edge of the periople. The boundary between the periople and the stratum medium is marked by an epidermal fold (the perioplic fold) that, in life, projects into the adjacent dermis, forming a groove demarcating perioplic from coronary dermis. The perioplic and coronary grooves are pitted with tapering sockets that, in life, contain dermal papillae. Similar to the *stratum medium*, the *stratum externum* (periople) consists of tubular and intertubular horn, generated from continuous proliferation of the epidermal basal cells that line its inner surface. The feet in the photograph have been soaked in water to make the periople more noticeable. Perioplic horn absorbs water, swells, and becomes opaque. The tubular nature of the periople is lost distally where it dries out and becomes a shiny, thin layer (the *stratum tectorium*) that covers a few millimeters of the proximal hoof wall. More distally, the *stratum tectorium* is worn away by abrasion from the environment.

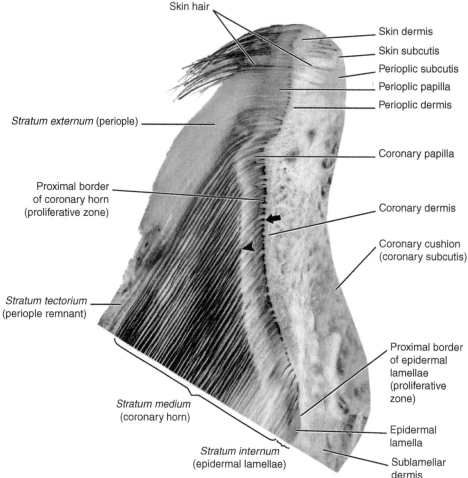

Skin hair

Skin dermis

Skin subcutis

Perioplic subcutis

Perioplic papilla

Perioplic dermis

Stratum externum (periople)

Coronary papilla

Proximal border
of coronary horn
(proliferative zone)

Coronary dermis

Coronary cushion
(coronary subcutis)

Stratum tectorium
(periople remnant)

Proximal border
of epidermal
lamellae
(proliferative
zone)

Stratum medium
(coronary horn)

Epidermal
lamella

Stratum internum
(epidermal lamellae)

Sublamellar
dermis

• **Figure 2.17** The coronary band of the pigmented hoof of a normal adult horse. The junction between skin and hoof is called the limbus and contains the perioplic epidermis, dermis, and subcutis. Like the *stratum medium*, the periople is a tubular epidermis (*stratum externum*), but instead of cornifying with hard keratins, it does so with soft, flexible, skinlike keratins. The papillae of the perioplic dermis are short and fine, compared with coronary papillae and support the production of tubular perioplic horn. The coronary band is distal to the limbus and includes the coronary epidermis (*stratum medium*), coronary dermis, and coronary subcutis. The epidermal basal cells of the proximal 2-4 mm of the *stratum medium* proliferate throughout the life of the horse, producing populations of cells that cornify into hard tubular and intertubular horn. Pigment-producing melanocytes are interspersed among the coronary basal cells and give the most proximal coronary epidermis a dark-colored border (*arrow*). The melanocytes extend their cytoplasm between keratinocytes and use these tubular processes to deposit melanin into cells at the point of cornification. Melanin accumulating in cornifying keratinocytes forms a second, more distal, dark zone (*arrowhead*) in the coronary epidermis. The *stratum medium* appears striped because melanin is deposited into intertubular horn and not the tubules themselves, producing an alternating dark-and-light pattern. The coronary dermis is densely packed with a meshwork of white collagen bundles continuous proximally with the perioplic dermis and distally with the lamellar dermis. Coronary papillae are long, tapering extensions of the coronary dermis that fit tightly into the sockets of the coronary epidermis. Dermal collagen bundles extend into the coronary papillae where they attach to the basement membrane, lining the entire surface of the coronary epidermis. Deep to coronary dermis is the loose, spongy, coronary subcutis that bulges forward in life as the coronary cushion.

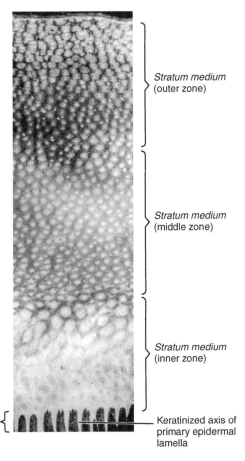

Stratum medium
(outer zone)

Stratum medium
(middle zone)

Stratum medium
(inner zone)

White line

Keratinized axis of
primary epidermal
lamella

• **Figure 2.18** Hoof wall tubule zonation. The tubules of the equine hoof wall are not arranged randomly. The tubules of the *stratum medium* are arranged in three distinct zones based on the density of tubules in the intertubular horn.[4] The zone of highest tubule density is the outermost layer and the density declines stepwise toward the internal lamellar layer. Because the force of impact with the ground (the ground reaction force) is transmitted proximally up the wall,[12] the tubule density gradient across the wall appears to be a mechanism for smooth energy transfer, from the rigid (high tubule density) outer wall to the more plastic (low tubule density) inner wall, and ultimately to the distal phalanx. The gradient in tubule density mirrors the gradient in water content across the hoof wall, and together these factors represent an optimum design for equine hoof wall.

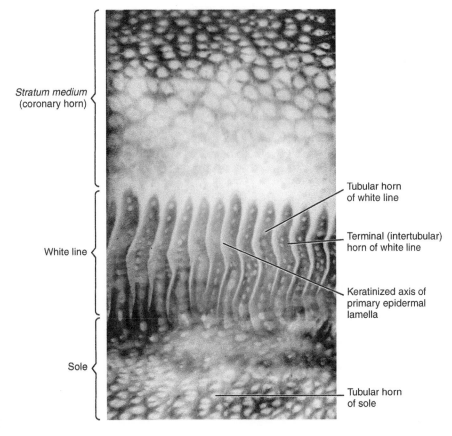

Stratum medium
(coronary horn)

White line

Sole

Tubular horn
of white line

Terminal (intertubular)
horn of white line

Keratinized axis of
primary epidermal
lamella

Tubular horn
of sole

• **Figure 2.19** Macro photograph of the inner *stratum medium*, white line, and dorsal sole; the wall and sole junction. Both the hoof wall (*stratum medium*) and the sole are darkly pigmented—note the pigment is confined to the intertubular horn and is absent in the tubules themselves. The non-pigmented keratinized axes of the primary epidermal lamellae are continuous with the tubular inner hoof wall, also devoid of pigment. In between each lamella are cross-sections of the tubular horn generated by the terminal papillae. The epidermal lamellae, visible on the ground surface of the hoof, arose on the shoulders of the coronary groove eight to nine months previously and have been pushed downward, past the dorsal surface of the distal phalanx, by continual growth from above.

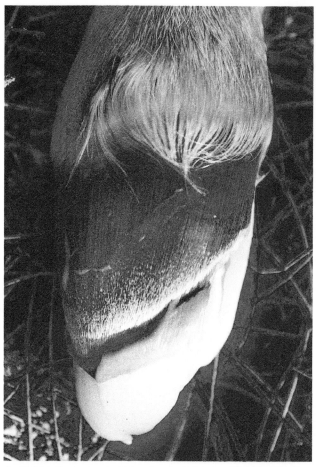

• **Figure 2.20** Newborn foal's foot. Foals stand within minutes of birth on hooves developed in utero. At the time of birth, the hard, pigmented hoof is capped with soft, unpigmented hoof, derived mainly from the frog and sole. During the latter half of pregnancy, the soft deciduous hoof capsule (*capsula ungulae decidua*) is continually being replaced by newly forming, cornified permanent hoof capsule.[5] The soft, blunt cap is thought to lessen the possibility of a foal hoof damaging the uterus. When the foal stands, the cap separates along a preformed break-line, and is soon shredded and lost. Note the obvious tubular structure of the hoof wall.

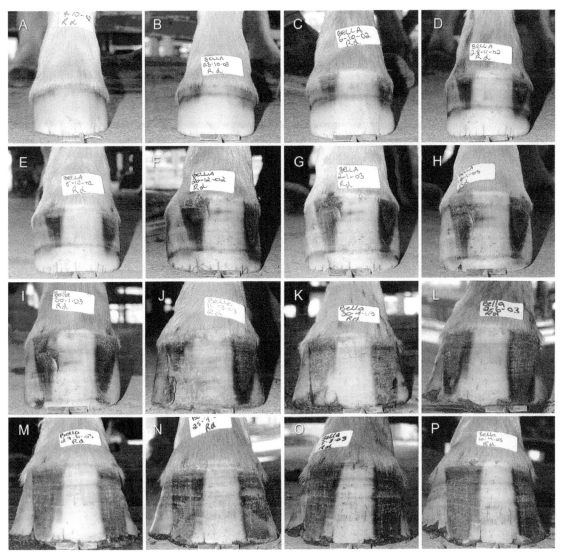

• **Figure 2.21** The right front foot of a Thoroughbred horse was photographed weekly, from the day it was born, for 11 months. The panel of 16 images records the dynamic changes in hoof shape and size as the filly matured from foal to yearling. The filly was barefoot throughout the study period; the substrate was shale-covered hills with pasture in the valleys. There was no supplementary feeding. The hoof at birth was manufactured in utero when the fetus was non–weight bearing. It is sometimes referred to as the "foal hoof" but in fact should be referred to as the fetal hoof. The foal hoof is the hoof grown by the foal after it is born.[1] In the first photograph (**A**) the medial and lateral wall of the hoof are vertical and the hoof capsule resembles a cylinder. Four weeks later (**C**) the distal fetal hoof remains the same shape and size, but the hoof above it is larger. Now the hoof resembles an inverted cone—the coronary band is larger than the bearing border. The border between fetal and foal hoof is marked by a circumferential, blood-stained ring, perhaps a signature of coronary band trauma at first weight bearing. The ring is also known as the foal hoof crease.[7] By five months (**J**) the fetal hoof has grown out, and the foot begins to adopt an adult appearance—a bearing border greater in circumference than the coronary band. The shape is that of a "truncated cone"—a cone with its apex cut off. Note the two ermine marks in the skin of the dorsal coronet at birth (**A**). No pigment had been delivered for incorporation into the coronary hoof in utero. Hoof pigmentation commenced at birth and followed the foal hoof boundary to the bearing border. At 8 weeks (**F**) the lateral coronary band was injured and tubular hoof production was arrested until the lesion healed. The deficit in the hoof wall, corresponding to the period of zero hoof production, moved distally down the hoof wall and "grew out" five months later. The 30-mm scale in each photograph enabled calibrated measurements—at birth the dorsal hoof wall measured 39.5 mm. Eleven months later, it was 615.0 mm. The foal hoof boundary grew 50.8 mm in 113 days, approximately 2 mm/day. The adult hoof grows at 0.2 mm/day or 6 mm/month.[1] However, the hoof growth rate incorporates the rapid growth of the foal itself, increasing in body weight from 42 kg at birth to 380 kg at the end of the study period. Nevertheless, this result tends to confirm the observation that the hooves of young horses grow faster than older horses.[6] (Photograph by Tracy Soward-Amalfi and the author)

References

1. Adams, O. R., & Stashak, T. S. (1987). *Adams' lameness in horses.* (4th ed.). (pp. xiii, 906). Philadelphia, PA: Lea & Febiger.

2. Bertram, J. E. A., & Gosline, J. M. (1986). Fracture toughness design in horse hoof keratin. *Journal of Experimental Biology, 125,* 29–47.

3. Bertram, J. E. A., & Gosline, J. M. (1987). Functional design of horse hoof keratin: The modulation of mechanical properties through hydration effects. *Journal of Experimental Biology, 130,* 121–136.

4. Bolliger, C., & Geyer, H. (1992). Morphology and histochemistry of the equine hoof. *Pferdeheilkunde, 8*(5), 269–286.

5. Bragulla, H. (1991). The deciduous hoof capsule *(Capsula ungulae decidua)* of the equine fetus and newborn foal. *Anatomia, Histologia, Embryologia, 20*(1), 66–74.

6. Butler, K. D., & Hintz, H. F. (1977). Effect of level of feed intake and gelatin supplementation on growth and quality of hoofs of ponies. *Journal of Animal Science, 44,* 257–261.

7. Curtis, S., Martin, J., & Hobbs, S. (2014). Hoof renewal time from birth of Thoroughbred foals. *Vet J, 201,* 116–117.

8. Dyhre-Poulsen, P., Smedegaard, H. H., Roed, J., et al. (1994). Equine hoof function investigated by pressure transducers inside the hoof and accelerometers mounted on the first phalanx. *Equine Veterinary Journal, 26,* 362–366.

9. Hampson, B. A., de Laat, M. A., Mills, P. C., Pollitt, C. C. (2013). The feral horse foot. Part A: Observational study of the effect of environment on the morphometrics of the feet of 100 Australian feral horses. *Australian Veterinary Journal, 91,* 14–22.

10. Leach, D. H. (1980). *The structure and function of the equine hoof wall.* PhD, University of Saskatchewan. Saskatoon, Saskatchewan, Canada.

11. Reilly, J. D., Cottrell, D. F., et al. (1996). Tubule density in equine hoof horn. *Biomimetics, 4,* 23–36.

12. Thomason, J. J., Biewener, A. A., et al. (1992). Surface strain on the equine hoof wall in vivo: Implications for the material design and functional morphology of the wall. *Journal of Experimental Biology, 166,* 145–165.

3 The Dermis

The highly vascular dermis, or corium, underlies the hoof wall and consists of a dense matrix of tough, connective tissue (tendonlike collagen) containing a network of arteries, veins, and capillaries, and sensory and vasomotor nerves. All parts of the hoof dermis, except for the lamellar corium, have papillae that fit tightly into the holes in the adjacent hoof. The lamellar corium has dermal lamellae that interlock with the epidermal lamellae of the inner hoof wall and bars. The dermis provides the hoof with nourishment, and its dense matrix of connective tissue connects the basement membrane of the dermal-epidermal junction to the parietal surface of the distal phalanx and thus suspends the distal phalanx from the inner wall of the hoof capsule— the suspensory apparatus of the distal phalanx.

THE CORONARY DERMIS

The coronary dermis fills the coronary groove and blends with the lamellar dermis of the inner hoof wall. The coronary dermis is connected to the lamellar and sublamellar dermis and firmly attached to the extensor tendon and the cartilages of the distal phalanx. Thus wherever the distal phalanx goes, the coronary band goes with it. This fact becomes important when laminitis precipitates a downward displacement of the distal phalanx. Collectively, the coronary dermis and subcutis and the germinal epidermal cells that rest upon its basement membrane are known as the coronary band. A feature of the coronary dermis is the large number of hairlike papillae projecting from its surface. In life each tapering papilla fits snugly into a hole on the surface of the epidermal coronary groove. Each papilla is responsible for nurturing an individual hoof wall tubule.

The basement membrane of coronary and terminal papillae is folded into numerous ridges parallel with the long axis of the papilla. These longitudinal ridges on the surface of the papillae, are analogous to the secondary dermal lamellae (SDLs) and likely share the similar role of increasing the surface area of attachment between the epidermal hoof and the connective tissue on the parietal surface of the distal phalanx. They may also act as guides or channels, directing columns of maturing keratinocytes in a correctly oriented proximodistal direction. The density of coronary papillae is greatest at the periphery and least adjacent to the lamellae, mirroring the arrangement of the hoof wall tubules of the stratum medium in zones based on tubule size and density.

THE SOLE CORIUM

As in the coronet, each dermal papilla of the sole corium fits into a socket in the epidermal sole. At the distal end of each dermal lamella are the terminal papillae. The epidermis surrounding the terminal papillae is nonpigmented and forms the inner part of the white zone (white line). The white zone is soft and flexible and effectively "seals" the sole to the hoof wall. It is sometimes subject to degeneration and infection, usually described as "seedy toe" or "white line disease."

● **Figure 3.1** Dorsal coronary papillae and proximal dermal lamellae from the pigmented hoof of a normal horse. The photograph was taken underwater to float the individual papillae and prevent them from sticking together. They appear pigmented, suggesting melanocytes from the epidermal basal cell layer detached with the dermis during hoof exungulation. The papillae are fine, hairlike, tapering projections of the coronary dermis that, in life, fit into complementary sockets in the coronary groove of the stratum medium. Distal to the papillae, in remarkably straight, uniform rows, are the dermal lamellae that also, in life, fit between complementary epidermal lamellae.

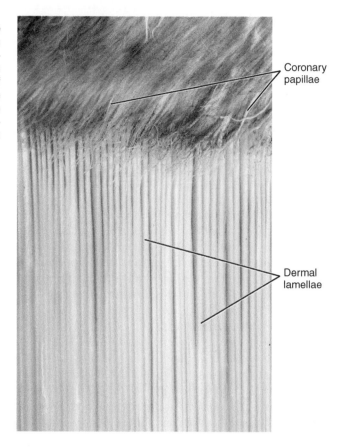

Coronary papillae

Dermal lamellae

● **Figure 3.2** Dorsal dermal lamellae and terminal papillae from the normal hoof of a horse. The photograph was taken underwater to float the individual papillae and prevent them from sticking together. On the dorsal, distal border of the dermal lamellae is a fringe of very fine cap horn papillae. Distal to the cap horn papillae are the large terminal papillae and, more distal still, the sole papillae. Five to seven papillae terminate the distal border of each dermal lamella, hence the name. Thus rows of terminal papillae line up with rows of dermal lamellae. Terminal papillae fit into epidermal sockets between the most distal primary epidermal lamellae and nourish the production of the tubular terminal horn (white line).

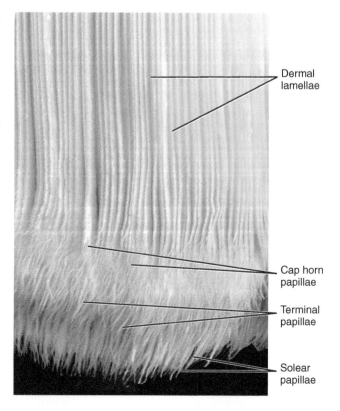

Dermal lamellae

Cap horn papillae

Terminal papillae

Solear papillae

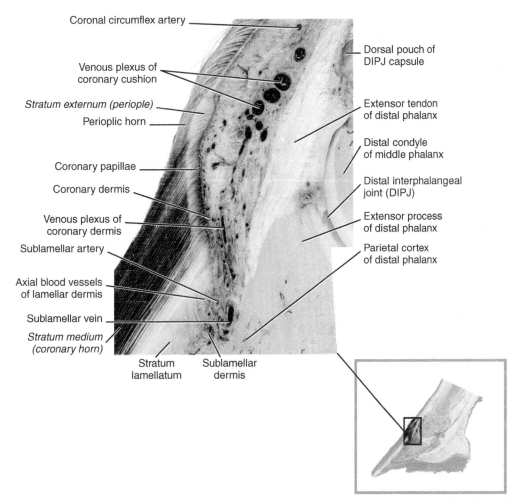

Coronal circumflex artery

Venous plexus of coronary cushion

Stratum externum (periople)

Perioplic horn

Coronary papillae

Coronary dermis

Venous plexus of coronary dermis

Sublamellar artery

Axial blood vessels of lamellar dermis

Sublamellar vein

Stratum medium (coronary horn)

Stratum lamellatum

Sublamellar dermis

Dorsal pouch of DIPJ capsule

Extensor tendon of distal phalanx

Distal condyle of middle phalanx

Distal interphalangeal joint (DIPJ)

Extensor process of distal phalanx

Parietal cortex of distal phalanx

• **Figure 3.3** Macrophotograph of an unstained, sagittal section of dorsal coronary band and proximal lamellae with blood vessels previously perfused with liquid methyl methacrylate (MMA). The MMA has polymerized, resulting in a vascular cast. The arterial system contains red-pigmented MMA and the venous system, blue. The viscosity of the MMA mixtures was deliberately kept high so that only major vessels were perfused. Veins are more prominent than arteries, especially the large venous plexus of the coronary subcutis (coronary cushion), a feature familiar to radiologists performing foot venograms where these veins are particularly prominent. Branches from the many small arteries in the coronary dermis enter the numerous coronary papillae. The near-vertical angle of the axial blood vessels of the lamellar dermis replicates the similar angle of the suspensory apparatus of the distal phalanx in this region. The box in the inset shows the provenance of the specimen.

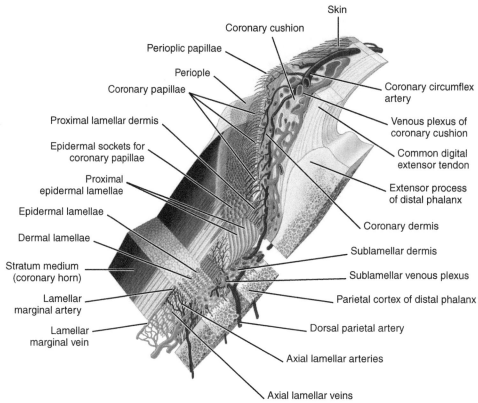

Skin

Coronary cushion

Perioplic papillae

Periople

Coronary papillae

Proximal lamellar dermis

Epidermal sockets for coronary papillae

Proximal epidermal lamellae

Epidermal lamellae

Dermal lamellae

Stratum medium (coronary horn)

Lamellar marginal artery

Lamellar marginal vein

Coronary circumflex artery

Venous plexus of coronary cushion

Common digital extensor tendon

Extensor process of distal phalanx

Coronary dermis

Sublamellar dermis

Sublamellar venous plexus

Parietal cortex of distal phalanx

Dorsal parietal artery

Axial lamellar arteries

Axial lamellar veins

• **Figure 3.4** Artistic representation of the coronary region of a normal horse foot. Designed by the author, the coronary diagram was digitally painted by Richard Tibbetts and was constructed from the study of numerous dissections, vascular casts, radiographic images, and photographs of specimens of normal adult horse feet. It went through much iteration before agreement was reached. For clarity many structures are enlarged and reduced in number for illustrative purposes.

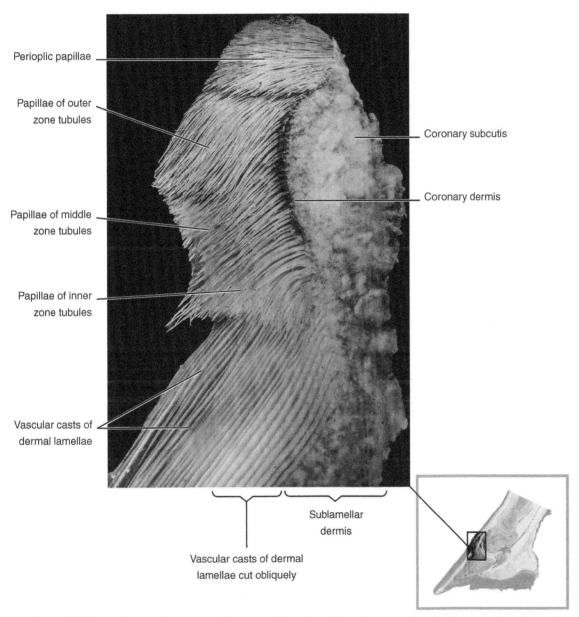

Perioplic papillae

Papillae of outer
zone tubules

Coronary subcutis

Coronary dermis

Papillae of middle
zone tubules

Papillae of inner
zone tubules

Vascular casts of
dermal lamellae

Sublamellar
dermis

Vascular casts of dermal
lamellae cut obliquely

• **Figure 3.5** Macro photograph of an unstained, sagittal section of dorsal coronary band and proximal lamellae with arterial vessels previously perfused with red-pigmented, liquid polyurethane. The polyurethane has polymerized, resulting in vascular casts of coronary papillae and dermal lamellae. The specimen was macerated in 10% sodium hydroxide to remove epidermis. Note the large number of papillae, each one associated with a single hoof wall tubule. The papillae vary in size with the inner one third the largest and longest, as are the inner hoof wall tubules they nurture. The lamellae are in uniform parallel rows.

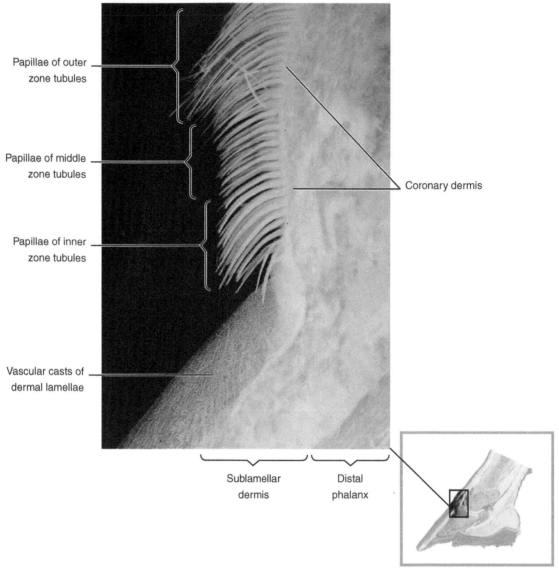

Papillae of outer
zone tubules

Papillae of middle
zone tubules

Papillae of inner
zone tubules

Vascular casts of
dermal lamellae

Coronary dermis

Sublamellar
dermis

Distal
phalanx

• **Figure 3.6** Macro photograph of an unstained, sagittal section of dorsal coronary band and a single proximal lamella with arterial vessels previously perfused with blue-pigmented, liquid polyurethane. The polyurethane has polymerized, resulting in vascular casts of coronary papillae and the dermal lamella. The specimen was macerated in 10% sodium hydroxide to remove epidermis. Note the papillae correspond in size to the tubules that they nurture. The hoof wall papillae and their corresponding tubules are arranged in three distinct zones based on the density of tubules in the intertubular horn.[1] The zone of highest tubule density is the outermost layer, and the density declines stepwise toward the internal lamellar layer. The axial vessels in the lamella parallel the near-vertical arrangement of the collagen bundles of the suspensory apparatus of the distal phalanx.

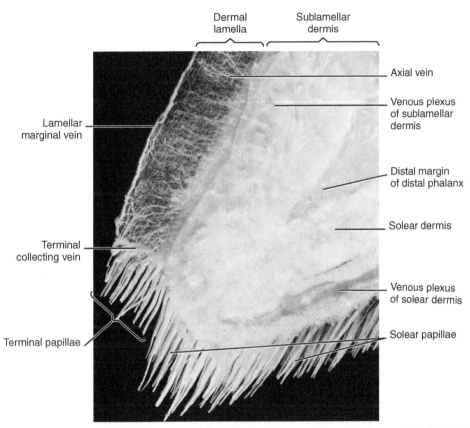

Dermal
lamella

Sublamellar
dermis

Axial vein

Venous plexus
of sublamellar
dermis

Lamellar
marginal vein

Distal margin
of distal phalanx

Solear dermis

Terminal
collecting vein

Venous plexus
of solear dermis

Solear papillae

Terminal papillae

• **Figure 3.7** Partially macerated distal toe of normal equine foot. The circulation was perfused with liquid blue poly-urethane, which polymerized within arteries, veins, and capillaries, creating a vascular cast. The large veins of the sublamellar and solear plexi, embedded in white connective tissue, are adjacent to the dorsal and palmar margin of the distal phalanx, respectively. A single dermal lamella (bracket) with its terminal papillae have been dissected free of its neighbors and projects dorsally from the sublamellar dermis. Axial arteries and veins traverse the lamella oriented at right angles to the dorsal surface of the distal phalanx. Multiple fine capillaries, oriented parallel to the long axis of the lamella, are just visible in the semitransparent dermal lamella. The marginal vein, the largest and most peripheral (abaxial) lamellar vessel, merges with the large collecting vein at the base of the 8 to 12 terminal papillae. Terminal papillae merge with sole papillae, but are separated by a step.

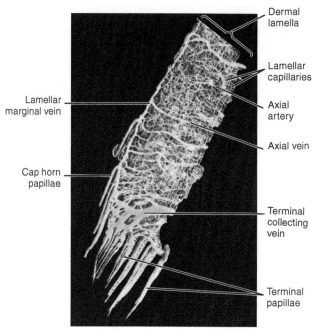

Dermal
lamella

Lamellar
capillaries

Axial
artery

Axial vein

Terminal
collecting
vein

Terminal
papillae

Lamellar
marginal vein

Cap horn
papillae

• **Figure 3.8** A single dermal lamella and its terminal papillae, partially macerated after the arterial blood supply was injected with blue polyurethane. Axial arteries and veins traverse the lamellae oriented at right angles to the long axis of the lamella. Multiple fine capillaries are oriented parallel to the long axis of the lamella, along with the marginal vein. The marginal vein, the largest and most peripheral (abaxial) lamellar vessel, merges with the large collecting vein at the base of the terminal papillae. The terminal collecting vein drains into the circumflex marginal vein and the sublamellar venous plexus.

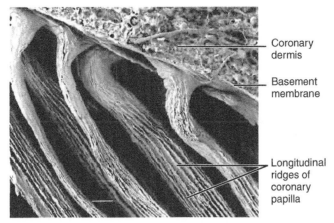

Coronary
dermis

Basement
membrane

Longitudinal
ridges of
coronary
papilla

• **Figure 3.9** Coronary papillae; scanning electron microscopic (SEM) image. The coronary papillae have been gently released from their sockets in the epidermal coronary groove. Between the bases of the papillae is the basement membrane associated with the intertubular horn. The basement membrane of each coronary papilla is folded into numerous longitudinal ridges, all parallel to the long axis of the papilla.

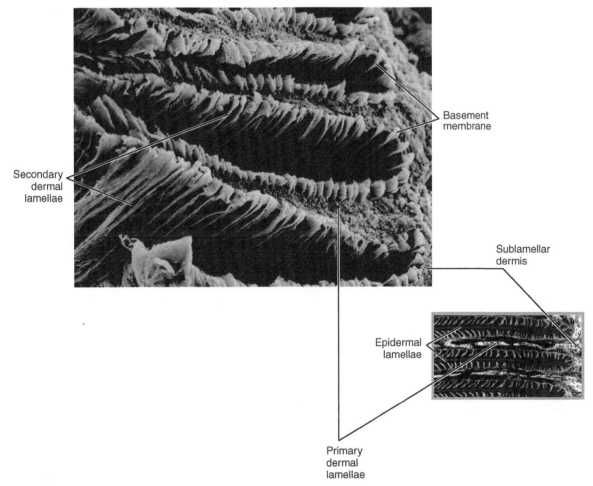

Basement
membrane

Secondary
dermal
lamellae

Sublamellar
dermis

Epidermal
lamellae

Primary
dermal
lamellae

• **Figure 3.10** Dermal lamellae and lamellar basement membrane; scanning electron micrographic (SEM) image of transverse section. The epidermal lamellae are absent, having been gently dissected free of their attachments to the blue-colored lamellar basement membrane. The empty spaces retain an epidermal lamellar shape bordered by fabric-like basement membrane. The primary dermal lamellae and the sublamellar dermis consist of densely packed bundles of collagen fibers. The inset shows a Masson's trichrome stained histologic section with the primary and secondary epidermal lamellae in place; it is the red-stained epidermal lamellae that have been removed from SEM image, leaving behind the blue-stained basement membrane and lamellar dermis.

References

1. Bolliger, C., & Geyer, H. (1992). Morphology and histochemistry of the equine hoof. *Pferdeheilkunde, 8*(5), 269-286.

4 The Mimics Anatomic Models

The author acknowledges that Simon Collins created the Mimics models (Mimics Innovation Suite, Materialise) using magnetic resonance (MR) and computed tomography (CT) data in this and the sections that follow from material we jointly acquired, prepared, and scanned. We planned the tissue segmentation and color scheme together. The author arranged the virtual dissections, added the labeling, and designed the page layouts.

Comprehending anatomy in three dimensions is a difficult but essential task for the student of the horse's foot. Traditionally two-dimensional diagrams, freeze-dried and plastinated sagittal sections, and fiberglass models based on dissected specimens and artistic imagination have been the best aids available. More recently, virtual models that can be manipulated in three dimensions and dissected via the computer monitor have become available. 3D models can be printed using additive technology, rendering anatomically correct, life-size models that can be held in the hand and viewed from all sides (available at www.3dvetanatomize.com). Foot anatomy can be imaged by both magnetic resonance (MR) or computed tomography (CT) technology. MR gives excellent soft tissue resolution, whereas CT is superior for bones (Fig. 4-1).

Each modality results in a stack of multiple 2D layers resolved in monochrome grayscale. Tissues are recognized based on the intensity of their contrast in shades of gray and their proximity to other structures. With appropriate computer software, the stacked 2D data (pixels) can be combined into 3D data (*voxels* = a pixel with volume). By painstaking analysis and hours of computer time, each tissue can be reconstructed as a virtual solid object until a structure (such as the deep digital flexor tendon or distal sesamoidean impar ligament), built from its component tissues, emerges on the computer monitor. The software allows enlargement and rotation of the model and switching on and off of various components to allow virtual dissection.

To prepare the 3D models shown here we took a normal Standardbred stallion cadaver limb and placed it in a wooden, nonmagnetic jig in the loaded stance phase. Thus locked in place, it was MR scanned in a high resolution (3T) scanner for soft tissue data and then transported to a CT scanner where high-resolution bone data were obtained. Using Materialise Mimics Innovation Suite (MIS) software, the two sets of data were coregistered to produce an accurate, multicomponent anatomic model of the horse's

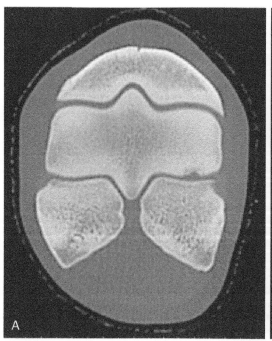 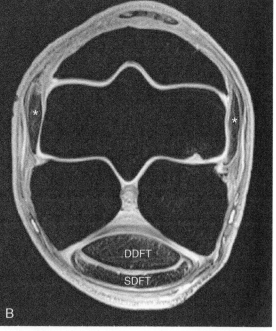

• **Figure 4.1** Computed tomography (CT) and magnetic resonance (MR) transverse images of the same region compared. CT scans result in excellent bone but poor soft tissue images, whereas MR gives the opposite: poor bone but good soft tissue resolution. CT of the fetlock joint region (**A**) shows the third metacarpal, proximal phalanx, and the proximal sesamoid bones, but little soft tissue. The MR image (**B**) resolves no bone detail but clearly shows the deep digital flexor tendon (DDFT) and superficial digital flexor tendon (SDFT) as well as the collateral ligaments of the metacarpophalangeal (fetlock) joint (asterisks).

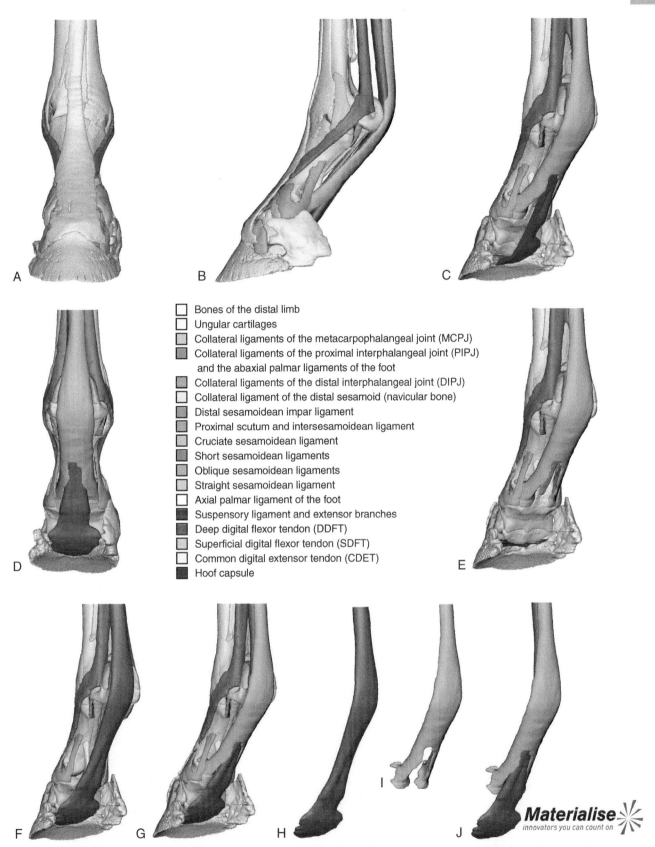

A   B   C

Bones of the distal limb
Ungular cartilages
Collateral ligaments of the metacarpophalangeal joint (MCPJ)
Collateral ligaments of the proximal interphalangeal joint (PIPJ)
  and the abaxial palmar ligaments of the foot
Collateral ligaments of the distal interphalangeal joint (DIPJ)
Collateral ligament of the distal sesamoid (navicular bone)
Distal sesamoidean impar ligament
Proximal scutum and intersesamoidean ligament
Cruciate sesamoidean ligament
Short sesamoidean ligaments
Oblique sesamoidean ligaments
Straight sesamoidean ligament
Axial palmar ligament of the foot
Suspensory ligament and extensor branches
Deep digital flexor tendon (DDFT)
Superficial digital flexor tendon (SDFT)
Common digital extensor tendon (CDET)
Hoof capsule

D   E

F   G   H   I   J

Materialise
innovators you can count on

• **Figure 4.2** Mimics modeled horse foot showing anatomic relationships between ligaments, tendons, and bones. In the dorsal and lateral views (**A** and **B**) the common digital extensor tendon inserts partially on the proximal and middle phalanges and finally on the broad extensor process of the distal phalanx; the lateral extensor tendon inserts on the lateral proximal phalanx. Note the supporting, dorsal extensor branches of the suspensory ligament (interosseous muscle) merging dorsally into the extensor tendon. In **C, D,** and **E,** the superficial digital flexor tendon bifurcates into two branches that insert on the distal extremity of the proximal phalanx and the proximal extremity of the middle phalanx just palmar to the collateral ligaments of the proximal interphalangeal joint (PIPJ). The deep digital flexor tendon descends between the two branches of the superficial digital flexor tendon and inserts on the semilunar flexor surface of the distal phalanx. In **F, G, H, I,** and **J,** the flexor tendons and adjacent tissues are isolated to show the relationships between them.

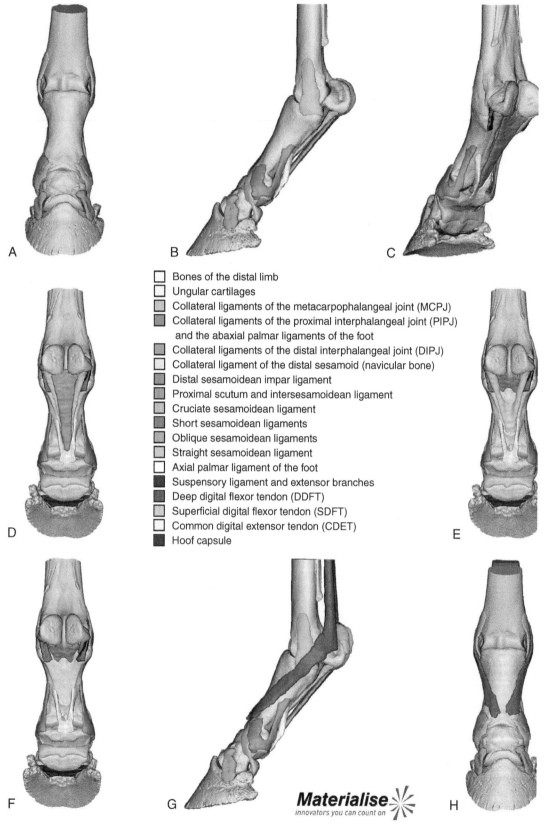

Bones of the distal limb
Ungular cartilages
Collateral ligaments of the metacarpophalangeal joint (MCPJ)
Collateral ligaments of the proximal interphalangeal joint (PIPJ)
   and the abaxial palmar ligaments of the foot
Collateral ligaments of the distal interphalangeal joint (DIPJ)
Collateral ligament of the distal sesamoid (navicular bone)
Distal sesamoidean impar ligament
Proximal scutum and intersesamoidean ligament
Cruciate sesamoidean ligament
Short sesamoidean ligaments
Oblique sesamoidean ligaments
Straight sesamoidean ligament
Axial palmar ligament of the foot
Suspensory ligament and extensor branches
Deep digital flexor tendon (DDFT)
Superficial digital flexor tendon (SDFT)
Common digital extensor tendon (CDET)
Hoof capsule

Materialise
innovators you can count on

• **Figure 4.3** Mimics modeled horse foot showing anatomic relationships between ligaments and bones; the tendons are absent. The collateral ligaments show how the uniaxial, ginglymus saddle joints of the distal limb support movement in the dorsopalmar axis, minimizing mediolateral movement, and hold the digit together (**A** and **B**). Note the collateral ligaments are oriented vertically rather than parallel to the pastern axis (**B** and **G**). The axial palmar ligaments extend from the trigone (the triangular rough surface on the proximal phalanx) to the palmar margin of the proximal extremity of the middle phalanx (**C,D, E** and **F**). The abaxial medial and lateral palmar ligaments pass from the borders of the proximal phalanx to the palmar surface of the proximal extremity of the middle phalanx, where they blend with the insertion of the superficial digital flexor tendon (**B,C** and **D**).

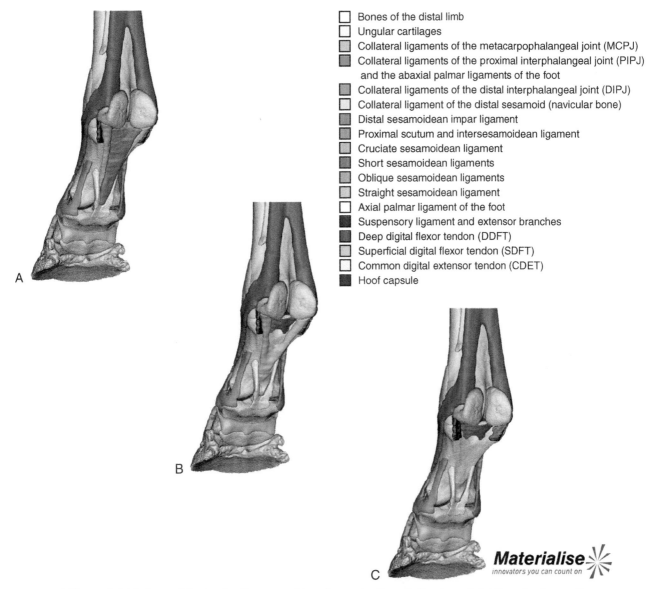

□ Bones of the distal limb
□ Ungular cartilages
□ Collateral ligaments of the metacarpophalangeal joint (MCPJ)
□ Collateral ligaments of the proximal interphalangeal joint (PIPJ)
   and the abaxial palmar ligaments of the foot
□ Collateral ligaments of the distal interphalangeal joint (DIPJ)
□ Collateral ligament of the distal sesamoid (navicular bone)
□ Distal sesamoidean impar ligament
□ Proximal scutum and intersesamoidean ligament
□ Cruciate sesamoidean ligament
□ Short sesamoidean ligaments
□ Oblique sesamoidean ligaments
□ Straight sesamoidean ligament
□ Axial palmar ligament of the foot
□ Suspensory ligament and extensor branches
□ Deep digital flexor tendon (DDFT)
□ Superficial digital flexor tendon (SDFT)
□ Common digital extensor tendon (CDET)
□ Hoof capsule

Materialise
innovators you can count on

• **Figure 4.4** Mimics models showing the sesamoidean ligaments. Beneath the deep digital flexor tendon are three distal sesamoidean ligaments attaching the two proximal sesamoid bones to the palmar pastern (**A** and **B**). The superficial straight sesamoidean ligament attaches distally to the plate of the fibrocartilaginous middle scutum on the proximal extremity of the palmar middle phalanx (**A**); the triangular oblique sesamoidean ligament attaches distally to a rough trigone on the palmar surface of the proximal phalanx (**B**). The pair of deep cruciate ligaments cross and attach distally to the proximal extremity of the proximal phalanx (**C**). The short medial and lateral sesamoidean ligaments attach the base of each proximal sesamoid bone to the palmar edge of the articular surface of the proximal phalanx.

foot. Colors were ascribed to each of the 26 components for anatomic cross-referencing in various views. In the figures that follow, structures are not labeled; instead, the reader is encouraged to utilize the color codes. Shown from different points of view, each structure will have the same color and working through the figures, the reader will come to comprehend the important relationships between the various elements that make the foot function. The outcome should be a three-dimensional mental picture of the horse's foot, invaluable whenever a foot is examined clinically.

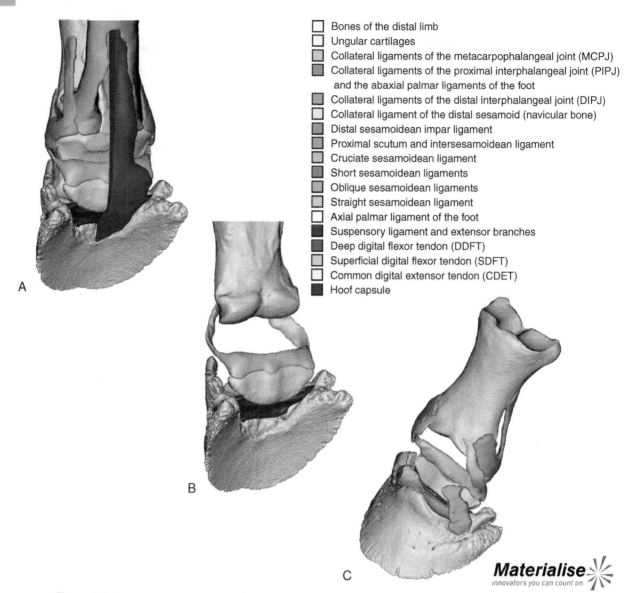

☐ Bones of the distal limb
☐ Ungular cartilages
▢ Collateral ligaments of the metacarpophalangeal joint (MCPJ)
▢ Collateral ligaments of the proximal interphalangeal joint (PIPJ)
   and the abaxial palmar ligaments of the foot
▢ Collateral ligaments of the distal interphalangeal joint (DIPJ)
☐ Collateral ligament of the distal sesamoid (navicular bone)
▢ Distal sesamoidean impar ligament
▢ Proximal scutum and intersesamoidean ligament
☐ Cruciate sesamoidean ligament
▢ Short sesamoidean ligaments
☐ Oblique sesamoidean ligaments
☐ Straight sesamoidean ligament
☐ Axial palmar ligament of the foot
■ Suspensory ligament and extensor branches
■ Deep digital flexor tendon (DDFT)
☐ Superficial digital flexor tendon (SDFT)
☐ Common digital extensor tendon (CDET)
■ Hoof capsule

A

B

C

Materialise
innovators you can count on

● **Figure 4.5** Mimics modeled horse foot showing anatomic relationships between the distal sesamoid (navicular) bone and the middle and distal phalanges. The articular surface of the navicular bone makes contact with the distal articular surface of the middle phalanx (removed in **C** to show the articulation). Three ligaments make up the navicular suspensory apparatus. The collateral ligament of the distal sesamoid bone (suspensory navicular ligament) arises on each side of the distal end of the proximal phalanx, blending with the collateral ligaments of the proximal interphalangeal joint (PIPJ) and the abaxial palmar ligaments (**A** and **C**). The two collateral sesamoidean ligaments cross the pastern joint obliquely and unite on the proximal border of the navicular bone (**A** and **B**). The distal sesamoidean impar ligament attaches the distal border of the navicular bone to the flexor surface of the distal phalanx (**A** and **B**). The distal articular surface of the middle phalanx, the articular surface of the distal phalanx, and the two articular surfaces of the navicular bone form the coffin joint, a ginglymus (a joint that allows movement in one plane, forward and backward, as does a door hinge) of limited action.

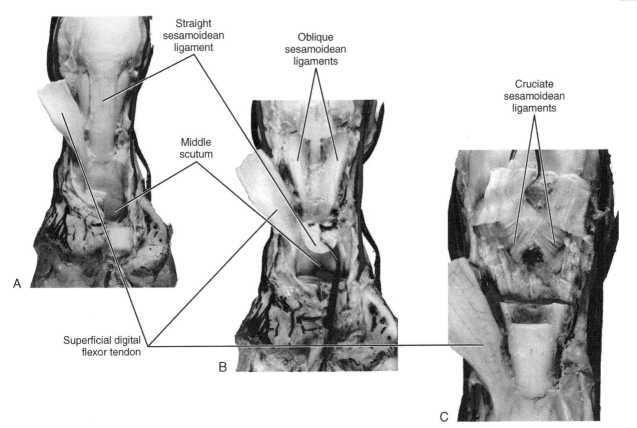

Straight sesamoidean ligament

Oblique sesamoidean ligaments

Cruciate sesamoidean ligaments

Middle scutum

A

Superficial digital flexor tendon

B

C

• **Figure 4.6** The sesamoidean ligaments dissected. The sesamoidean ligaments are really the distal continuation of the suspensory (interosseus) ligament. The proximal sesamoid bones are embedded in the ligament and contribute to the suspensory apparatus of the distal limb. When the fetlock receives its maximum load and is severely overextended, it is the proximal sesamoid bones that receive the thrust of the descending metacarpal (cannon) bone. The sesamoids are held in place by the palmar annular ligament and distally by the three sesamoidean ligaments. In **A,** the deep and superficial flexor tendons have been cut and reflected to show the straight sesamoidean ligament. Deeper dissections show the triangular, medial, and lateral oblique sesamoidean ligaments (**B**) and the cruciate sesamoidean ligaments (**C**) on the palmar surface of the proximal phalanx. The straight sesamoidean ligament inserts onto a special fibrocartilagenous extension on the proximal extremity of the palmar surface of the middle phalanx (the middle scutum). The medial and lateral oblique sesamoidean ligaments insert on the trigone, the roughened triangular region on the palmar surface of the proximal phalanx.

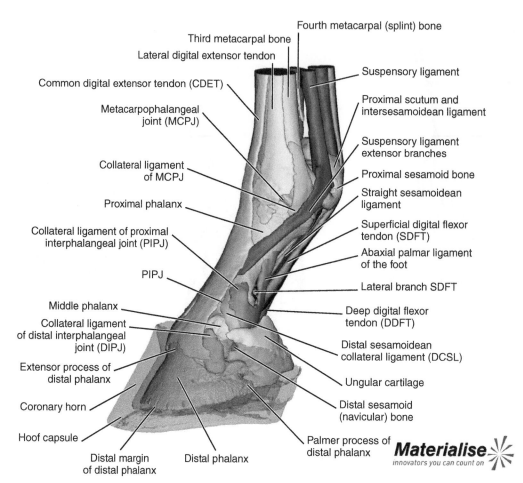

Third metacarpal bone

Fourth metacarpal (splint) bone

Lateral digital extensor tendon

Common digital extensor tendon (CDET)

Metacarpophalangeal joint (MCPJ)

Collateral ligament of MCPJ

Proximal phalanx

Collateral ligament of proximal interphalangeal joint (PIPJ)

PIPJ

Middle phalanx

Collateral ligament of distal interphalangeal joint (DIPJ)

Extensor process of distal phalanx

Coronary horn

Hoof capsule

Distal margin of distal phalanx

Distal phalanx

Suspensory ligament

Proximal scutum and intersesamoidean ligament

Suspensory ligament extensor branches

Proximal sesamoid bone

Straight sesamoidean ligament

Superficial digital flexor tendon (SDFT)

Abaxial palmar ligament of the foot

Lateral branch SDFT

Deep digital flexor tendon (DDFT)

Distal sesamoidean collateral ligament (DCSL)

Ungular cartilage

Distal sesamoid (navicular) bone

Palmer process of distal phalanx

Materialise
innovators you can count on

• **Figure 4.7** Mimics distal limb with transparent hoof. The one third of the ungular cartilage that projects above the proximal border of the hoof wall is palpable. Most of the collateral ligament (CL) of the distal interphalangeal joint (DIPJ) is below the proximal hoof wall and thus difficult to examine by radiography or ultrasound. However, DIPJ CL desmitis is the second most common reason for lameness and requires magnetic resonance imaging (MRI) for efficient identification.

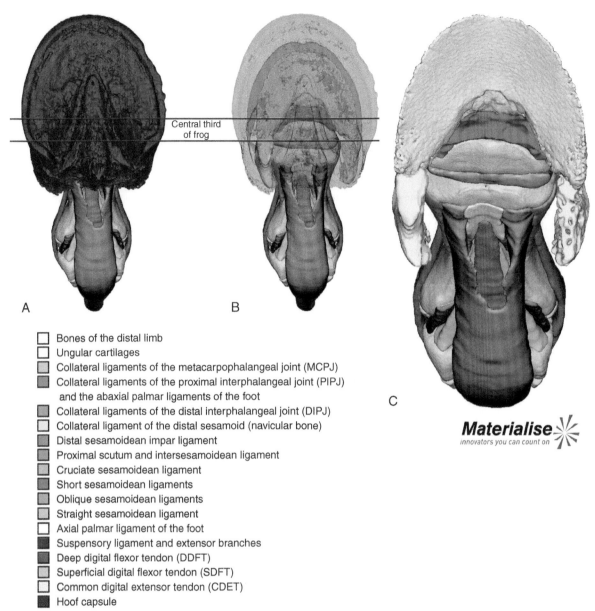

Central third
of frog

A

B

C

Bones of the distal limb
Ungular cartilages
Collateral ligaments of the metacarpophalangeal joint (MCPJ)
Collateral ligaments of the proximal interphalangeal joint (PIPJ)
  and the abaxial palmar ligaments of the foot
Collateral ligaments of the distal interphalangeal joint (DIPJ)
Collateral ligament of the distal sesamoid (navicular bone)
Distal sesamoidean impar ligament
Proximal scutum and intersesamoidean ligament
Cruciate sesamoidean ligament
Short sesamoidean ligaments
Oblique sesamoidean ligaments
Straight sesamoidean ligament
Axial palmar ligament of the foot
Suspensory ligament and extensor branches
Deep digital flexor tendon (DDFT)
Superficial digital flexor tendon (SDFT)
Common digital extensor tendon (CDET)
Hoof capsule

Materialise
innovators you can count on

• **Figure 4.8** The transparent frog. Mimics modeled left forefoot viewed from the ground surface. The hoof capsule is opaque in **A** and transparent in **B.** Note the location of the distal sesamoid (navicular) bone in relation to the frog. The central third of the frog directly overlies the navicular bone. Hoof tester pressure applied to the central third of the frog acts on the navicular bone and its attached soft tissue (**C**) and is a sensitive test for evoking navicular pain.

5 Planar Anatomy

ANATOMIC TERMS

Precise and unambiguous terms that describe the position and relationship of body parts are essential if anatomy is to be understood and discussed between colleagues. Based on Latin and Greek, the terms are universal. Those pertaining to the horse's foot are illustrated in Figure 5-1. The nomenclature used throughout the text follows Nomina Anatomica Veterinaria[1] and the Illustrated Veterinary Anatomical Nomenclature.[2]

Planar Anatomy

Three planes of section are utilized in MR and CT scanning and analyzing planar images enables three-dimensional comprehension (Fig. 5-2). Anatomic sections can be cut in the same planes as in MR and CT imaging, and working through gross anatomic sagittal, transverse, and frontal sections, structure by structure is instructive. Images in this chapter are gross sections of normal adult horse feet cut in the sagittal (parasagittal), transverse, and frontal planes to

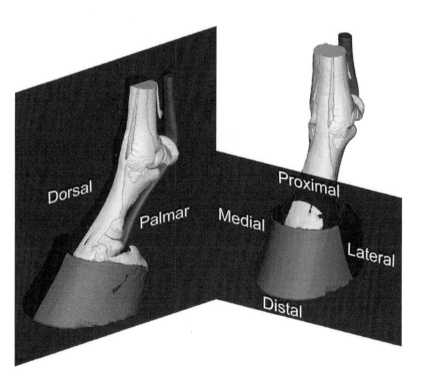

• **Figure 5.1** The anatomic terms for describing the left front foot of a horse. *Plantar* is substituted for *palmar* in the case of a left hind foot. *Medial* and *lateral* would be swapped if the right foot were pictured.

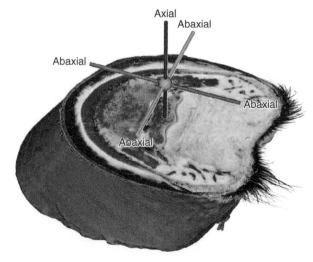

• **Figure 5.2** The axis of the horse foot is an imaginary plumb line through its center. All points away from the axial plumb line are abaxial. Thus the axial and abaxial surfaces of the ungular cartilages, whether medial or lateral, can be referred to with certainty. Also, a single epidermal lamella has an axial end (that closest to the distal phalanx) and an abaxial end (that closest to the *stratum medium* of the hoof wall whether at the toe, quarters, or heels).

assist CT and MR image analysis and to better understand the horse's foot in the third dimension.

Sagittal and Parasagittal Anatomy

Images of the sagittal plane are commonly used to illustrate the anatomy of the horse foot. The sagittal image, whether drawn or photographed, appears in textbooks and charts dating back through the centuries. It is a good place to start, as the dead center midline cut contains nearly all of the key structures of the foot (Fig. 5-3). However, studying the adjacent parasagittal cuts adds to the picture in the mind's eye and begins to reveal complexities not comprehended in a single plane. This is reinforced by studying images made in the transverse and frontal planes.

GROSS ANATOMY FROM SECTIONS

The gross anatomy sections were from the feet of euthanized, normal Standardbred and Thoroughbred horses and were cut frozen, using a high-speed, professional band saw. Each section was approximately 15 mm in thickness, and after washing in water was photographed immediately, still partially frozen, using fluorescent studio lighting. Despite washing, major blood vessels retained frozen clotted blood, thus enabling subsequent identification and labeling from the photographic image.

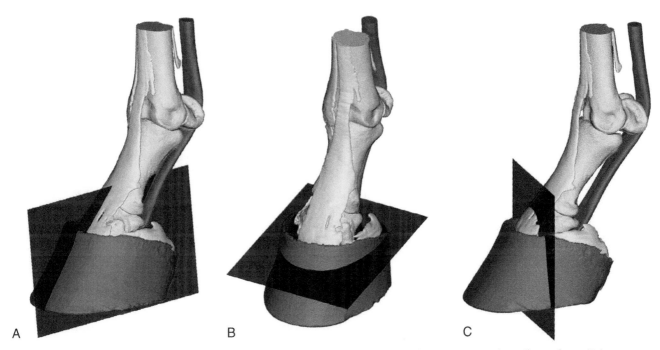

A   B   C

• **Figure 5.3** The three planes of section utilized to analyze the accompanying gross anatomic sections. **A,** sagittal plane, **B,** transverse plane, and **C,** frontal plane. Sections on either side of the sagittal plane are parasagittal sections (medial to lateral). Transverse sections are distal to proximal and frontal sections are dorsal to palmar-plantar.

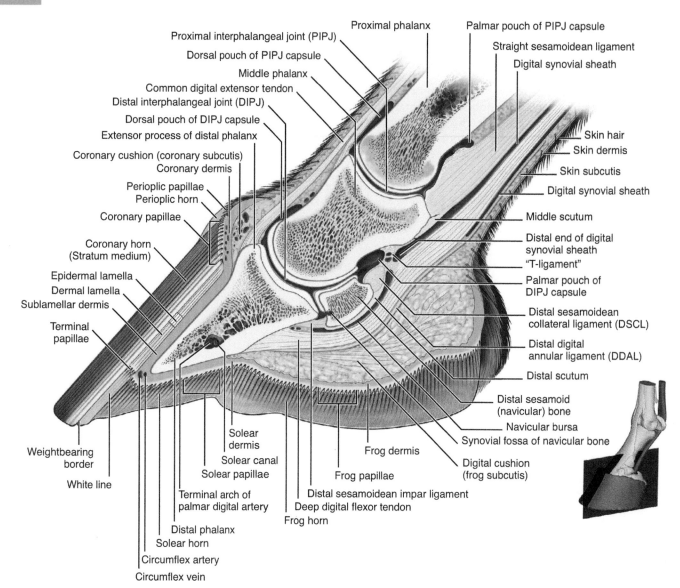

Figure 5.4 A current artistic representation of the sagittal section of a normal horse's foot. Designed by the author, the sagittal diagram was digitally painted by Richard Tibbetts and was constructed from the study of numerous scanned and photographed sagittal sections of normal adult horse feet. It went through much iteration before agreement was reached. Some structures are shown enlarged and reduced; thus only a few coronary, perioplic, solear, and frog papillae and their associated hoof tubules are shown. For clarity, only a few blood vessels are labeled and many structures are enlarged and reduced in number for illustrative purposes. The inset shows the plane of the section.

SAG 05

SAG 04

SAG 03

SAG 02

SAG 01

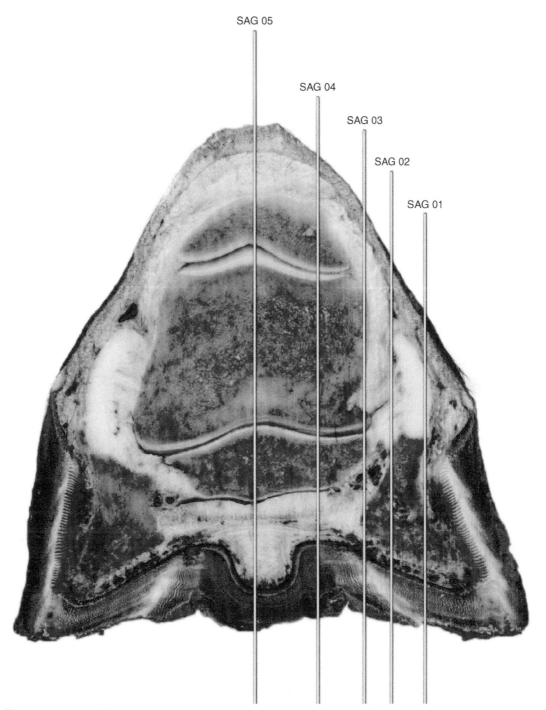

• **Figure 5.5** Gross anatomy sagittal and parasagittal sections. The vertical lines superimposed on a midfoot frontal section show the planes of the five parasagittal and sagittal cuts used to prepare the specimens that follow (Figures 5.6 - 5.10). In addition, each section is accompanied by a diagram of the plane of section superimposed on a model of the foot. The aim of these guides is to assist three-dimensional comprehension of horse foot anatomy. *SAG* = sagittal and parasagittal section.

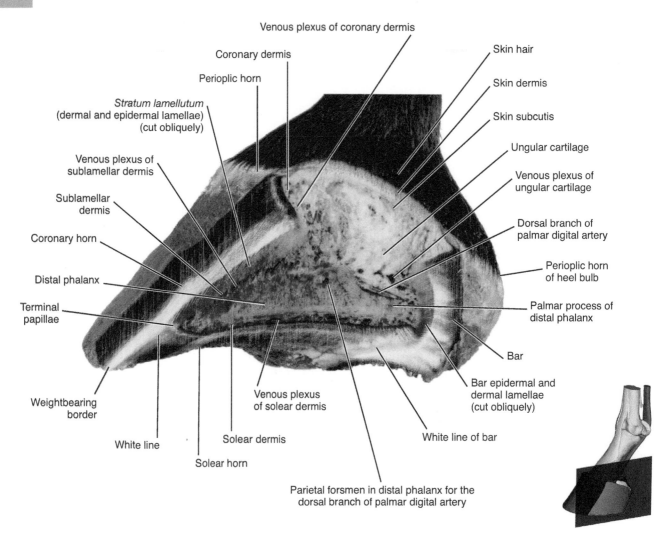

Venous plexus of coronary dermis

Coronary dermis

Perioplic horn

Stratum lamellutum
(dermal and epidermal lamellae)
(cut obliquely)

Venous plexus of
sublamellar dermis

Sublamellar
dermis

Coronary horn

Distal phalanx

Terminal
papillae

Weightbearing
border

White line

Solear horn

Solear dermis

Venous plexus
of solear dermis

Parietal forsmen in distal phalanx for the
dorsal branch of palmar digital artery

White line of bar

Bar epidermal and
dermal lamellae
(cut obliquely)

Bar

Palmar process of
distal phalanx

Perioplic horn
of heel bulb

Dorsal branch of
palmar digital artery

Venous plexus of
ungular cartilage

Ungular cartilage

Skin subcutis

Skin dermis

Skin hair

• **Figure 5.6** Gross anatomy of a parasagittal section from a normal, adult Standardbred forefoot. The first cut in this series of five is through the toe and heel and has removed the quarter (see Figure 5.5 cut SAG 01). The dorsal hoof and the bar lamellae are cut obliquely and show as fine overlapping striations. The palmar process of the distal phalanx and a portion of the ungular cartilage are also sectioned. Note the dorsal branch of lateral digital artery running on the abaxial surface of the distal phalanx in the parietal groove. It enters the body of the distal phalanx through the parietal foramen. The inset shows the plane of section.

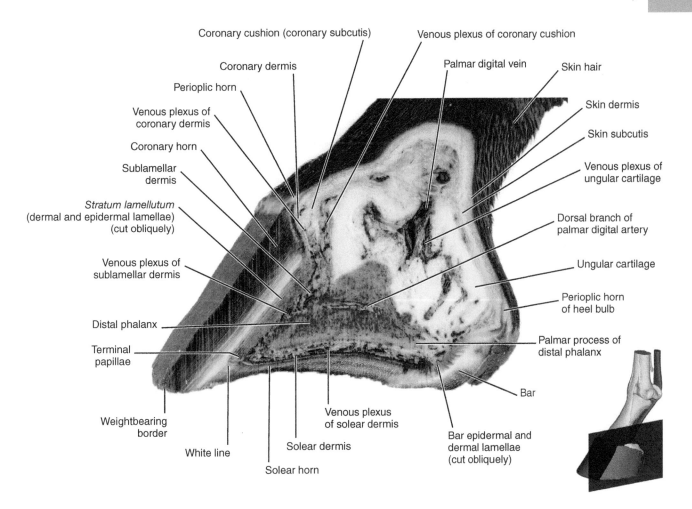

Coronary cushion (coronary subcutis)

Coronary dermis

Perioplic horn

Venous plexus of
coronary dermis

Coronary horn

Sublamellar
dermis

Stratum lamellutum
(dermal and epidermal lamellae)
(cut obliquely)

Venous plexus of
sublamellar dermis

Distal phalanx

Terminal
papillae

Weightbearing
border

White line

Solear horn

Solear dermis

Venous plexus
of solear dermis

Bar epidermal and
dermal lamellae
(cut obliquely)

Bar

Palmar process of
distal phalanx

Perioplic horn
of heel bulb

Ungular cartilage

Dorsal branch of
palmar digital artery

Venous plexus of
ungular cartilage

Skin subcutis

Skin dermis

Skin hair

Venous plexus of coronary cushion

Palmar digital vein

• **Figure 5.7** Gross anatomy of a parasagittal section from the same foot as in Figure 5-6. The cut is now through the lateral pastern and the hoof capsule (see Figure 5.5 cut SAG 02). The lamellae are cut obliquely and the distal sesamoid (navicular) bone is not yet in the plane of section. The dorsal and palmar borders of the ungular cartilage dominate the picture. The large palmar digital vein contains dark clotted blood, and the lateral border of the distal phalanx has been sectioned through the groove that accommodates the dorsal branch of the palmar digital artery.

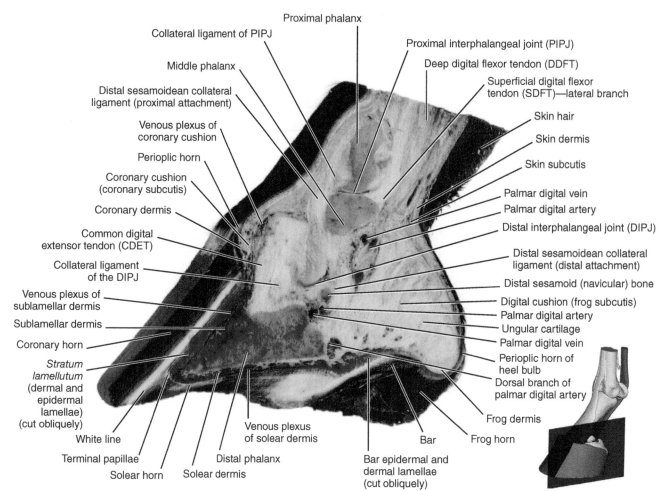

Proximal phalanx

Collateral ligament of PIPJ

Proximal interphalangeal joint (PIPJ)

Middle phalanx

Deep digital flexor tendon (DDFT)

Distal sesamoidean collateral ligament (proximal attachment)

Superficial digital flexor tendon (SDFT)—lateral branch

Venous plexus of coronary cushion

Skin hair

Perioplic horn

Skin dermis

Coronary cushion (coronary subcutis)

Skin subcutis

Coronary dermis

Palmar digital vein

Palmar digital artery

Common digital extensor tendon (CDET)

Distal interphalangeal joint (DIPJ)

Collateral ligament of the DIPJ

Distal sesamoidean collateral ligament (distal attachment)

Venous plexus of sublamellar dermis

Distal sesamoid (navicular) bone

Sublamellar dermis

Digital cushion (frog subcutis)

Coronary horn

Palmar digital artery

Ungular cartilage

Stratum lamellutum (dermal and epidermal lamellae) (cut obliquely)

Palmar digital vein

Perioplic horn of heel bulb

Dorsal branch of palmar digital artery

White line

Venous plexus of solear dermis

Frog dermis

Terminal papillae

Distal phalanx

Bar

Frog horn

Solear horn

Solear dermis

Bar epidermal and dermal lamellae (cut obliquely)

• **Figure 5.8** Gross anatomy of a parasagittal section from the same foot as in Figure 5-6. The cut is now deeper into the lateral pastern and hoof capsule (see Figure 5.5 cut SAG 03). The lamellae are cut obliquely, and the distal sesamoid (navicular) bone has a circular profile being cut close to its lateral extremity. At the level of the middle phalanx the palmar digital artery is cut longitudinally; note the lumen and thick muscular wall. At the level of the distal sesamoid bone the palmar digital artery is cut transversely before it enters the distal phalanx to form the terminal arch. The collateral ligaments of both the distal interphalangeal joint (DIPJ) and proximal interphalangeal joint (PIPJ) and the ungular cartilage and its venous plexus appear in the section.

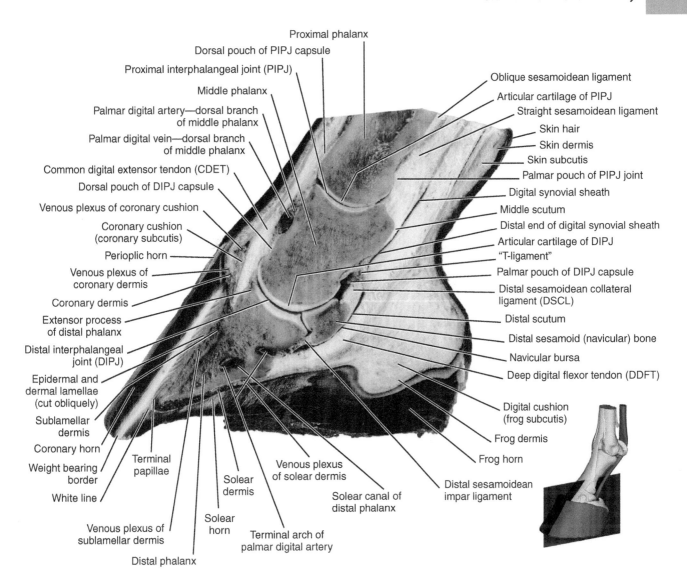

Proximal phalanx

Dorsal pouch of PIPJ capsule

Proximal interphalangeal joint (PIPJ)

Middle phalanx

Palmar digital artery—dorsal branch of middle phalanx

Palmar digital vein—dorsal branch of middle phalanx

Common digital extensor tendon (CDET)

Dorsal pouch of DIPJ capsule

Venous plexus of coronary cushion

Coronary cushion (coronary subcutis)

Perioplic horn

Venous plexus of coronary dermis

Coronary dermis

Extensor process of distal phalanx

Distal interphalangeal joint (DIPJ)

Epidermal and dermal lamellae (cut obliquely)

Sublamellar dermis

Coronary horn

Weight bearing border

White line

Terminal papillae

Venous plexus of sublamellar dermis

Distal phalanx

Solear horn

Solear dermis

Venous plexus of solear dermis

Terminal arch of palmar digital artery

Solear canal of distal phalanx

Oblique sesamoidean ligament

Articular cartilage of PIPJ

Straight sesamoidean ligament

Skin hair

Skin dermis

Skin subcutis

Palmar pouch of PIPJ joint

Digital synovial sheath

Middle scutum

Distal end of digital synovial sheath

Articular cartilage of DIPJ

"T-ligament"

Palmar pouch of DIPJ capsule

Distal sesamoidean collateral ligament (DSCL)

Distal scutum

Distal sesamoid (navicular) bone

Navicular bursa

Deep digital flexor tendon (DDFT)

Digital cushion (frog subcutis)

Frog dermis

Frog horn

Distal sesamoidean impar ligament

• **Figure 5.9** Gross anatomy of a parasagittal section from the same foot as in Figure 5-6. Not being parallel proximodistally, the dorsal hoof wall lamellae are cut obliquely, giving a striated appearance. The distal phalanx shows more of the solear canal and the terminal arch of the palmar digital artery. The oblique sesamoidean ligament of the proximal sesamoid bones is now within the section (see Figure 5.5 cut SAG 04).

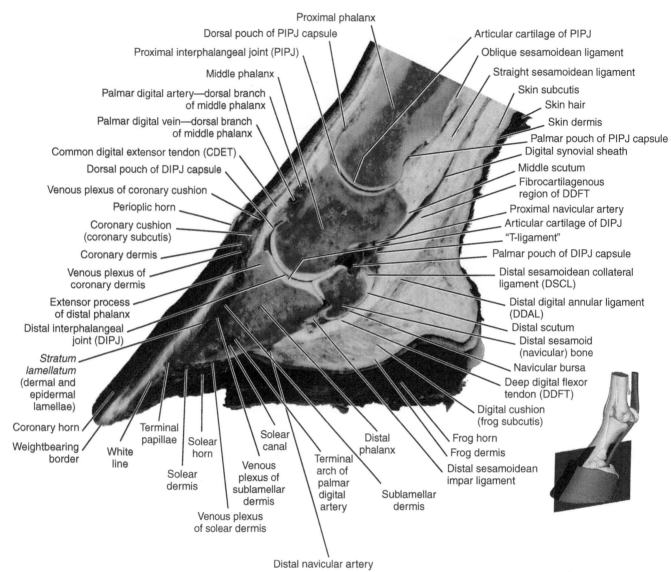

● **Figure 5.10** Gross anatomy of a sagittal section from the same foot as in Figure 5-6. The midline center cut shows most of the structures of the foot but without the ungular cartilages and the collateral ligaments of the two interphalangeal joints (see Figure 5.5 cut SAG 05). Palmar to the proximal phalanx are the straight sesamoidean and oblique sesamoidean ligaments; the insertion of the superficial digital flexor tendon is absent being abaxial to the cut. Opposite the middle scutum on the proximal palmar aspect of the middle phalanx is the fibrocartilaginous pad of the deep digital flexor tendon. The pad accepts pressure from the middle scutum when loading brings the middle phalanx and tendon into contact. The fibrocartilagenous gliding surface for the tendon is lubricated by fluid from the digital synovial sheath.

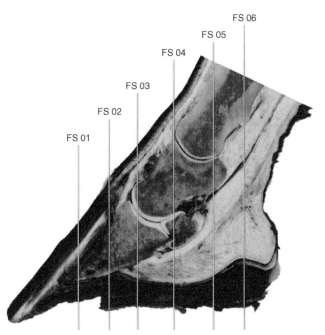

FS 01   FS 02   FS 03   FS 04   FS 05   FS 06

• **Figure 5.11** Gross anatomy frontal sections. The vertical lines superimposed on a foot sagittal section show the planes of the six frontal cuts used to prepare the specimens that follow (Figures 5.12 - 5.17). In addition, each section is accompanied by a diagram of the plane of section superimposed on a model the foot. The aim of these guides is to assist three-dimensional comprehension of horse foot anatomy. FS = frontal section..

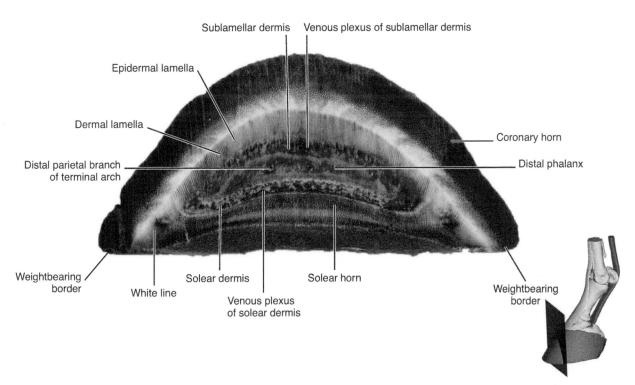

Sublamellar dermis   Venous plexus of sublamellar dermis

Epidermal lamella

Dermal lamella

Coronary horn

Distal parietal branch
of terminal arch

Distal phalanx

Weightbearing
border

Weightbearing
border

White line   Solear dermis   Solear horn

Venous plexus
of solear dermis

• **Figure 5.12** Gross anatomy of a frontal section from a normal, adult Standardbred forefoot. The first cut in this series of seven is through the toe (see Figure 5.11 cut FS 01). The distal margin of the distal phalanx (DP) has been removed showing the sublamellar dermis proximal and solear dermis distal to the DP. The distal parietal arteries branch from the terminal arch and exit through foramina in the dorsal parietal cortex of the DP just proximal to the margin of the DP. The epidermal lamellae appear much longer than in the more familiar transverse section because they are cut obliquely along their long axis.

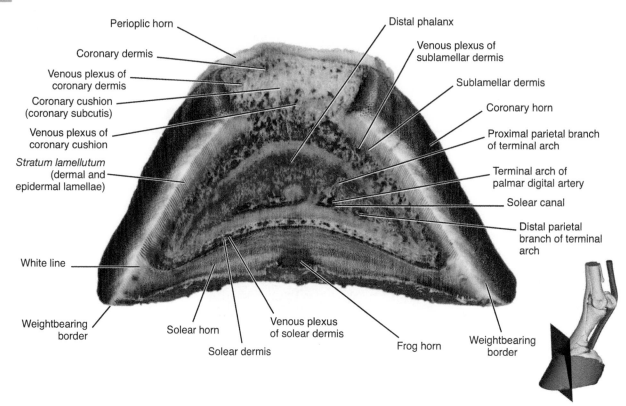

Figure 5.13 Gross anatomy of a frontal section from the same foot as in Figure 5-12. The plane of section is through the coronary cushion proximally and the apex of the frog distally (see Figure 5.11 cut FS 02). The section is through the solear canal and shows the terminal arch of the medial and lateral digital arteries. Branching from the terminal arch are the proximal and distal parietal arteries, medial and lateral, on either side of the midline. These major arteries supply the obliquely cut proximal and distal lamellae. Note how the concave sole follows the profile of the equally concave solear cortex of the distal phalanx. Ground contact is made principally at the weight bearing border of the distal *stratum medium*, the white line (terminal horn), and abaxial margins of the sole. Excess wear of the bearing border or misguided removal with nippers or rasp creates painful pathology between the sole and the margin of the distal phalanx.

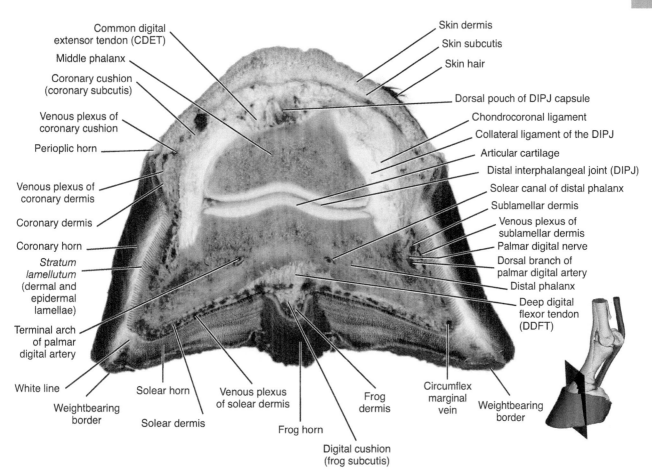

Common digital extensor tendon (CDET)
Middle phalanx
Coronary cushion (coronary subcutis)
Venous plexus of coronary cushion
Perioplic horn
Venous plexus of coronary dermis
Coronary dermis
Coronary horn
Stratum lamellutum (dermal and epidermal lamellae)
Terminal arch of palmar digital artery
White line
Weightbearing border
Solear horn
Solear dermis
Venous plexus of solear dermis
Frog horn
Digital cushion (frog subcutis)
Frog dermis
Circumflex marginal vein
Weightbearing border
Skin dermis
Skin subcutis
Skin hair
Dorsal pouch of DIPJ capsule
Chondrocoronal ligament
Collateral ligament of the DIPJ
Articular cartilage
Distal interphalangeal joint (DIPJ)
Solear canal of distal phalanx
Sublamellar dermis
Venous plexus of sublamellar dermis
Palmar digital nerve
Dorsal branch of palmar digital artery
Distal phalanx
Deep digital flexor tendon (DDFT)

• **Figure 5.14** Gross anatomy of a frontal section from the same foot as in Figure 5-12. Now the distal interphalangeal joint (DIPJ) is sectioned at the level of the strong collateral ligaments of the DIPJ (see Figure 5.11 cut FS 04). Note how the collateral ligament attachment zones are recessed deeply into the bone commensurate with their importance in mediolateral stabilization of the DIPJ. The section includes the solear canal of the distal phalanx and the terminal arch of the palmar digital arteries within its lumen. The apex of the frog and the most dorsal part of the digital cushion are aligned proximodistally with the insertion of the deep digital flexor tendon.

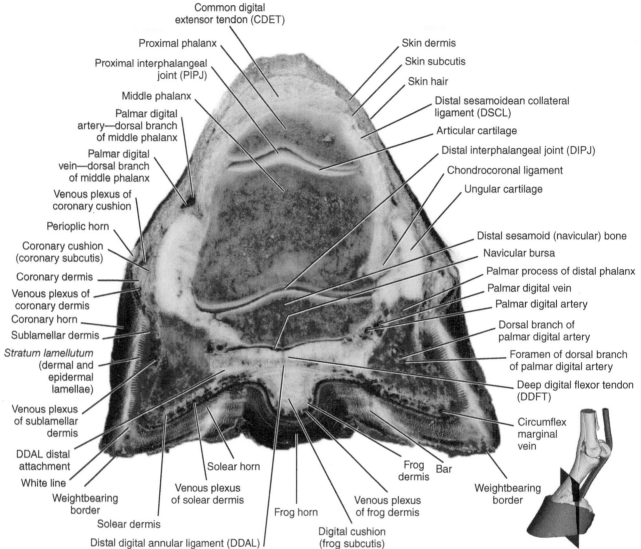

Common digital extensor tendon (CDET)
Proximal phalanx
Proximal interphalangeal joint (PIPJ)
Middle phalanx
Palmar digital artery—dorsal branch of middle phalanx
Palmar digital vein—dorsal branch of middle phalanx
Venous plexus of coronary cushion
Perioplic horn
Coronary cushion (coronary subcutis)
Coronary dermis
Venous plexus of coronary dermis
Coronary horn
Sublamellar dermis
Stratum lamellutum (dermal and epidermal lamellae)
Venous plexus of sublamellar dermis
DDAL distal attachment
White line
Weightbearing border
Solear dermis
Distal digital annular ligament (DDAL)

Skin dermis
Skin subcutis
Skin hair
Distal sesamoidean collateral ligament (DSCL)
Articular cartilage
Distal interphalangeal joint (DIPJ)
Chondrocoronal ligament
Ungular cartilage
Distal sesamoid (navicular) bone
Navicular bursa
Palmar process of distal phalanx
Palmar digital vein
Palmar digital artery
Dorsal branch of palmar digital artery
Foramen of dorsal branch of palmar digital artery
Deep digital flexor tendon (DDFT)
Circumflex marginal vein
Weightbearing border

Solear horn
Venous plexus of solear dermis
Frog horn
Frog dermis   Bar
Venous plexus of frog dermis
Digital cushion (frog subcutis)

• **Figure 5.15** Gross anatomy of a frontal section from the same foot as in Figure 5-12. The section transects all three phalangeal bones and the distal sesamoid (navicular) bone (see Figure 5.11 cut FS 04). The distal sesamoid (navicular) bone contacts the distal phalanx (DP) proximally (as part of the distal interphalangeal joint) and the deep digital flexor tendon distally. Between the fibrocartilagenous flexor surface of the navicular bone (the distal scutum) and deep digital flexor tendon is the navicular bursa. Note the dorsal edge of the ungular cartilages attached to the proximal borders palmar processes of the DP and the proximity of the palmar digital artery and vein to the abaxial borders of the distal sesamoid bone and the insertion of the deep digital flexor tendon on the distal phalanx. The medial and lateral palmar digital arteries and veins are sectioned just before they enter or exit the solear canal of the distal phalanx.

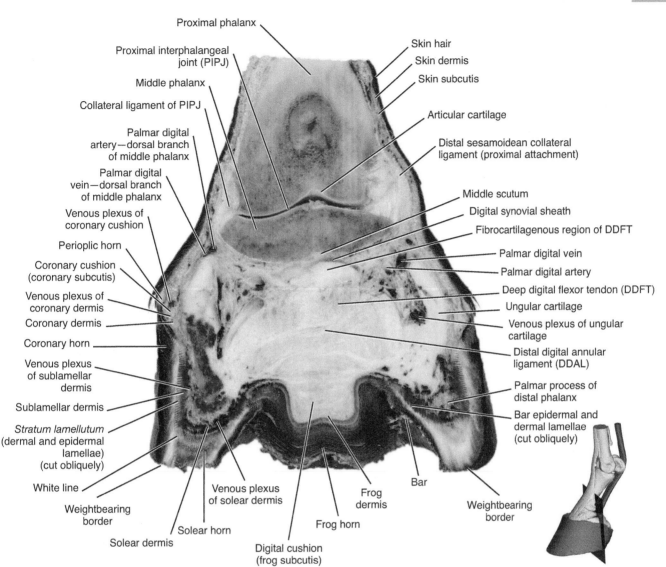

Proximal phalanx

Proximal interphalangeal joint (PIPJ)

Middle phalanx

Collateral ligament of PIPJ

Palmar digital artery—dorsal branch of middle phalanx

Palmar digital vein—dorsal branch of middle phalanx

Venous plexus of coronary cushion

Perioplic horn

Coronary cushion (coronary subcutis)

Venous plexus of coronary dermis

Coronary dermis

Coronary horn

Venous plexus of sublamellar dermis

Sublamellar dermis

Stratum lamellutum (dermal and epidermal lamellae) (cut obliquely)

White line

Weightbearing border

Solear dermis

Solear horn

Venous plexus of solear dermis

Digital cushion (frog subcutis)

Frog horn

Frog dermis

Bar

Skin hair

Skin dermis

Skin subcutis

Articular cartilage

Distal sesamoidean collateral ligament (proximal attachment)

Middle scutum

Digital synovial sheath

Fibrocartilagenous region of DDFT

Palmar digital vein

Palmar digital artery

Deep digital flexor tendon (DDFT)

Ungular cartilage

Venous plexus of ungular cartilage

Distal digital annular ligament (DDAL)

Palmar process of distal phalanx

Bar epidermal and dermal lamellae (cut obliquely)

Weightbearing border

• **Figure 5.16** Gross anatomy of a frontal section from the same foot as in Figure 5-12. The palmar aspect of the bilobed deep digital flexor tendon is partitioned from the digital cushion by the distal digital annular ligament (see Figure 5.11 cut FS 05). The distal part of digital synovial sheath is sectioned just palmar to the middle scutum on the palmar aspect of the middle phalanx and ensheaths only the dorsal surface of the deep digital flexor tendon in this section plane. Note the change in the appearance of the dorsal deep digital flexor tendon compared with the more distal sections. Here the tendon is a fibrocartilaginous pad that accepts loading pressure from the transverse prominence on the proximopalmar aspect of the middle phalanx 3.[3] This prominence is the middle scutum, providing a fibrocartilagenous gliding surface for the tendon, lubricated by fluid from the digital synovial sheath. The axial surface of each ungular cartilage has an extensive venous plexus. Note the proximal attachment of the distal sesamoidean collateral ligament on the distal condyle of the proximal phalanx.

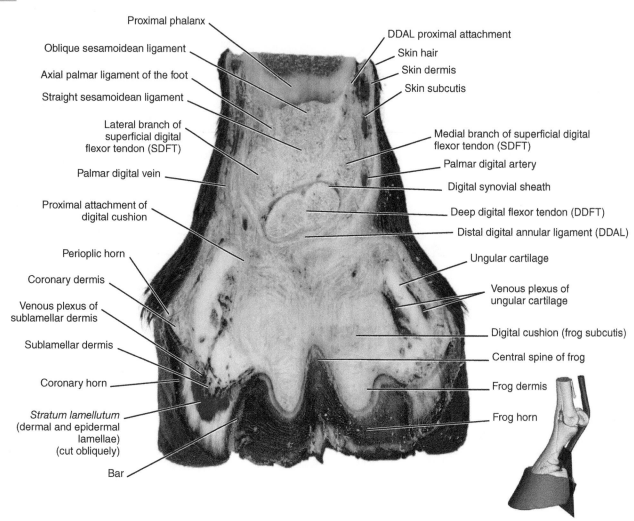

Proximal phalanx

Oblique sesamoidean ligament

Axial palmar ligament of the foot

Straight sesamoidean ligament

Lateral branch of
superficial digital
flexor tendon (SDFT)

Palmar digital vein

Proximal attachment of
digital cushion

Perioplic horn

Coronary dermis

Venous plexus of
sublamellar dermis

Sublamellar dermis

Coronary horn

Stratum lamellutum
(dermal and epidermal
lamellae)
(cut obliquely)

Bar

DDAL proximal attachment

Skin hair

Skin dermis

Skin subcutis

Medial branch of superficial digital
flexor tendon (SDFT)

Palmar digital artery

Digital synovial sheath

Deep digital flexor tendon (DDFT)

Distal digital annular ligament (DDAL)

Ungular cartilage

Venous plexus of
ungular cartilage

Digital cushion (frog subcutis)

Central spine of frog

Frog dermis

Frog horn

• **Figure 5.17** Gross anatomy of a frontal section from the same foot as in Figure 5-12. The only bone in this palmar section is the proximal phalanx sectioned close to the attachments of the oblique sesamoidean ligament, the straight sesamoidean ligament, and the axial palmar ligament of the foot (see Figure 5.11 cut FS 06). Also transected are the medial and lateral branches of the superficial digital flexor tendon on either side of the bilobed deep digital flexor tendon. Trace the distal digital annular ligament (DDAL) from its proximal attachment on the proximal phalanx as it wraps around the deep digital flexor tendon. Note the large veins on the axial and abaxial surfaces of both medial and lateral ungular cartilages; compression of these veins against the flexible cartilages during foot loading, assists in the return of venous blood to the heart.

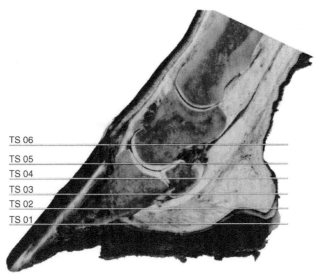

• **Figure 5.18** Gross anatomy transverse sections. The horizontal lines superimposed on a sagittal section show the planes of the six transverse cuts used to prepare the specimens that follow (Figures 5.19 - 5.24). In addition, each section is accompanied by a diagram of the plane of section superimposed on a model of the foot. The aim of these guides is to assist three-dimensional comprehension of horse foot anatomy. TS = transverse section.

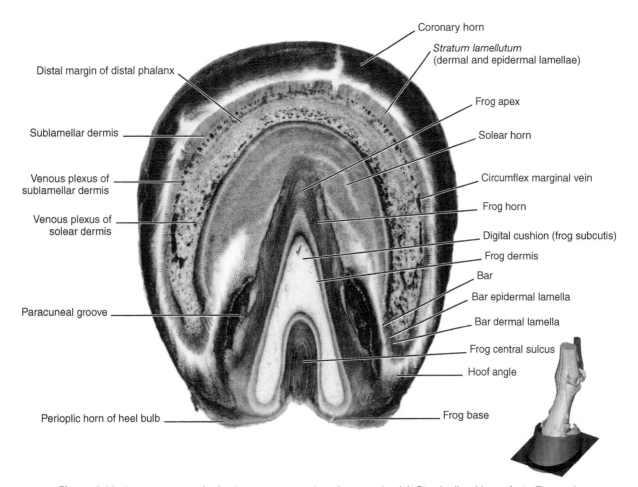

• **Figure 5.19** Gross anatomy of a fresh transverse section of a normal, adult Standardbred horse foot. The cut has removed the bearing border of the hoof wall and sectioned the distal margin of the distal phalanx (see Figure 5.18 cut TS 01). The sublamellar and solear dermis (and their prominent veins) are on both the abaxial and axial borders of the bone. Digital photographs in this plane of section are used to count the number of epidermal lamellae of the hoof wall and bars (approximately 560). Note how the lamellae follow the contours of the angles of the sole and bars.

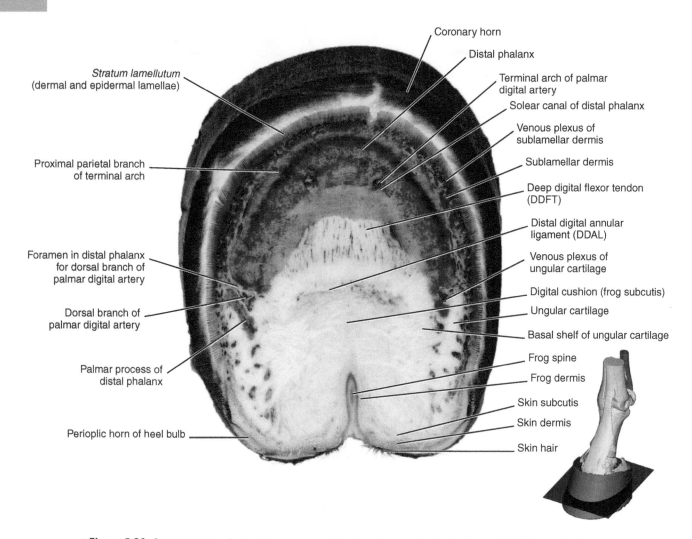

Stratum lamellutum
(dermal and epidermal lamellae)

Proximal parietal branch
of terminal arch

Foramen in distal phalanx
for dorsal branch of
palmar digital artery

Dorsal branch of
palmar digital artery

Palmar process of
distal phalanx

Perioplic horn of heel bulb

Coronary horn

Distal phalanx

Terminal arch of palmar
digital artery

Solear canal of distal phalanx

Venous plexus of
sublamellar dermis

Sublamellar dermis

Deep digital flexor tendon
(DDFT)

Distal digital annular
ligament (DDAL)

Venous plexus of
ungular cartilage

Digital cushion (frog subcutis)

Ungular cartilage

Basal shelf of ungular cartilage

Frog spine

Frog dermis

Skin subcutis

Skin dermis

Skin hair

• **Figure 5.20** Gross anatomy of a fresh transverse section from the same foot as in Figure 5-19. The section transects the distal phalanx and the deep digital flexor tendon at its semilunar insertion on the distal phalanx (see Figure 5.18 cut TS 02). The lamellae of the inner hoof wall are cut in transverse section along with the sublamellar dermis and its extensive array of veins (the sublamellar plexus). Note the dorsal branch of the palmar digital artery in the sectioned foramen in the palmar process of the distal phalanx. The medial and lateral digital arteries are sectioned in the solear canal of the distal phalanx, proximal to where they unite to form the terminal arch.

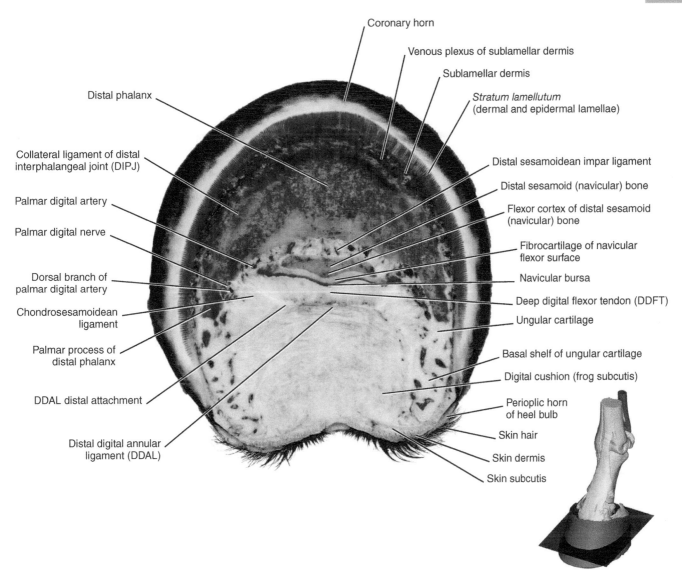

Coronary horn

Venous plexus of sublamellar dermis

Sublamellar dermis

Stratum lamellutum
(dermal and epidermal lamellae)

Distal phalanx

Collateral ligament of distal
interphalangeal joint (DIPJ)

Palmar digital artery

Palmar digital nerve

Dorsal branch of
palmar digital artery

Chondrosesamoidean
ligament

Palmar process of
distal phalanx

DDAL distal attachment

Distal digital annular
ligament (DDAL)

Distal sesamoidean impar ligament

Distal sesamoid (navicular) bone

Flexor cortex of distal sesamoid
(navicular) bone

Fibrocartilage of navicular
flexor surface

Navicular bursa

Deep digital flexor tendon (DDFT)

Ungular cartilage

Basal shelf of ungular cartilage

Digital cushion (frog subcutis)

Perioplic horn
of heel bulb

Skin hair

Skin dermis

Skin subcutis

● **Figure 5.21** Gross anatomy of a fresh transverse section from the same foot as in Figure 5-19. The section transects the distal phalanx, the distal interphalangeal joint (DIPJ), and the distal border of the distal sesamoid (navicular) bone (see Figure 5.18 cut TS 03). The deep digital flexor tendon is cut close to its insertion on the distal phalanx and is separated from the distal sesamoid by the navicular bursa. The tendon is juxtaposed to the fibrocartilagenous distal scutum of the distal sesamoid. The section is just proximal to the distal sesamoidean impar ligament (DSIL) and therefore within the DIPJ. The thick, white, collagenous bundles of the DSIL connect the distal sesamoid bone to the distal phalanx. The medial and lateral palmar digital arteries and veins are sectioned just before they enter-exit the solear canal of the distal phalanx. Note the sectioned dorsal branches of the palmar digital arteries and the palmar digital nerves are axial to the palmar processes of the distal phalanx, that is, sectioned before they enter the foramen (or grooves) in the palmar processes of the distal phalanx. The lamellae of the inner hoof wall are cut in transverse section along with the sublamellar dermis and its extensive array of veins (the sublamellar plexus). The collateral ligaments of the distal interphalangeal joint are cut close to their attachment site on the distal phalanx; note how deeply they are set into the bone.

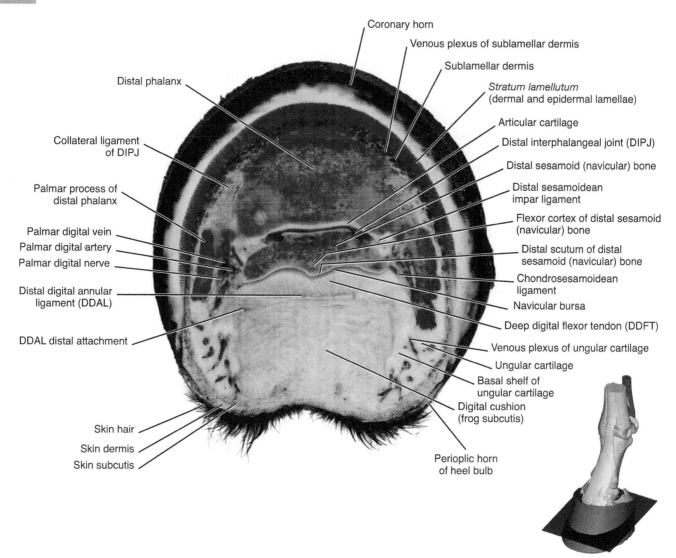

Coronary horn

Venous plexus of sublamellar dermis

Sublamellar dermis

Stratum lamellutum
(dermal and epidermal lamellae)

Articular cartilage

Distal interphalangeal joint (DIPJ)

Distal sesamoid (navicular) bone

Distal sesamoidean
impar ligament

Flexor cortex of distal sesamoid
(navicular) bone

Distal scutum of distal
sesamoid (navicular) bone

Chondrosesamoidean
ligament

Navicular bursa

Deep digital flexor tendon (DDFT)

Venous plexus of ungular cartilage

Ungular cartilage

Basal shelf of
ungular cartilage

Digital cushion
(frog subcutis)

Perioplic horn
of heel bulb

Distal phalanx

Collateral ligament
of DIPJ

Palmar process of
distal phalanx

Palmar digital vein

Palmar digital artery

Palmar digital nerve

Distal digital annular
ligament (DDAL)

DDAL distal attachment

Skin hair

Skin dermis

Skin subcutis

• **Figure 5.22**   Gross anatomy of a fresh transverse section from the same foot as in Figure 5-19. The section transects the distal phalanx, the distal interphalangeal joint (DIPJ), and the distal sesamoid (navicular) bone through its distal articular surface (see Figure 5.18 cut TS 04). The deep digital flexor tendon is adjacent to the fibrocartilagenous distal scutum of the distal sesamoid bone. The white medial and lateral extremities of the distal sesamoidean impar ligament connect the distal sesamoid bone to the distal phalanx. The collateral ligaments of the DIPJ are cut through their attachments on the distal phalanx. The medial and lateral palmar digital veins, arteries, and nerves are sectioned proximal to their entry or exit into the solear canal of the distal phalanx. The lamellae of the inner hoof wall are cut in transverse section along with the sublamellar dermis and its extensive array of veins (the sublamellar plexus). Note the extensive array of veins criss-crossing the basal shelf of the ungular cartilage.

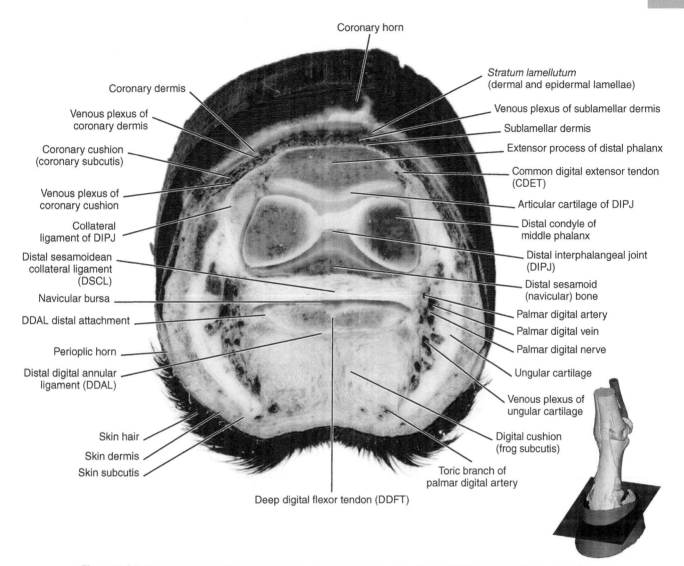

Coronary horn

Coronary dermis

Venous plexus of
coronary dermis

Coronary cushion
(coronary subcutis)

Venous plexus of
coronary cushion

Collateral
ligament of DIPJ

Distal sesamoidean
collateral ligament
(DSCL)

Navicular bursa

DDAL distal attachment

Perioplic horn

Distal digital annular
ligament (DDAL)

Skin hair

Skin dermis

Skin subcutis

Deep digital flexor tendon (DDFT)

Stratum lamellutum
(dermal and epidermal lamellae)

Venous plexus of sublamellar dermis

Sublamellar dermis

Extensor process of distal phalanx

Common digital extensor tendon
(CDET)

Articular cartilage of DIPJ

Distal condyle of
middle phalanx

Distal interphalangeal joint
(DIPJ)

Distal sesamoid
(navicular) bone

Palmar digital artery

Palmar digital vein

Palmar digital nerve

Ungular cartilage

Venous plexus of
ungular cartilage

Digital cushion
(frog subcutis)

Toric branch of
palmar digital artery

• **Figure 5.23** Gross anatomy of a fresh transverse section from the same foot as in Figure 5-19. The section transects the distal phalanx, middle phalanx, the distal interphalangeal joint (DIPJ), and the distal sesamoid (navicular) bone through its collateral ligament (see Figure 5.18 cut TS 05). The collateral ligaments of the DIPJ are cut through their central part between the middle and distal phalanges. The dorsal lamellae of the inner hoof wall are cut in transverse section along with the sublamellar dermis. Note the veins adjacent to the ungular cartilage are mainly axial at this level.

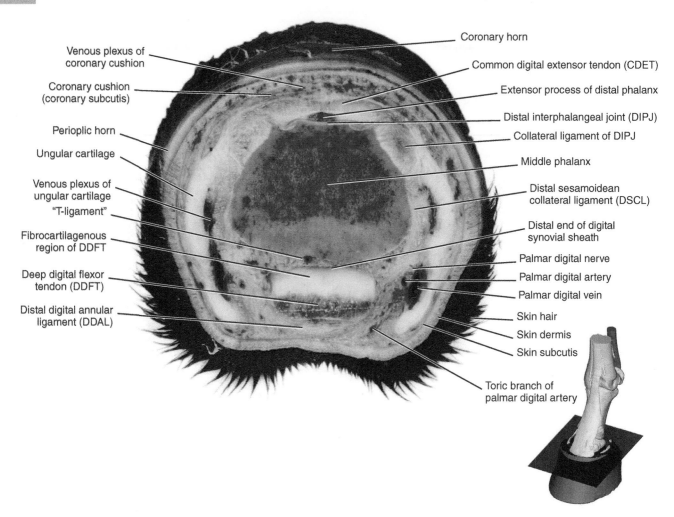

Venous plexus of
coronary cushion

Coronary cushion
(coronary subcutis)

Perioplic horn

Ungular cartilage

Venous plexus of
ungular cartilage

"T-ligament"

Fibrocartilagenous
region of DDFT

Deep digital flexor
tendon (DDFT)

Distal digital annular
ligament (DDAL)

Coronary horn

Common digital extensor tendon (CDET)

Extensor process of distal phalanx

Distal interphalangeal joint (DIPJ)

Collateral ligament of DIPJ

Middle phalanx

Distal sesamoidean
collateral ligament (DSCL)

Distal end of digital
synovial sheath

Palmar digital nerve

Palmar digital artery

Palmar digital vein

Skin hair

Skin dermis

Skin subcutis

Toric branch of
palmar digital artery

● **Figure 5.24** Gross anatomy of a fresh transverse section from the same foot as in Figure 5-19. The section transects the foot through the proximal apex of the extensor process of the distal phalanx and the common digital extensor tendon on either side of it (see Figure 5.18 cut TS 06). The extensor tendon thins in the midline, palpable in life as a soft depression in the coronet. The proximal extent of the distal interphalangeal joint (DIPJ) is abaxial to the extensor process. There are no hoof lamellae at this level; the cut is through the periople, middle phalanx, and palmar pastern above the distal sesamoid (navicular) bone. However, the collateral ligaments of the distal sesamoid bone are attached to the middle phalanx. The collateral ligaments of the DIPJ are cut through their attachment to the distal middle phalanx. The palmar digital vein is prominent, having received blood from the coronary plexus and thus virtually all the venous blood distal to this level. The palmar digital artery and nerve can be palpated near this level, and this is important clinically, to assess arterial pulse quality and for perineural anesthesia of the palmar digital nerve. Note the change in the appearance of the deep digital flexor tendon compared with the more distal sections. The dorsal tendon is a fibrocartilaginous pad that accepts pressure from the transverse prominence (the middle scutum) on the proximo-palmar aspect of the middle phalanx.

References

1. Anon. (Ed.) (2005). *Nomina anatomica veterinaria*, Hannover. International Committee on Veterinary Gross Anatomical Nomenclature. (2005). *Nomina Anatomica Veterinaria*, (5th ed.). Hannover, Germany: World Association of Veterinary Anatomists.

2. Constantinescu G.M., Schaller O. (2012) *Illustrated Veterinary Anatomical Nomenclature*. Stuttgart, Germany: Enke Verlag.

3. Dyson, S. J. (2011). Primary lesions of the deep digtal flexor tendon within the hoof capsule in M. W. Ross and S. J. Dyson, *Diagnosis and management of lameness in the horse* (pp. 344-348). St Louis, MO: Elsevier.

6 The Suspensory Apparatus of the Distal Phalanx

In horses, the appendicular skeleton is suspended or slung within the hoof capsule by a unique anatomic structure: the suspensory apparatus of the distal phalanx (SADP). The horse walks on the bearing border of its hooves and is thus unguligrade, unlike digitigrade (dogs and cats) and plantigrade (bears and humans) animals where body weight is supported by digital and/or plantar cushions.

The SADP connects the distal phalanx to the inner lamellae (*stratum internum*) of the hoof wall. Because of the SADP, it is the hoof wall, not the distal phalanx, that acts as the principal weightbearing structure of the foot. Weightbearing forces are redirected from the distal phalanx to the bearing border of the hoof wall without involving the sole or digital cushion. Foot pain and lameness result if SADP suspensory anatomy is disrupted; a functional SADP is vital to the well-being of the horse. Laminitis is the principal cause of failure of the SADP, the osteopathology,[3] and the pain and suffering associated with laminitis, has ended the lives of numerous ponies and horses alike.

The SADP is a network of collagen bundles extending from the parietal surface of the distal phalanx, spanning the sublamellar dermis and inserting into the lamellar basement membrane. Transverse sections, cut perpendicular to the hoof wall and the dorsum of the distal phalanx, are often made to study lamellar anatomy. However, this transects the collagen bundles of the SADP across their lengths, and the resultant mass of rounded, disjoined shapes doesn't convey its suspensory function. However, sagittal sections of the toe reveal the true suspensory nature of the SADP; the collagen bundles are linearly arranged, extending from the parietal surface of the distal phalanx (DP) to the lamellar interface. The suspensory collagen bundles are near vertical proximally, but distally, where they insert into the terminal and dorsal sole papillae, approach the horizontal and resemble the spokes of a wheel.[2,5] The parietal surface of the distal phalanx is markedly ridged. Between the proximodistal bony ridges are numerous large and small foramina through which blood vessels pass. The collagen bundles of the SADP insert only on the crests of the bone ridges and are absent in the intervening channels.

We used new sectioning planes and histologic stains to study the SADP.[6] Instead of sectioning across the collagen bundles of the SADP, we sectioned along their lines of tension, and this illustrated the suspensory nature of the SADP.

In transverse sections made proximally, at 70 degrees to the dorsal hoof wall (instead of perpendicular), the SADP collagen bundles were linear (in straight lines) and resembled elastic bands connecting two anchor points: the distal phalanx and the hoof lamellae. SADP collagen bundles entering between epidermal lamellae progressively diminished in size abaxially. Within each primary dermal lamella, collagen fibers arborized and, branching from the axial collagen bundles into progressively smaller fibers, entered between secondary epidermal lamellae to insert into the lamellar basement membrane. Here the smallest collagen fibers of the terminal SADP (collagen I and III) unite with the anchoring fibrils (collagen VII) projecting from the lamina densa on the dermal side of the basement membrane. The epidermal basal cells are attached to the other side of the basement membrane via the anchoring filaments (Laminin-332) of the hemidesmosome. The basal cells are connected via their adhesion plaques and cytoskeleton to the increasingly keratinized *stratum internum* and *stratum medium,* thus forming a structural continuum from basement membrane to hoof wall. In this way, hoof wall, dermis, and bone are united into a single functional unit, whereby the entire body weight is suspended from the hoof wall. There was a concentration of fiber insertion around secondary epidermal lamellae tips, suggesting lamellar tips encounter greater strain.

In transverse sections made distally, at 30 degrees to the dorsal hoof wall, the SADP collagen bundles were also linear but now connected the distal margin of the distal phalanx to distal lamella, terminal and dorsal sole papillae.

Not only were the SADP collagen bundles linear as they crossed the sublamellar dermis, but they also aligned with the Sharpey's fibers that inserted the collagen bundles into the surface of the distal phalanx. The Sharpey's fibers were 50 to 100 microns long and, typical of elastin (collagen III), silver stained strongly. The insertion of the SADP onto the parietal surface of the distal phalanx resembled classical entheses where tendon inserts onto bone. However, SADP insertion was achieved, not by a single chondral-apophyseal junction as in tendon to bone but also by a myriad of miniature tendonlike insertions over the entire ridged, parietal surface of the distal phalanx. Unlike nonextensible collagen, elastin is flexible, stretching and recoiling under load: a property well suited to the SADP. The combination of elastin and cartilage at the SADP insertion sites likely prevents stress concentration during loading, as occurs in tendon–bone attachments. Stress is progressively dissipated across noncalcified to calcified fibrocartilage, thus mitigating the risk of traumatic tearing and/or avulsion.

The functional importance of the SADP to the well-being of the horse should not be underestimated. The SADP enables the forces associated with static and dynamic weightbearing to be accommodated and ultimately resisted by the foot. Approximately 67% of the impact vibrations that occur during initial ground impact are dissipated by the lamellar region, thus protecting the distal phalanx and the phalangeal joints from concussive damage.[7] During weightbearing, the distal phalanx descends into the hoof capsule and results in compression of the underlying solar dermis and stretching of dermal and epidermal lamellae. This generates tensile forces within the SADP that enables the distal phalanx to return to its original anatomic location as the foot is unloaded. Controlled movement of the distal phalanx plays a major role in maintaining effective blood circulation and energy delivery to the foot during limb cycling.[4]

A correctly functioning SADP prevents the pain associated with excessive tissue strain, tissue damage, and vascular occlusion. When galloping at 120 strides per minute, up to 1.7 times the horse's body weight is painlessly transferred between ground and skeleton by the SADP.[7] This exceptional feat of bioengineering, seamlessly connecting bone to hoof, is a prime example of adaptive evolution to the running lifestyle of the horse. Evidence of SADP damage (e.g., the clinical signs of laminitis) is of major clinical significance, demanding urgent veterinary and farriery intervention to stabilize and support the foot. Laminitis viewed as disintegration of the SADP is logical,[1] and appreciating the pathologic consequences of this should instruct more rational therapeutic strategies.

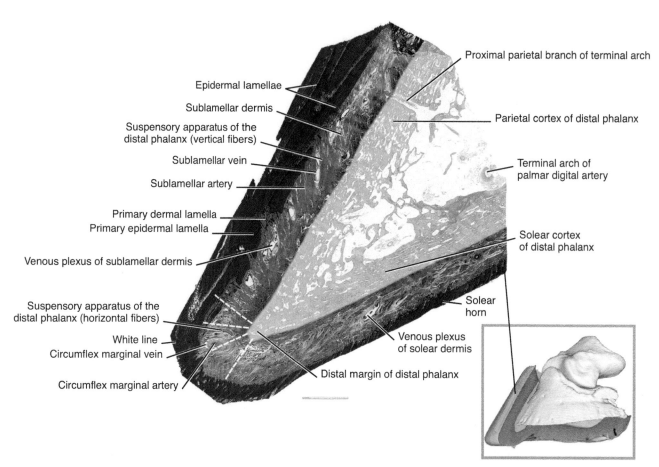

Proximal parietal branch of terminal arch

Epidermal lamellae

Sublamellar dermis

Suspensory apparatus of the distal phalanx (vertical fibers)

Parietal cortex of distal phalanx

Sublamellar vein

Sublamellar artery

Terminal arch of palmar digital artery

Primary dermal lamella
Primary epidermal lamella

Solear cortex of distal phalanx

Venous plexus of sublamellar dermis

Suspensory apparatus of the distal phalanx (horizontal fibers)

Solear horn

White line
Circumflex marginal vein

Venous plexus of solear dermis

Distal margin of distal phalanx

Circumflex marginal artery

• **Figure 6.1** Sagittal section of normal horse toe stained with Masson's trichrome to show collagen connective tissue blue and hoof keratin red. The section is slightly oblique, and the surfaces of two to three adjacent dermal and epidermal lamellae overlap. The bone of the distal phalanx has been decalcified and stains blue instead of the usual red. The outline of the distal phalanx has been lightened to highlight the blue-staining, adjacent collagen of the suspensory apparatus of the distal phalanx (SADP). Note the orientation of the SADP collagen bundles; they are near vertical proximally and horizontal distally. SADP collagen bundles originate on the parietal cortex of the distal phalanx, penetrate between epidermal lamellae as dermal lamellae, and insert over the surface of the epidermal basement membrane. Distally, collagen bundles are arranged like the spokes of a wheel (represented by four dotted lines), centered on the distal margin of the distal phalanx (DP). Collagen bundles, originating proximal to the DP margin, extend dorsoproximally and enter between the distal lamellae. Some extend dorsally, parallel to the ground surface (horizontal), and merge into the terminal papillae of the white line. Others are oriented distally toward solear papillae. Collagen bundles beneath the DP solear cortex are aligned parallel to the sole and are sandwiched between it and the hoof DP. (Stain = Masson's trichrome. Scale = 20 mm.) The inset shows the provenance and plane of section of the specimen.

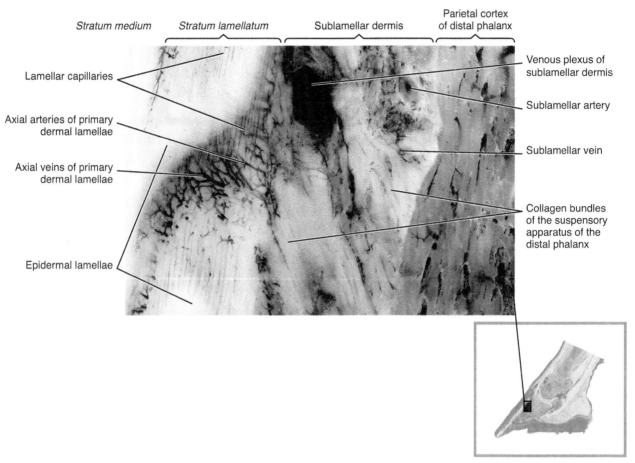

Stratum medium   Stratum lamellatum   Sublamellar dermis   Parietal cortex of distal phalanx

Lamellar capillaries

Axial arteries of primary dermal lamellae

Axial veins of primary dermal lamellae

Epidermal lamellae

Venous plexus of sublamellar dermis

Sublamellar artery

Sublamellar vein

Collagen bundles of the suspensory apparatus of the distal phalanx

• **Figure 6.2** Macro photograph of an unstained section of dorsal midline lamellae with blood vessels previously perfused with a low viscosity mixture of India Ink and 7% gelatin dissolved in warm, 45 C° saline. After the gelatin sets the circulation, including the lamellar capillaries are filled with a semirigid, black gel. The specimen was dissected and photographed under water, and the white collagen bundles of the suspensory apparatus of the distal phalanx (SADP) stand out against the large, dark veins in the sublamellar dermis. In this proximal lamellar region (see inset), the SADP is oriented near vertically. Two epidermal lamellae are cut obliquely and have lifted away, exposing the axial arteries and veins in the translucent primary dermal lamellae beneath. Note these vessels are oriented at the same oblique angle as the SADP collagen bundles. Lamellar capillaries are still embedded between secondary lamellae and are oriented differently—proximodistally, parallel to the hoof wall. The inset shows the provenance of the specimen.

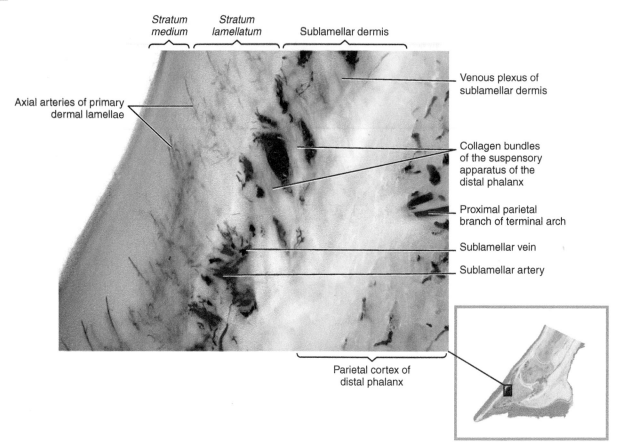

Stratum medium   *Stratum lamellatum*   Sublamellar dermis

Axial arteries of primary dermal lamellae

Venous plexus of sublamellar dermis

Collagen bundles of the suspensory apparatus of the distal phalanx

Proximal parietal branch of terminal arch

Sublamellar vein

Sublamellar artery

Parietal cortex of distal phalanx

• **Figure 6.3** Macro photograph of an unstained section of dorsal midline lamellae with blood vessels previously perfused with liquid methyl methacrylate (MMA). The MMA has polymerized, resulting in a vascular cast. Most of the *stratum medium* of the hoof wall has been removed. The arterial system contains red-pigmented MMA and the venous system blue. The viscosity of the MMA mixtures was deliberately kept high so that only the major vessels were perfused. The white collagen bundles of the suspensory apparatus of the distal phalanx are highlighted against the large, dark-blue veins of the sublamellar venous plexus. In this proximal lamellar region (see inset), the SADP is oriented near vertically. The proximal parietal artery passes through a foramen in the parietal cortex of the distal phalanx and branches in the sublamellar dermis. Sublamellar arteries and veins are located in the spaces between the collagen bundles of the SADP. Small axial lamellar arteries branch from the sublamellar arteries and enter the primary dermal lamellae at the same oblique angle as the SADP. The inset shows the provenance of the specimen.

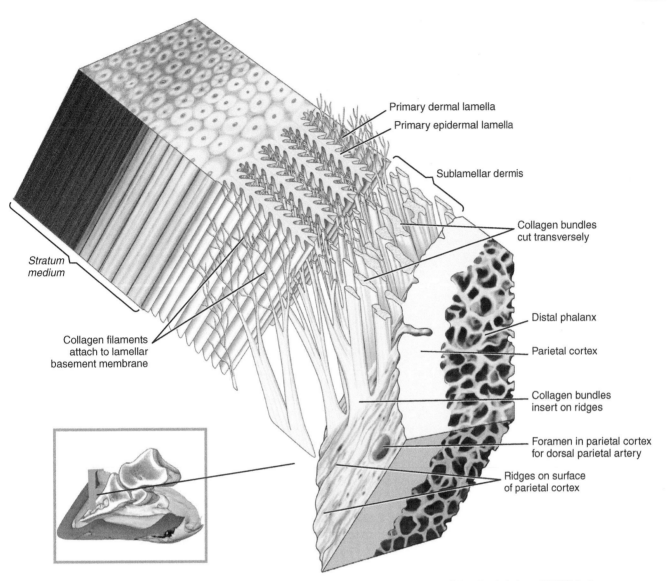

Primary dermal lamella
Primary epidermal lamella
Sublamellar dermis
Collagen bundles cut transversely
Distal phalanx
Parietal cortex
Collagen bundles insert on ridges
Foramen in parietal cortex for dorsal parietal artery
Ridges on surface of parietal cortex
Stratum medium
Collagen filaments attach to lamellar basement membrane

• **Figure 6.4** Diagram of the white collagen bundles of the suspensory apparatus of the distal phalanx (SADP) in the proximal lamellar region, where the collagen bundles are oriented near vertically. The collagen bundles arise on ridges on the parietal surface of the distal phalanx and cross the sublamellar dermis to insert as fine filaments on the lamellar basement membrane. When sectioned transversely, the collagen bundles have rounded and ovoid profiles (as in Figs. 8-8 & 8-13). When sectioned at 70 degrees to the horizontal, the collagen bundles are aligned parallel to the long axes of the suspensory apparatus, and the collagen bundles have linear profiles (as in Fig. 6-6 & 6-6). The inset shows the provenance of the specimen. (Diagram designed by the author.)

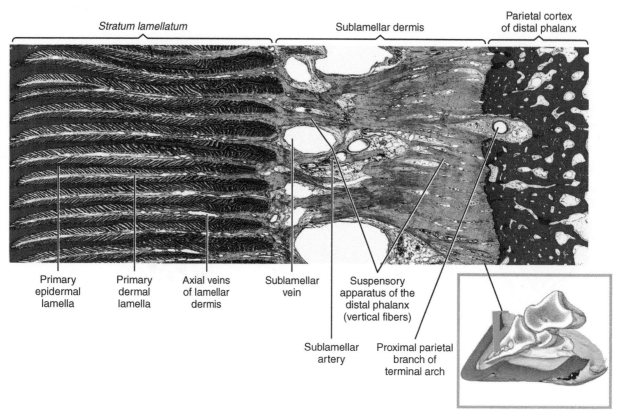

Stratum lamellatum   Sublamellar dermis   Parietal cortex of distal phalanx

Primary epidermal lamella   Primary dermal lamella   Axial veins of lamellar dermis   Sublamellar vein   Suspensory apparatus of the distal phalanx (vertical fibers)

Sublamellar artery   Proximal parietal branch of terminal arch

• **Figure 6.5** Photomicrograph proximal transverse plane (see inset) showing blue-staining bundles of collagen fibers crossing the the sublamellar dermis between red-staining epidermal lamellae and the light-red-staining parietal surface of the distal phalanx. When sectioned at 70 degrees to the horizontal, the collagen bundles are aligned parallel to the long axes of the suspensory apparatus of the distal phalanx. The collagen bundles of the sublamellar dermis are linear, separated by blood vessels, and insert on the parietal surface of the DP. The collagen bundles branch and enter primary dermal lamellae between red-staining epidermal lamellae. In this plane of section, the lamellae are transected obliquely and measure (mean ± s.e.) 5.24 ± 0.02 mm. Located in the loose connective tissue between collagen bundles are numerous veins, arteries, and nerves. Note the number and large size of the sublamellar veins. They anastomose freely with each other forming an extensive sublamellar venous plexus. (Stain = Masson's trichrome.) The insert shows the provenance of the specimen and the plane of section.

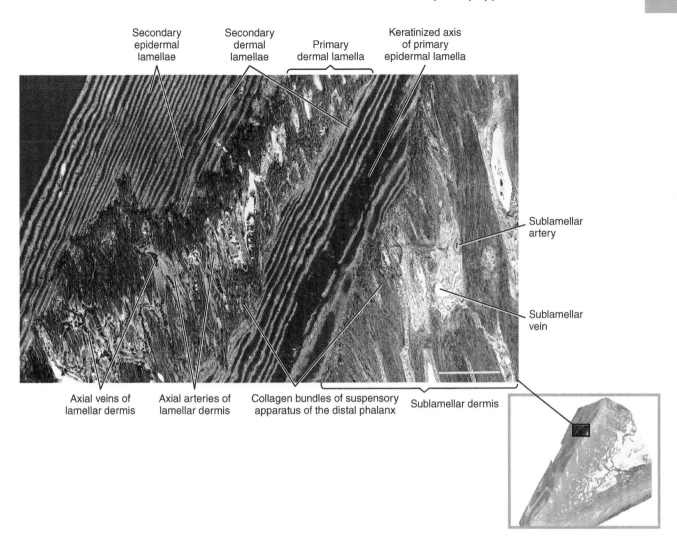

• **Figure 6.6** Longitudinal section of red-staining epidermal lamellae and the blue-staining collagen bundles of the suspensory apparatus of the distal phalanx (SADP). This unique plane of section transects obliquely from the sublamellar dermis, across a primary dermal lamella and through several secondary epidermal lamellae. The angle of the SADP collagen bundles in this proximal specimen is about 70° to the horizontal. Note the large number of axial vessels in the primary dermal lamella oriented at the same angle as the SADP collagen bundles. The large vessels are veins, and between them are thick-walled arteries. Likewise, in the sublamellar dermis, feeder arteries deliver blood to the lamellar axial vessels; collecting veins drain it away. The inset shows the provenance of the section. (Bar = 1000 microns [1 mm]. Stain = Masson's trichrome.)

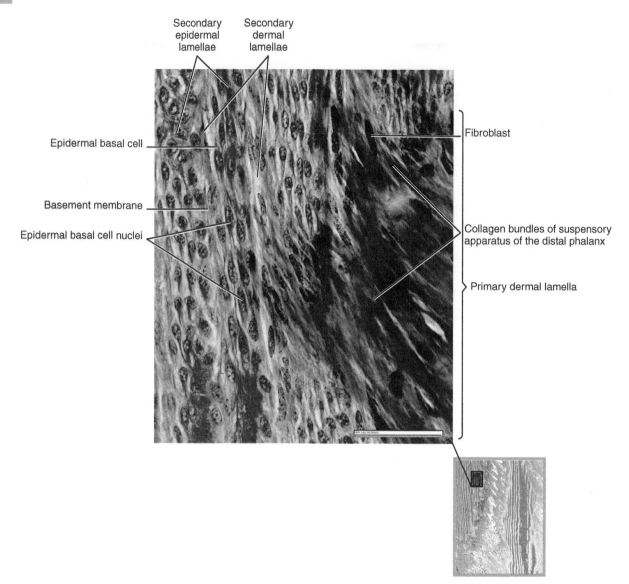

Secondary epidermal lamellae

Secondary dermal lamellae

Epidermal basal cell

Basement membrane

Epidermal basal cell nuclei

Fibroblast

Collagen bundles of suspensory apparatus of the distal phalanx

Primary dermal lamella

• **Figure 6.7** Longitudinal section of red-staining epidermal lamellae and the blue-staining terminal fibers of the suspensory apparatus of the distal phalanx (SADP). This unique plane of section transects obliquely across a primary dermal lamella and through several secondary epidermal lamellae. Note the oblique angle of the SADP collagen bundles that originated distally on the parietal cortex of the distal phalanx and are now inserting on the basement membrane covered surface of the secondary epidermal lamellae. The lamellar epidermal basal cells (LEBCs) are fusiform, and the long axes of the LEBCs are aligned proximodistally similar to the load-bearing collagen bundles of the SADP. The LEBC nuclei are also fusiform and suspended between the poles of the cells by the dark, red-staining keratin cytoskeleton. The inset shows the provenance of the section. (Bar = 50 microns [0.05 mm]. Stain = Masson's trichrome.)

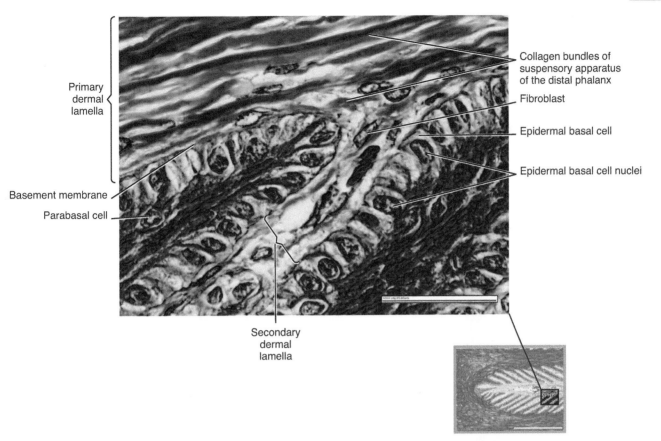

Primary dermal lamella

Collagen bundles of suspensory apparatus of the distal phalanx

Fibroblast

Epidermal basal cell

Epidermal basal cell nuclei

Basement membrane

Parabasal cell

Secondary dermal lamella

● **Figure 6.8** Photomicrograph of 70-degree transverse section of red-staining epidermal lamellae and the blue-staining collagen bundles of the suspensory apparatus of the distal phalanx. Branches from the linear collagen bundles in the primary dermal lamella enter the secondary dermal lamellae. Diminishing in size, they fuse to the secondary epidermal lamellar (SEL) basement membrane. In particular, there is a focus of collagen fiber attachment at the SEL tip. The inset shows the provenance of the section. (Bar = 25 microns [0.025 mm]. Stain = Masson's trichrome.)

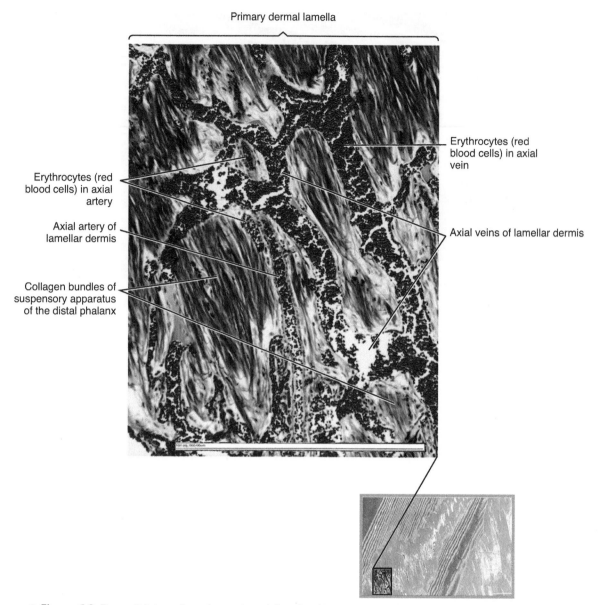

Primary dermal lamella

Erythrocytes (red blood cells) in axial vein

Erythrocytes (red blood cells) in axial artery

Axial veins of lamellar dermis

Axial artery of lamellar dermis

Collagen bundles of suspensory apparatus of the distal phalanx

● **Figure 6.9** Figure 6.9 Lamellar primary dermal lamellar blood vessels. The epidermal lamellae have a high requirement for glucose, and this is delivered to the lamellar capillary network by axial arteries and arterioles, where it becomes available for lamellar metabolism. Thus, many arteries cross the sublamellar dermis and, after branching, deliver blood to the axial lamellar arteries in the primary dermal lamellae. This longitudinal (parasagittal) section is through a single primary dermal lamella (PDL) and shows an artery and numerous veins between the blue-staining collagen bundles of the suspensory apparatus of the distal phalanx (SADP). The section bisects the artery along its length showing its lumen packed with erythrocytes and its relatively thick wall. The veins also contain numerous erythrocytes, but, in contrast to the unbranching artery, the thin walled veins branch (anastomose) extensively. In life, the veins are laterally compressed (flat and ribbon-like) and the section is along the length of the veins showing the multiple channels along which blood returning from the capillary blood may flow. Compare the profiles of the lamellar veins in this section with those sectioned transversely in Figure 6.5. Each load cycle of the SADP compresses the lamellar veins delivering blood to the adjacent, sublamellar venous plexus. (Bar = 500 μm [0.5 mm]. Stain = Masson's trichrome.) The inset box shows the provenance of the specimen.

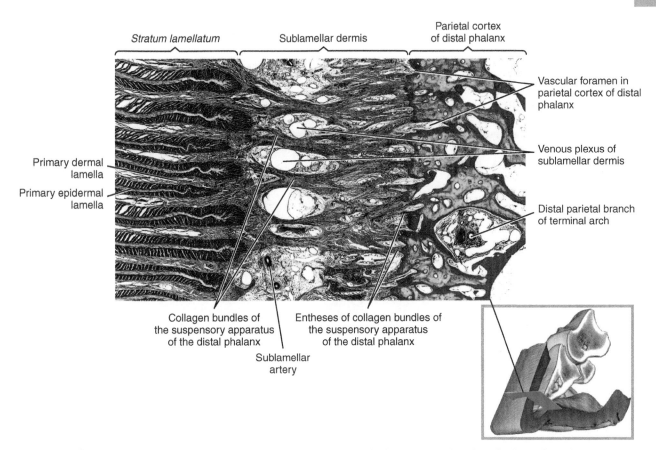

Stratum lamellatum   Sublamellar dermis   Parietal cortex of distal phalanx

Vascular foramen in parietal cortex of distal phalanx

Primary dermal lamella

Primary epidermal lamella

Venous plexus of sublamellar dermis

Distal parietal branch of terminal arch

Collagen bundles of the suspensory apparatus of the distal phalanx

Entheses of collagen bundles of the suspensory apparatus of the distal phalanx

Sublamellar artery

● **Figure 6.10** Photomicrograph distal transverse plane (see inset) of blue-staining bundles of collagen fibers in the sublamellar dermis, between red-staining epidermal lamellae and the light-red-staining parietal surface of the distal phalanx (DP). When sectioned at 30 degrees to the horizontal, the collagen bundles are aligned parallel to the long axes of the suspensory apparatus of the DP. The collagen bundles are linear, separated by blood vessels, and insert on prominent ridges on the parietal surface of the DP. Between the ridges are foramina traversed by blood vessels. The collagen bundles branch and enter primary dermal lamellae between red-staining epidermal lamellae. Located in the loose connective tissue between collagen bundles are numerous veins, arteries, and nerves. (Stain = Masson's trichrome.) The inset shows the provenance and plane of section of the specimen.

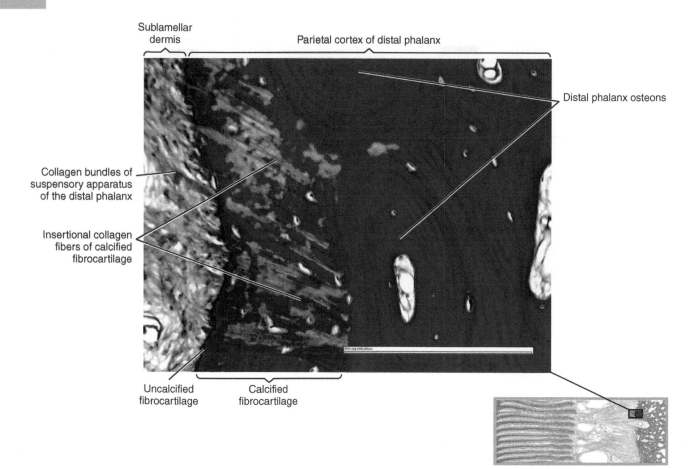

• Figure 6.11 Photomicrograph of 70-degree transverse section of the chondral-apophyseal interface between the suspensory apparatus and the parietal cortex of the distal phalanx. Bundles of tendonlike collagen fibers cross the sublamellar dermis and insert on a thin layer of blue-staining uncalcified fibrocartilage (the tide-mark). Blue staining, linear collagen fibers (50–100 microns long) cross the zone of calcified cartilage and merge into the adjacent osteons of the parietal cortex of the distal phalanx. The blue structures are likely fibers of elastin and collagen type III and are thus Sharpey's fibers. Stain = Masson's trichrome. Bar = 200 μm (0.20 mm). The insert shows the provenance of the specimen.

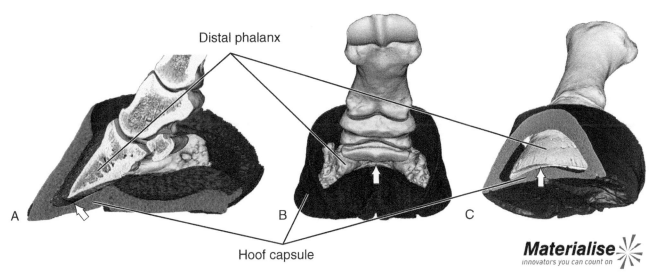

Distal phalanx

A B C

Hoof capsule

Materialise
innovators you can count on

• **Figure 6.12** Mimics model of a normal front foot showing the anatomic relationship between the distal phalanx (DP) and the hoof capsule. The suspensory apparatus of the DP maintains the DP in a fixed position relative to the hoof capsule; this applies not only to the wall but also to the sole. The DP margin is never in contact with the sole and always a uniform distance from it. The arrows in **A, B,** and **C** are beneath the dermis normally present between the margin of the distal phalanx and the horny sole. The dermis is not shown in the model so the clearance between bone and hoof appears as a space.

References

1. Budras, K. D., Hinterhofer, C., Hirschberg, R., Polsterer, E., & Konig, H. E. (2009a). The suspensory apparatus of the coffin bone. Part 2: Clinical relevance of the suspensory apparatus and its fan-shaped reinforcement in chronic equine laminitis with coffin bone or hoof capsule rotation. *Pferdeheilkunde, 25,* 198–204.

2. Budras, K. D., Hirschberg, R., Hinterhofer, C., Polsterer, E., & Konig, H. E. (2009b). The suspensory apparatus of the coffin bone. Part 1: The fan-shaped reinforcement of the suspensory apparatus at the tip of the coffin bone in the horse. *Pferdeheilkunde, 25,* 96–104.

3. Engiles, J. B., Galantino-Homer, H. L., Boston, R., McDonald, D., Dishowitz, M. & Hankenson, K. D. (2015). Osteopathology in the equine distal phalanx associated with the development and progression of laminitis. *Veterinary Pathology, 52,* 928–944.

4. Medina-Torres, C. E., Pollitt, C. C., Underwood, C., Castro-Olivera, E. M., Collins, S. N., Allavena, R. E., et al. (2014). Equine lamellar energy metabolism studied using tissue microdialysis. *Veterinary Journal, 201,* 275–282.

5. Pellmann, R., Budras, K. D., & Bragulla, H. (1997). Structure and function of the suspensory apparatus of the coffin bone in the horse. *Pferdeheilkunde, 13,* 53–64.

6. Pollitt, C. C. & S. N. Collins (2015). The suspensory apparatus of the distal phalanx in normal horses. *Equine Veterinary Journal.* Advance online publication. doi:10.1111/evj.12459.

7. Setterbo, J. J., Garcia, T. C., Campbell, I. P., Reese, J. L., Morgan, J. M., Kim, S. Y., et al. (2009). Hoof accelerations and ground reaction forces of Thoroughbred racehorses measured on dirt, synthetic, and turf track surfaces. *American Journal of Veterinary Research, 70,* 1220–1229.

8. Willemen, M. A., Jacobs, M. W., & Schamhardt, H. C. (1999). In vitro transmission and attenuation of impact vibrations in the distal forelimb. *Equine Veterinary Journal, 30*(Suppl.), 245–248.

The overriding priority of the vascular system of the foot is to deliver energy to the lamellar interface of the suspensory apparatus of the distal phalanx (SADP). Having evolved into the ultimate ungulate with a distal phalanx attached within a single hoof, it is not surprising to find a vast array of capillaries adjacent to every square millimeter of lamellar epidermis. Attachment of surfaces in biological systems requires energy, and the source of that energy is the glucose delivered by the blood vascular system. The epidermis itself is avascular and relies on capillaries in the adjacent dermis to deliver the requirements needed to maintain attachment and a multiplicity of other functions. Significantly, lamellar capillaries are located only in secondary dermal lamellae (SDLs) and are absent in the primary dermal lamellae and sublamellar dermis. This means that the capillaries are extremely close to the target of energy delivery: the secondary epidermal lamellae. Arteries and veins serve to get blood to and away from the capillary bed, but it is the capillaries that deliver the goods.

On the arterial, afferent side of the circulation, thin-walled capillaries flow with nutrient-rich plasma and oxygen-loaded red blood cells (erythrocytes). However, what the epidermal lamellae require most is blood sugar (glucose), without which the lamellar interface disintegrates.[1] The normal equine foot consumes glucose and produces lactate, and one foot has a glucose consumption exceeding that of the horse's head.[2] Since the hoof doesn't store glycogen, glucose consumption reflects glycolysis and oxidation; the high concentration of lactate in the digital veins indicates that most of the glucose is metabolized anaerobically to lactate.

The glucose-hungry lamellar epidermal cells do not rely on insulin to transport glucose across their cell membranes into their cytoplasm. Instead, like the brain, lamellar epidermal cells are enriched with a glucose transport molecule called *GLUT-1*. Glucose is a small molecule and readily diffuses through tissues. Glucose delivered by the porous lamellar capillaries to the dermal tissue fluid, outside the target epidermal cells, is rapidly sequestered by GLUT-1 and transported to the epidermal cell interior. Here it is trapped by conversion to glucose 6-phosphate, a phosphorylation reaction requiring adenosine triphosphate (ATP). Thus an efficient diffusion gradient is maintained, drawing glucose from outside the lamellar epidermal cell to its interior.

After the capillary network has delivered its payload of energy, blood exits to veins in the primary dermal lamellae that in turn deliver it to large veins in the sublamellar plexus, draining into the even larger veins of the coronary plexus. Without contractile muscle in the foot, compression of foot veins to return blood to the heart is achieved by cyclic loading and unloading of soft tissues (especially the ungular cartilages) massaged between bone, hoof, and skin. The arteries also encounter large fluctuations in pressure during cyclic loading and unloading, and backflow, in the wrong direction, is a detrimental possibility. However, built-in at specific points along the arterial tree are valve-like structures preventing retrograde flow and ensuring onward delivery of arterial blood to the foot at all times.

The design of the horse foot and its vasculature is complex as befits an athletic ungulate equipped with a single hoof, the most highly evolved integumentary structure among all the mammals.[3] For the most part, the vascular system of the foot serves the horse well, contributing to pain-free athletic performance in normal circumstances. However, evolution to the single-digit lifestyle has its drawbacks. The foot depends on a single, major artery for blood delivery below the fetlock. Compromise to this artery (the median or common digital artery) or its superficial fetlock and pastern branches can lead to severe ischemic, even gangrenous, complications. As if anticipating such problems, the arterial tree is equipped with circular anatomic arrangements that ensure blood can reach key structures from more than one direction. Medial branches encircle the tissue they serve and unite with the lateral branch of the same artery, giving off nutrient branches along the way. Thus if trauma obliterates blood flow on one side, the encircling artery can restore blood flow from the other side. The five major circumflex arteries are the proximal phalangeal, middle phalangeal, coronal, terminal arch, and circumflex marginal.

The distal limb arteries have thick muscular walls well innervated with nerves controlling tone for dilation and constriction when required. The arteries are markedly resilient, capable of withstanding considerable stretching and compression during the wide range of flexion and extension encountered by the horse distal limb during extremes of locomotory activity. The veins that run beside the arteries are thin walled, lightly innervated, and equipped with valves to prevent retrograde blood flow and ensure efficient venous return. However, within and around the hoof capsule, the very large venous network is completely without valves and anastomoses extensively in all directions. During a foot load cycle, soft tissue compression promotes blood outflow from the solear, lamellar, coronal, bulbar venous plexi without hindrance, in all or any direction—following lines of least resistance. The lack of valves in and around the venous system of the foot also accommodates potentially dangerous peaks of hydraulic pressure[4]; blood can escape rapidly from the confines of the hoof capsule and the axial skeleton, thus dissipating the impact of hoof strike and ameliorating the risk of small vessel rupture and edema. The fluid in the blood vascular system serves to dampen concussive forces encountered during locomotion; 30% to 60% of the shock encountered during foot ground contact is primarily attenuated by the lamellar interface.[5]

THE TERMINAL ARCH—THE SOURCE

The conventional way to describe the circulation of the horse foot is to start with the major arteries of the leg and work down its branches to the foot. For just such a classical description of the circulation see the next section; the Arterial System. For students of the horse's foot, another way to consider the blood circulation of the foot is to start inside the foot with the terminal arch of the medial and lateral digital arteries. This vessel, as its name suggests, is the terminus and distribution center for a significant proportion of the output of blood from the heart. The horse at rest has about 40 liters of blood in its blood vascular system. At rest the horse heart pumps about 70 liters per minute into the aorta and major vessels and, via the median artery, delivers a proportion of this to the foot. The output of blood by the Thoroughbred heart can increase eightfold at the gallop reaching 300 l/min delivered at a heart rate of 220 beats/min.[6] For a horse weighing 450 kg this corresponds to 150 to 475 ml/min/kg. Based on a horse foot from the fetlock joint down weighing 1.5 kg, this means that at rest 225 ml of blood per minute are flowing through the foot, increasing to 712 ml per minute during exercise. As arterial blood is delivered to the foot, almost 15% of the glucose is consumed, in contrast to the head, which consumes just 8%.[7] In comparison, the human brain consumes 20% of the glucose delivered, remarkable since the brain is only 2% of the body weight.[8]

The terminal arch is located deep inside the distal phalanx housed in a tunnel called the *solear canal* or sometimes the *semilunar arch* because of its shape. Inside the distal phalanx, this vital blood vessel is protected from outside trauma—important for an animal that may strike its feet onto rocky terrain when galloping at high speed. The solear cortex of the distal phalanx is particularly dense compared with the porous parietal cortex that faces the hoof wall.

Nine to ten branches of the terminal arch exit the parietal cortex of the distal phalanx via natural tunnels called *foramina*. Plain radiographs of the distal phalanx show the parietal foramina resembling the spokes of a wheel (Fig 12.2). Four to five of the terminal arch branches (proximal parietal branches of the terminal arch) exit via dorsal foramina located around the base of the extensor process of the distal phalanx. These arteries supply the proximal lamellae and the papillae of the proximal coronary hoof. The remaining five to six (distal parietal branches of the terminal arch) exit the parietal cortex close to the distal margin of the distal phalanx and supply branches to the distal lamellae and the terminal papillae. They also anastomose with each other to form the well-known arterial circle called the *circumflex marginal artery*, which is peripheral to the distal margin of the distal phalanx and borders the distal inner hoof wall (sole wall junction). Branches from the circumflex marginal artery are directed inward beneath the distal margin of the distal phalanx and its palmar cortex to branch and ramify the solear dermis and supply the solear epidermis.

Collectively, the parietal arteries branch and arborize into smaller vessels that cross the sublamellar dermis and ramify into fine arterioles that supply the entire lamellar interface. They pass between the primary epidermal lamellae as axial arteries at angles corresponding to the collagen bundles of the suspensory apparatus of the distal phalanx (SADP)—near vertical proximally and horizontal distally. From terminal arterioles, tufts of capillaries arise that, in a direction different to the axial vessels and exclusively within the SDLs, form a vast interconnected system of thin-walled vessels fulfilling the destiny of their anatomy, delivering energy to the lamellar epidermal basal cells. The circulation is completed by the capillaries merging into venules in the primary dermal lamellae that anastomose into larger axial veins that drain to the large plexus of veins in the sublamellar dermis. Venous blood exits the sublamellar and solar plexi with each compressive loading cycle via a multitude of anastomosing routes. There are veins beside arteries in the parietal foramina and solear canal that aid in the multidirectional return of blood to the heart.

Thus lamellar capillaries supply the energy required to maintain the attachment of the suspensory apparatus of the distal phalanx at the lamellar interface. Equally important is the blood supplied to the growth areas of the tubular hoof epidermis. Arteries in the coronary and sole dermis branch into smaller arterioles that enter each dermal papilla. Within the dermis of the papilla they branch farther, giving rise to the tufts of anastomosing capillaries adjacent to the epidermal basal cell lined surface of each tubular hoof socket. Here they supply energy to maintain not only attachment but also the constant proliferation of new wall, periople, terminal horn, and sole. Veins adjacent to each papillary artery collect blood exiting the capillaries and feed it into the adjacent venous plexus. The dermis adjacent to intertubular horn production is equally well invested with blood vessels large and small to maintain constant intertubular horn production.

THE ARTERIAL SYSTEM (FORELIMB): A CLASSICAL DESCRIPTION

The blood supply to the forelimb occurs via the axillary branch of the subclavian artery. At the shoulder joint the axillary artery gives rise to several arterial branches supplying the cephalic and thoracic regions before progressing distally along the forearm as the brachial artery. The brachial artery provides branches to the triceps, biceps, cranial extensor muscles, and also a collateral ulnar branch.

At the elbow joint, the brachial artery gives rise to the common interosseous artery before progressing distad in the forearm (antebrachium) as the median artery. Several arterial branches are given off from the median artery, including the palmar branch of the medial artery that anastomoses with the collateral ulnar artery to form the lateral palmar artery. Immediately proximad to the carpus, the median artery gives rise to the radial artery before progressing distally.

It is the median artery (the proper common digital artery) that represents the major arterial supply to the forefoot. Immediately distal to the carpus, the proximal palmar arterial arch unites the terminus of the radial artery with the lateral artery and gives rise to the lateral and medial metacarpal arteries.

At the level of the fetlock, the median artery, lateral artery, and lateral and medial metacarpal arteries anastomose to form the distal palmar arterial arch. It is from this arterial arch that the medial and lateral palmar digital arteries arise and continue distally to the foot, where the digital arteries enter the solear canal of the distal phalanx and anastomose to form the terminal arch of the arterial circulation of the distal limb.

The medial and lateral digital arteries branch at various levels between the fetlock and the foot to provide the arterial supply to tendons, ligaments and integumentary structures of the pastern region and foot, and the bones of the phalangeal axis.

The major arterial branches are:

1. The dorsal and palmar branches of the proximal phalanx, which form a bifurcating, circumflex arterial complex that encircles the entire proximal region of the pastern.

2. The dorsal and palmar branches of the middle phalanx, which form a circumflex arterial supply to the distal region of the pastern. The dorsal branch bifurcates to form a distinct, proximal circumflex loop deep to the common digital extensor tendon, and the distal coronal circumflex artery superficial to the common digital extensor tendon. The palmar branches anastomose deep to the flexor tendons and give rise to a series of axial vessels that ascend into the proximal dorsal border of the middle phalanx immediately distad to the middle scutum. The palmar anastomosis, deep to the digital flexor tendons, forms the proximal navicular artery (contained within the connective tissue of the "T-ligament"), which supports the arterial circulation to the proximal aspect of the distal sesamoidean (navicular) bone. A series of descending axial vessels arise from the proximal navicular artery, passing over the dorsal aspect of the collateral sesamoidean ligament before finally entering into the proximal border of the distal sesamoid bone. A second series of axial arterial vessels arise from the proximal navicular artery to form a distinct arterial circulation to the deep digital flexor tendon in the region of the flexor surface of the distal sesamoid.

Three additional branches occur before the palmar digital arteries enter the solear canal of the distal phalanx. Immediately distad to the circumflex branches of the middle phalanx, the toric branch arises, providing the arterial supply to the palmar structures of the foot, including the bars and frog. The toric branch further divides into a major axial and abaxial branch on both sides of the foot, with the axial branches of the medial and lateral circulation anastomosing to form the cuneal artery of the frog. The abaxial branches further subdivide to provide an extensive circulation to the heel and bars. In addition, a connecting branch unites the abaxial toric branch to the coronal circumflex artery. In this way a continuous arterial supply is formed between the medial and lateral aspect of the foot immediately distad to the coronary band.

Further distad, at the level of the distal sesamoid, the dorsal branch of the palmar digital artery arises. This branch passes through the foramen, or notch, of the palmar process of the distal phalanx and further subdivides to provide the arterial supply to the quarters of the foot. It then continues along the parietal sulcus (parietal groove) of the distal phalanx dorsally before entering into the distal phalanx, through the parietal foramen to anastomose with the terminal arch of the palmar digital artery within the solear canal. Immediately proximad to the solear canal, a final anastomotic branch occurs between the medial and lateral digital artery, which passes through the distal sesamoid impar ligament to form the distal navicular artery. This artery gives off a series of ascending axial vessels, which enter the distal border of the distal sesamoid (navicular) bone dorsal to the foramina of the synovial invaginations of the distal interphalangeal joint (DIPJ) capsule.

Within the solear canal the palmar digital artery gives off several parietal arterial branches that emerge through foramina on the proximal and distal parietal surface of the distal phalanx. The proximal arterial vessels further subdivide and send axial vessels proximad to anastomose with a corresponding series of axial vessels that descend from the coronal circumflex artery and its connecting branch with the abaxial toric artery.

The distal parietal arteries anastomose to form the circumflex marginal artery from which a series of radial arteries traverse inward across the solear aspect of the foot, providing the arterial supply to the solear dermis, to finally anastomose with the cuneal artery. In addition, the circumflex marginal artery gives rise to a parallel array of arterial vessels, which ascend within the sublamellar dermis. The arterial circulation of the sublamellar dermis gives rise to a complex array of axial arterial vessels, which supplies the dermal lamellar tissues. This complex array is described in detail within the microcirculation section of this chapter.

THE ARTERIAL SYSTEM OF THE HINDLIMB: A CLASSIC DESCRIPTION

The arterial system of the hindlimb follows a pattern broadly similar to the forelimb, with arterial branching to support the different topographic regions of the limb. However, it differs from the forelimb in the following aspects of detail.

The hindlimb circulation arises from the external iliac artery, which merges into the femoral artery. Following numerous arterial branching that provides arterial supply to the musculature of the thigh, it continues distad as the popliteal artery. The popliteal artery divides into the cranial and plantar tibial artery, continues distad, and at the level of the hock, forms the dorsal pedal artery, which passes between the third and fourth metatarsal bone as the dorsal metatarsal artery. It is this artery, the dorsal metatarsal, that serves as the principal artery to the foot. The smaller plantar tibial artery continues distad and immediately below the hock, forms the deep plantar arch from which the small medial and lateral plantar arteries and the medial and lateral metatarsal arteries arise. These arteries continue distad on the plantar aspect of the third metatarsal bone and unite with the dorsal metatarsal artery to form the distal plantar arterial arch, from which the medial and lateral plantar digital arteries arise immediately proximad to the fetlock.

The medial and lateral plantar arteries continue distally and finally anastomose to form the terminal arch within the solear canal of the distal phalanx. A similar pattern of arterial branching occurs within the region of the pastern as seen in the forelimb, characterized by anastomosing circular structures at the level of the proximal and middle phalanx. Likewise, the arterial circulation of the hind foot is identical to that described for the forelimb.

THE VENOUS SYSTEM OF THE FOOT

The venous vessels of the foot and distal limb serve as a portal system by which blood depleted of glucose, gases, and other nutrients/minerals and containing the by-products of metabolic activity is returned from the periphery to the central circulation. Failure to achieve this venous return leads to vascular stasis, characterized by depleted nutrient supply and the toxic build-up of harmful metabolic by-products, which adversely affect normal cell function. Collectively, these events can lead to tissue damage and cell death.

Despite the fact that venography (retrograde delivery of contrast agent to the foot) is commonly used clinically to assess the competence of the venous side of the circulation, relatively little is known of the fine detail of the venous system, nor of the processes resulting in venous return from the foot itself.

The venous vessels within the foot of the forelimb can be considered as comprising two parts: one that returns blood from the deeper structures of the foot (including the distal phalanx and distal sesamoid [navicular] bone and their associated ligaments and tendons) and another that returns blood from the superficial dermal structures of the foot. However, this is an arbitrary simplification of the foot venous system as the venous return from deep and superficial structures are not independent of each other. The venous vasculature is interconnected throughout.

A complex array of venules (described in detail within the microcirculation section of this chapter) lead directly from the capillary networks contained within the coronary, lamellar, solear, bulbar, and cuneal dermal components of the foot to their respective venous plexi. These plexi are composed of a dense network of valveless, anastomotic veins, which, in the sublamellar and solear regions of the dermis, take on a characteristic reticular pattern. The sublamellar and solear plexi unite distally to form the circumflex marginal vein. This circumferential vein leads palmar from the distal parietal and peripheral margin of the sole to the major plexi of the ungular cartilages. Likewise, the venous plexus of the frog and the internal aspect of the solear plexus feed into the peripheral cuneal vein, which is continuous with the marginal circumflex vein. In this way

a single continuous "marginal" vein that extends around the entire distal margin of the foot is formed. This marginal vein serves as a direct portal to the plexi of the ungular cartilages located in the palmar foot.

The sublamellar plexus covers the entire parietal aspect of the distal phalanx. In its distal third, the sublamellar plexus is a single reticular layer. In its proximal two thirds, two distinct reticular layers are present, one superficial and the other deep. These unite with the venous plexus of the coronary dermis and the coronary subcutis, respectively. The sublamellar plexus, anastomosing with the plexi of the coronary region, forms the so-called "waterfall" evident venographically (bearing in mind that blood flows up the waterfall). The venous vessels of the coronary dermis and coronary subcutis feed into two major circumflex veins, which in turn unite and link with the venous vessels in the palmar aspect of the foot. This is described in further detail later within this section.

Venous return from the distal phalanx appears to follow one of two distinct routes. First, the parietal surface of the distal phalanx is perforated extensively by an array of microforamina through which venules (emanating from within the bone) emerge to unite with the venous plexus of the sublamellar dermis. In addition, the solear canal contains two or more anastomosing veins, forming the terminal arches of the palmar digital vein, which surround the terminal arch of the palmar digital artery. Numerous venous vessels also extend along the distal and proximal parietal formina, surrounding their arterial counterparts. Venographic studies however fail to provide evidence of their presence perhaps as an artifact of the technique. Decalcified histology of solear canal and distal and proximal parietal formina sections show numerous thin-walled venous vessels surrounding the arteries and emerging from the parietal surface of the distal phalanx. Two or more veins, associating closely with deep small arteries, such as the terminal arch and the parietal arteries, are known as *venae comitantes* or "accompanying veins." The veins, in close proximity to the artery and enclosed as they are within the bony canals of the distal phalanx, return venous blood to the heart, aided by the pulsations of the artery.

On emerging from the solear canal the medial and lateral palmar digital veins follow a reverse anatomic pathway to their arterial counterparts as they ascend the distal limb. Immediately distad to the solear canal, the medial and lateral palmar digital veins are joined by the distal navicular vein. This vein receives several venules, which emanate from the distal margin of the distal sesamoid (navicular bone). In a similar manner, the proximal navicular vein receives venules leading from the proximal border of the bone. At the proximal limit of the foot, the proximal navicular vein unites with the medial and lateral palmar digital veins, via the palmar branch of the middle phalanx. Meanwhile, dorsally, the two circumflex vessels of the coronary dermis and subcutis unite, forming the dorsal venous branch of the middle phalanx, and feed into the medial and lateral palmar digital veins. In this way, a circumferential venous portal is created around the middle phalanx leading to the palmar digital veins.

Immediately proximad to this major venous confluence, the deep and superficial venous plexi of the ungular cartilage unite with the palmar digital veins, and thereafter with the toric branch of the palmar digital vein that arises from venous convergence from within the bulbar regions of the foot. Unlike its arterial counterpart, the medial and lateral toric venous branches interconnect in the proximal aspect of the foot, thereby forming a complete circumferential venous drainage of the foot.

In the absence of musculature within the distal limb of the horse, venous return is solely dependent on mechanical forces associated with cyclic loading and weight bearing. To ensure controlled unidirectional venous return away from the foot, the venous system is extensively populated by a series of extracapsular semilunar valves. The distribution of these valves within the palmar aspect of the foot, the dorsal and palmar branch of the middle phalanx, and the palmar digital vein proximal to the pastern ensures a controlled pattern of blood flow up the limb as the foot takes weight and prevents retrograde blood flow due to the influence of gravity as weight is removed from the foot. The extensive presence of valves within the venous vessels of the palmar aspect of the foot suggests that this is the principal route of venous return.

The medial and lateral palmar digital vein follows the course of its arterial counterpart toward the fetlock, and a corresponding dorsal and palmar venous branch of the proximal phalanx unites with the digital veins (similar to that seen at the middle phalanx). At the level of the fetlock the digital veins converge with venous vessels from the proximal sesamoids at the distal palmar venous arch and continue proximally to the carpus. Here they unite with the third metacarpal veins to form the proximal palmar arch. Venous return from the proximal palmar venous arch occurs primarily via the median vein and also via the associated ulnar and radial veins. These in turn pass into the brachial and median cubital veins within the forearm, before passing into the axillary vein and, finally, the subclavian vein to join the central circulation.

The venous system of the hindlimb closely matches that seen in the forelimb, with the major veins being satellites of their arterial counterparts. There are, however, a few differences worthy of note. Proximal to the distal plantar arch, venous return occurs via the dorsal common digital vein along with collateral return via the plantar metatarsal veins. The dorsal common digital vein passes between the second and third metatarsal bones and continues proximally as the medial saphenous vein. This differs from its arterial counterpart, which passes between the third and fourth metatarsal bones. The plantar metatarsal veins similarly unite to form the proximal plantar arch before continuing proximally as the tibial vein. This in turn passes into the popliteal vein, where it unites with the saphenous vein. The popliteal vein passes into the femoral vein, before finally entering into the external iliac vein to join the central circulation.

THE MICROCIRCULATION

The microcirculation is organized to ensure that every cell in the foot is in close contact with a microvessel. This minimizes diffusion distances and facilitates the exchange of essential nutrients between blood and tissue, its most important function. The capillary beds adjacent to secondary epidermal lamellae (SELs) and proliferating tubular horn are particularly dense and conspicuous (when examined with the right modalities), thereby underlining their fundamental importance to foot structure and function. There are tens of thousands of microvessels per gram of tissue.

Components of the Microcirculation

The epidermal hoof is avascular and relies on an adjacent network of dermal capillaries to exchange nutrients, water, gases, hormones, and waste products between blood and the epidermal cells. The microcirculation begins with the smallest arteries, ends with the smallest veins; in between are arterioles, capillaries and venules. The lamellar microcirculation begins where arterioles branch from the lamellar axial arteries in the primary dermal lamellae (PDLs). Lamellar arterioles branch further in the PDLs and, decreasing in size but increasing in number, transition into the smallest unit of the circulation, the capillary and venules. Lamellar capillaries are located exclusively in the lamellar epidermal basal cells, where they form multiple looping anastomoses in close proximity (5–7 μm) to all faces of the SELs. Lamellar capillaries are extremely close to the target of energy delivery, the lamellar epidermal basal cells, where they deliver the nutrients essential for maintenance of attachment and a multiplicity of other functions. Capillaries are virtually absent in PDLs and the sublamellar dermis.

The capillaries exiting the SDLs merge with thin-walled venules that in turn join the axial veins in the PDL. In the nonlamellar dermis, small arteries branch in multiple directions from larger vessels until the entire hoof epidermis, from frog to periople, has a small artery adjacent to it. The papillary circulation begins with arterioles that branch from these arteries and enter the dermal papillae. Tufts of anastomosing capillaries arise from the arterioles and form a network of anastomosing capillaries that ensheaths the central arteriole. Adjacent to the central arteriole and entwined around it is a venule receiving blood from the capillaries. The venules join small veins that in turn join large veins to form the latticelike plexi of the solear and coronary dermis. The largest arterioles have an inner diameter of 100 to 400 μm, and the largest venules have a diameter of 200 to 800 μm.

The small sublamellar and axial lamellar arteries, combined with the lamellar arterioles of the microcirculation, are resistance blood vessels and, by constricting or dilating, are primarily responsible for regulating the flow of blood entering the capillary beds. Smooth muscle cells, encircling the vessel wall, shorten to achieve vasoconstriction, or relax and lengthen for vasodilation. The arteries and arterioles are innervated by autonomic (norepinephrine) and peptidergic nerves, which govern the activity of the vascular smooth muscle cells. Intense contraction of the encircling smooth muscle cells, which are arranged perpendicular to the long axis of the vessel, can completely shut arterioles down for brief periods. On the other hand, fully relaxed smooth muscle cells can nearly double the diameter of the vessel and increase blood flow dramatically.[9]

Together arteries and arterioles regulate about 70% to 80% of the total vascular resistance, with the remainder of the resistance equally divided between the capillary beds and venules.

Delivery of Glucose and Exchange of Water and Other Materials Occur Across Capillaries

Capillaries have inner diameters of between 4 and 8 μm and are the smallest vessels of the vascular system. A capillary is an endothelial tube enclosed by basement membrane (BM) with the same characteristics as the lamellar epidermal BM. Smooth muscle cells are absent, and they are unable to appreciably change their inner diameter. Pericytes (Rouget cells) are wrapped around the outside of the basement membrane and add structural integrity to the capillary. The capillary lumen is so small that red blood cells must fold to pass through a capillary; they virtually fill the entire lumen. A small diameter and a thin endothelial wall allow molecules inside the capillary lumen to rapidly diffuse to the interstitial fluid just outside the vessel. Most gases and inorganic ions pass through the capillary wall in less than 2 milliseconds.[9]

Molecules Pass Between and Through Capillary Endothelial Cells

The lipid components of capillary endothelial cell membranes allow lipid-soluble molecules, such as oxygen and carbon dioxide, to readily pass through the endothelial cell wall to the interstitial fluid outside the capillary. Small pores in the water-filled junctions between endothelial cells allow water, inorganic ions, glucose, amino acids, and similar small, water-soluble solutes to pass. The pores act as filters and permit only molecules with a radius <3 to 6 nm to pass through the vessel wall. Large molecules, such as serum albumin and the cellular components of blood, cannot pass and are retained within the capillary.

Diffusion of Molecules or Particles

Diffusion in biological systems means molecules or particles move passively—down concentration gradients, or in other words, molecules move from regions of high concentration to regions of low concentration. In the capillary beds of the foot, diffusion is the primary mechanism by which small molecules (glucose, amino acids, and oxygen) move from within the capillary to the interstitial fluid outside. There is no chemical energy involved, just simple diffusion. However, in the case of glucose a concentration gradient between capillary and epidermal basal cell is always present, as glucose is actively transported into the cytoplasm of epidermal basal cells by a special glucose transporter molecule (GLUT1). Epidermal basal cells of the foot integument stain strongly for the GLUT1 protein, thus confirming its

presence. Once inside the cell, glucose is rapidly converted to glucose-6-phosphate and is thus trapped, ready to participate in energy production for the cell's essential functions.[10] Conversely, carbon dioxide and other waste metabolites diffuse into the capillaries by the same process but in reverse.

Equilibrium in the Capillary Bed

As blood moves through the capillary bed losing water and small molecules but retaining large molecules (albumin and globular proteins), it becomes more concentrated, creating an osmotic gradient attracting water back into the capillary. Thus 90% of the water escaping the capillary on the arteriolar side is recovered by osmosis on the venular side. The remaining 10% is recovered by the lymphatic system and returned to the blood circulation as lymph. Thus edema is controlled and the interstitial fluid bathing cells, a filtrate of plasma, is kept in optimum condition. The lamellar interstitium resembles a gel that maintains a water reservoir facilitating water movement from capillary to cell. The interstitial gel is composed of proteoglycan filaments, a major component of the extracellular matrix of the lamellar, coronary, and solear dermis.[7] Proteoglycan forms large complexes with other proteoglycans and to dermal collagen and is able to bind electrolytes and water, thus regulating the movement of these molecules through the dermis. The amount of water in the gel reservoir increases if edema develops.

The net movement of fluid across capillary walls can be calculated by an equation (the Starling equation), which describes the interaction between the hydrostatic (blood) pressure and osmotic pressure both inside and outside the capillaries (Starling forces).

Venules Collect Blood from Capillaries and Act as A Blood Reservoir

After passing through the capillaries, blood enters the venules, which are larger-diameter endothelial tubes surrounded by small, long, vascular muscle cells. Venules operate at intravascular pressures of 10 to 16 mm Hg and do not need thick muscular walls. Unlike capillaries, the smallest venules are permeable to large and small molecules, and the exchange of large water-soluble molecules occurs as the blood passes through small venules. Approximately two thirds of the total blood volume is within the venous system and at least half of this is within venules. Thus a blood reservoir is formed through which blood moves slowly.

Arteriovenous Anastomoses

The microcirculation of the hoof integument contains direct connections between arteries and veins, which act as shunts (arterio-venous or AV shunts). There is no transfer of gases, nutrients, or wastes across the wall of an AV shunt. They are under the control of the nervous system and, by opening and closing, facilitate heat transfer through the hoof wall and thus thermoregulation.[4]

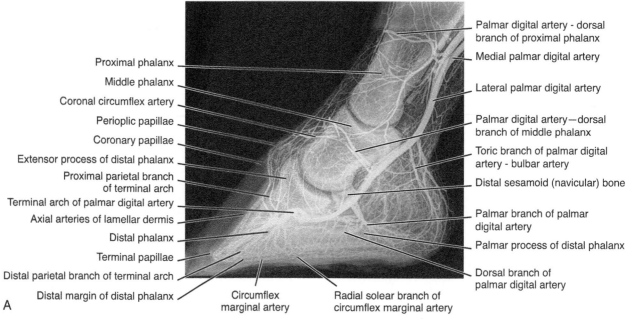

Proximal phalanx

Middle phalanx

Coronal circumflex artery

Perioplic papillae

Coronary papillae

Extensor process of distal phalanx

Proximal parietal branch of terminal arch

Terminal arch of palmar digital artery

Axial arteries of lamellar dermis

Distal phalanx

Terminal papillae

Distal parietal branch of terminal arch

Distal margin of distal phalanx

A

Circumflex marginal artery

Radial solear branch of circumflex marginal artery

Palmar digital artery - dorsal branch of proximal phalanx

Medial palmar digital artery

Lateral palmar digital artery

Palmar digital artery—dorsal branch of middle phalanx

Toric branch of palmar digital artery - bulbar artery

Distal sesamoid (navicular) bone

Palmar branch of palmar digital artery

Palmar process of distal phalanx

Dorsal branch of palmar digital artery

• **Figure 7.1 (A)** Lateromedial, contrast enhanced, radiographic image after infusion of the median artery of the left forelimb with the contrast medium barium sulfate (normal cadaver specimen). Within the arteries the radiopaque barium (a metal) highlights the vessels white against a gray-to-black background. This figure shows the four major branches that arise from the medial and lateral palmar digital arteries before they enter the body of the distal phalanx solear canal and unite to form the terminal arch. The first and most proximal is the artery of the proximal phalanx, which is divided into dorsal and palmar branches, both of which unite to complete a circle around the middle of the proximal phalanx. The dorsal branch passes beneath the extensor tendon, and the palmar branch passes between the flexor tendons and the proximal phalanx; they supply branches to the adjacent joints, synovial sheaths, ergot, and skin. The second branch is the toric branch of the palmar digital artery supplying the digital cushion (the pulvinus) and the dermis of the heels and frog. The third branch is the dorsal artery of the middle phalanx supplying branches to the skin, extensor tendon, distal interphalangeal joint (DIPJ), and coronary dermis of the quarters. Dorsally, the dorsal artery of the middle phalanx branches and, uniting with its opposite branch, completes the coronal circumflex artery. Branches of the coronal circumflex artery ramify the coronary dermis and anastomose with proximally directed branches of the proximal parietal arteries. The contour of the coronary groove of the proximal hoof wall is outlined by the distal and proximal branches of the coronal circumflex artery and the proximal parietal arteries, respectively. The fourth major artery is the dorsal branch of the palmar digital artery, with branches anastomosing above with the coronal circumflex artery, and below, with the circumflex marginal artery. The palmar branch of the palmar digital artery branches to the digital cushion and abaxial (outer) surface of the ungular cartilage. The proximal parietal branches of the terminal arch supply both the proximal lamellar dermis and the coronary dermis. The vertically oriented proximal parietal arteries anastomose with the downward branches of the coronal circumflex artery, thus connecting the terminal arch and the dorsal artery of the middle phalanx, ensuring an arterial supply from multiple sources. The distal parietal branches of the terminal arch unite to form the circumflex marginal artery from which radial solear branches curl inward under the distal margin of the distal phalanx to supply the solear dermis. From the circumflex marginal artery, branches enter the distal dermis of each of the 450 to 500 dermal lamellae. From these lamellar branches five to seven terminal papillae, at the distal extremity of each dermal lamella, receive individual arteries that extend to the distal tip of each papilla. In the radiograph, contrast has filled the arteries of the dorsal terminal papillae, and since they are aligned latero-medially, superimposition makes them visible. Similarly, the dorsal dermal lamellae are also superimposed latero-medially, and the lamellar axial arteries projecting from the numerous sublamellar arteries are also visible. Arteries of the coronary and perioplic papillae are also visible.

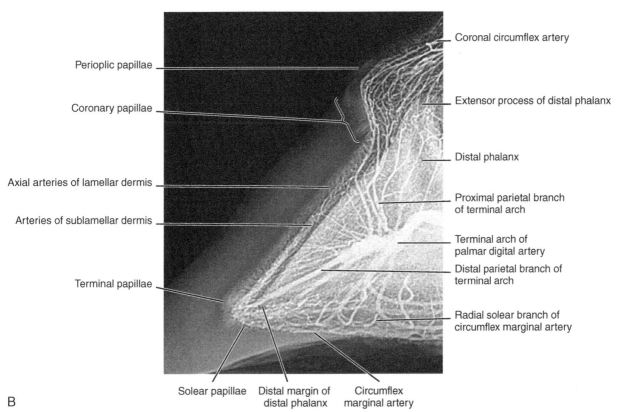

Perioplic papillae

Coronary papillae

Axial arteries of lamellar dermis

Arteries of sublamellar dermis

Terminal papillae

Coronal circumflex artery

Extensor process of distal phalanx

Distal phalanx

Proximal parietal branch
of terminal arch

Terminal arch of
palmar digital artery

Distal parietal branch of
terminal arch

Radial solear branch of
circumflex marginal artery

Solear papillae   Distal margin of   Circumflex
distal phalanx   marginal artery

B

• **Figure 7.1 (B)** Lateromedial, contrast enhanced, radiographic image after infusion of the median artery of the forelimb with the contrast medium barium sulfate (normal cadaver specimen). The radiograph shows the dorsal half of the foot with enhanced focus and contrast. Numerous proximal and distal parietal arteries branch from the terminal arch of the medial and lateral palmar digital arteries. The proximal parietal arteries freely anastomose with branches from the coronal circumflex artery but also supply the coronary dermis and the proximal lamellae. The contrast-filled arteries of the coronary papillae are of three different sizes conforming to the three-zone pattern of coronal hoof tubules. The distal parietal arteries unite outside the distal phalanx to form the circumflex marginal artery from which radial solear branches curl inward under the distal margin of the distal phalanx to supply the solear dermis. The terminal papillae are also supplied from the circumflex marginal artery and, filled with contrast, are clearly visible. The proximal and distal parietal arteries are the major branches of the terminal arch, but the radiograph shows numerous smaller branches exiting the parietal surface of the distal phalanx. These, along with the larger vessels, ramify the sublamellar dermis and supply innumerable smaller branches to the lamellar dermis. These are the lamellar axial arteries aligned between the connective tissue of the suspensory apparatus of the distal phalanx. Duplicating the orientation pattern of the collagen bundles of the suspensory apparatus of the distal phalanx, the proximal axial arteries are near vertical and the more distal arteries horizontal.

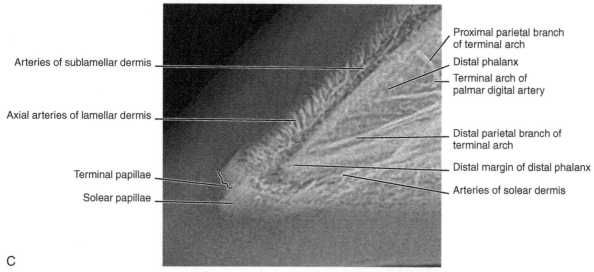

Arteries of sublamellar dermis

Axial arteries of lamellar dermis

Terminal papillae

Solear papillae

Proximal parietal branch
of terminal arch

Distal phalanx

Terminal arch of
palmar digital artery

Distal parietal branch of
terminal arch

Distal margin of distal phalanx

Arteries of solear dermis

C

• **Figure 7.1 (C)** Lateromedial, contrast-enhanced, radiographic image after infusion of the median artery of the left forelimb with barium sulfate (normal cadaver specimen). The specimen is a frozen, 15 mm sagittal slice, radiographed with the barium contrast still in situ. The alignment of terminal papillae parallels the angle of the parietal cortex of the distal phalanx and the hoof wall. The terminal papillae border the distal margin of each dermal lamella, and their filling is a guide to the location of the proximad lamellar zone. Proximad to the terminal papillae, traversing the lamellar zone, are the lamellar axial arteries. The lamellar axial arteries arise from sublamellar arteries, themselves branches of the parietal arteries from the terminal arch. The distal axial arteries are near horizontal and the dorsal near vertical as dictated by the orientation of the collagen bundles of the suspensory apparatus of the distal phalanx. Also clearly shown are the arteries of the dorsal sole papillae.

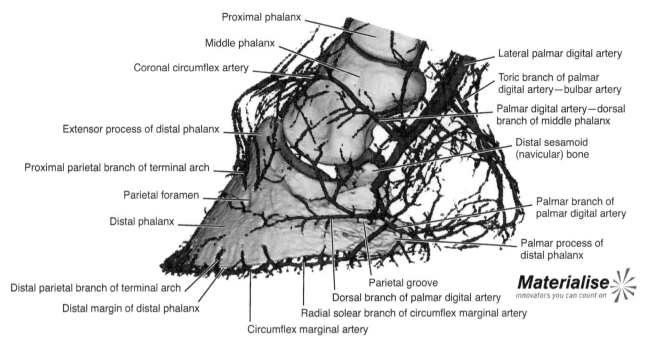

Proximal phalanx

Middle phalanx

Coronal circumflex artery

Extensor process of distal phalanx

Proximal parietal branch of terminal arch

Parietal foramen

Distal phalanx

Lateral palmar digital artery

Toric branch of palmar digital artery—bulbar artery

Palmar digital artery—dorsal branch of middle phalanx

Distal sesamoid (navicular) bone

Palmar branch of palmar digital artery

Palmar process of distal phalanx

Distal parietal branch of terminal arch

Distal margin of distal phalanx

Parietal groove

Dorsal branch of palmar digital artery

Radial solear branch of circumflex marginal artery

Circumflex marginal artery

Materialise
innovators you can count on

• **Figure 7.2** Lateral view of Mimics modeled computed tomography (CT) data of arteries and bones after infusion of the median artery of the left forelimb with the contrast-medium barium sulfate (normal cadaver specimen). This figure shows three major branches arising from the medial and lateral palmar digital arteries before they enter the foramina of the distal phalanx solear canal to form the terminal arch. The first and most proximad, level with the proximal border of the ungular cartilage and directed backward and down, is the toric branch of the palmar digital artery (the bulbar or pulvinus artery). This supplies the digital cushion (the pulvinus) and the dermis of the heels and frog. The second artery, branching forward at right angles to the palmar digital artery and beneath the ungular cartilage, is the dorsal artery of middle phalanx. It passes over the middle phalanx beneath the extensor tendon to unite with its opposite branch to complete a circle. It supplies branches to the skin, extensor tendon, the distal interphalangeal joint (DIPJ), and coronary dermis of the quarters. On the medial and lateral borders of the extensor tendon, the dorsal artery of the middle phalanx branches and the more dorsal branch passes above the tendon to unite with its opposite branch to complete an additional circle (the coronal circumflex artery) of the dorsal pastern. Multiple, distally directed branches of the coronal circumflex artery ramify the coronary dermis and anastomose with proximally directed branches of the proximal parietal arteries. In the Mimics model the shape of the dorsal coronary groove of the proximal hoof wall is outlined by the distal and proximal branches of the coronal circumflex artery and the proximal parietal arteries, respectively. The palmar artery of middle phalanx is smaller than the dorsal and passes above the distal sesamoid bone in the fascia of the "T-ligament" to unite with its opposite branch. This artery bridges the medial and lateral palmar digital arteries and sends from it numerous distally directed branches that pass over the dorsal aspect of the collateral sesamoidean ligament and enter the proximal border of the distal sesamoid through nutrient foramina. The third major artery, the dorsal branch of the palmar digital artery, arises opposite the distal sesamoid (navicular) bone and passes outward (abaxially) through the notch, or sometimes a foramen, in the palmar process of the distal phalanx. The dorsal branch (or dorsal artery of the distal phalanx) runs forward in a groove (the parietal groove) on the surface of the distal phalanx. It gives off branches, which anastomose above with the coronal circumflex artery, and below, with the circumflex marginal artery. The parietal groove terminates on the surface of the distal phalanx with the largest of the parietal foramina, and at this location, the dorsal branch of the palmar digital artery anastomoses with a dorsal parietal branch of the terminal arch. This is another example of multiple pathways of arterial blood delivery within the foot. Equivalent to the dorsal branch but directed in the opposite direction is the palmar branch of the palmar digital artery, which branches to the digital cushion and abaxial (outer) surface of the ungular cartilage. The arterial branches of the terminal arch exit through foramina in the parietal cortex of the distal phalanx. The proximal parietal branches of the terminal arch supply both the proximal lamellar dermis and the coronary dermis. Arteries from the coronal circumflex artery anastomose with branches of the proximal parietal branches of the terminal arch, ensuring that the growth zone of the proximal hoof wall receives blood from a multitude of directions. The distal parietal branches of the terminal arch unite to form the circumflex marginal artery from which radial solear branches curl inward under the distal margin of the distal phalanx to supply the solear dermis. Mimics model by Simon Collins.

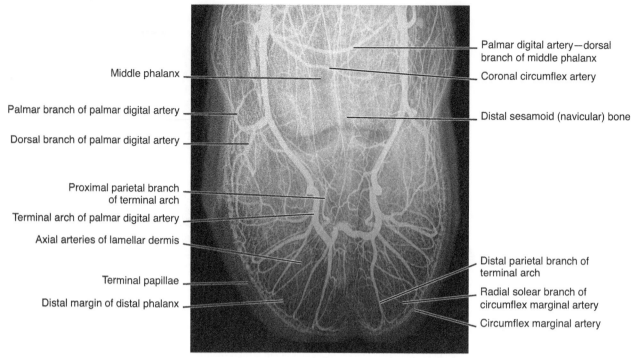

Middle phalanx

Palmar branch of palmar digital artery

Dorsal branch of palmar digital artery

Proximal parietal branch
of terminal arch

Terminal arch of palmar digital artery

Axial arteries of lamellar dermis

Terminal papillae

Distal margin of distal phalanx

Palmar digital artery—dorsal
branch of middle phalanx

Coronal circumflex artery

Distal sesamoid (navicular) bone

Distal parietal branch of
terminal arch

Radial solear branch of
circumflex marginal artery

Circumflex marginal artery

● **Figure 7.3** Dorsopalmar oblique (D45Pr-PaDiO) contrast-enhanced radiographic image after infusion of the median artery of the left forelimb with the contrast medium barium sulfate (normal cadaver specimen). The medial and lateral palmar digital arteries approach the solear canal of the distal phalanx on either side of the distal sesamoid (navicular) bone. Inside the distal phalanx the arteries unite to form the terminal arch. Arterial branches radiate from the terminal arch, exiting through foramina in the parietal cortex of the distal phalanx. The circumflex marginal artery is formed by the distal parietal branches of the terminal arch anastomosing in the dermis between the distal margin of the distal phalanx and the sole wall junction. From the circumflex marginal artery, the distal parietal branches curl inward under the distal margin of the distal phalanx. These radial solear branches of the circumflex marginal artery branch farther, ramifying the solear dermis, bringing fresh arterial blood to the entire dorsal sole. From the circumflex marginal artery, a branch enters the distal dermis of each of the 450 to 500 dermal lamellae. From this lamellar branch the five to seven terminal papillae at the distal extremity of each dermal lamella receive individual arteries that continue proximally up the lamella, anastomosing with other axial lamellar arteries. Because the lamellar branches and the terminal papillae are aligned in vertical rows, they show as a contrast-filled fringe peripheral to the circumflex marginal artery.

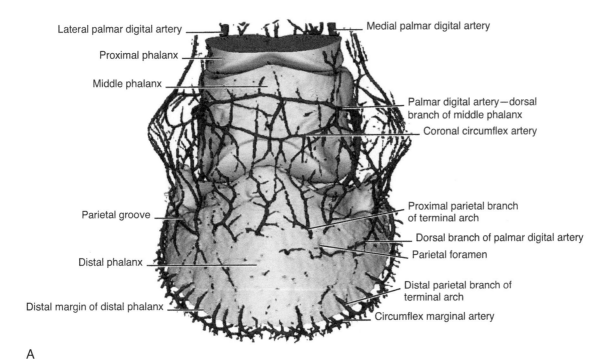

Lateral palmar digital artery

Proximal phalanx

Middle phalanx

Medial palmar digital artery

Palmar digital artery—dorsal branch of middle phalanx

Coronal circumflex artery

Parietal groove

Distal phalanx

Distal margin of distal phalanx

Proximal parietal branch of terminal arch

Dorsal branch of palmar digital artery

Parietal foramen

Distal parietal branch of terminal arch

Circumflex marginal artery

A

• **Figure 7.4 (A)** Frontal view of Mimics modeled computed tomography (CT) data of arteries and bones after infusion of the median artery of the left forelimb with the contrast medium barium sulfate (normal cadaver specimen). The terminal arch of the medial and lateral palmar digital arteries is invisible, deep within the distal phalanx. However, the arterial branches that radiate from the terminal arch exit through foramina in the parietal cortex of the distal phalanx and are visible. The proximal parietal branches of the terminal arch arborize in the proximal sublamellar dermis, and send branches to both the proximal lamellar dermis and the coronary dermis. Arteries from the coronal circumflex artery anastomose with branches of the proximal parietal branches of the terminal arch, ensuring that the growth zone of the proximal hoof wall receives blood from a multitude of directions. The distal parietal branches of the terminal arch exit just dorsal to the distal margin of the distal phalanx and unite to form the circumflex marginal artery. From the circumflex marginal artery, radial solear branches curl axially (inwards), under the distal margin of the distal phalanx, ramifying the solear dermis. Mimics model by Simon Collins

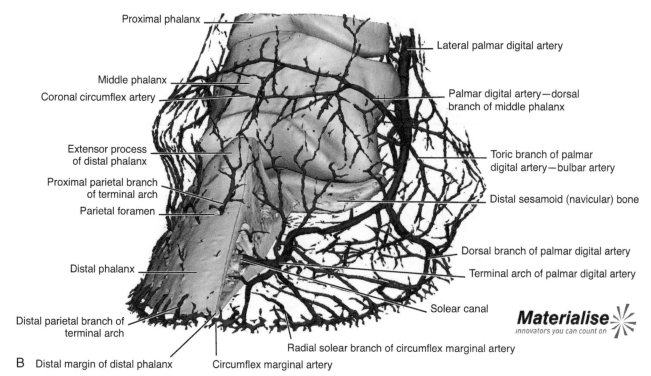

Proximal phalanx

Middle phalanx

Coronal circumflex artery

Extensor process
of distal phalanx

Proximal parietal branch
of terminal arch

Parietal foramen

Distal phalanx

Distal parietal branch of
terminal arch

B   Distal margin of distal phalanx

Lateral palmar digital artery

Palmar digital artery—dorsal
branch of middle phalanx

Toric branch of palmar
digital artery—bulbar artery

Distal sesamoid (navicular) bone

Dorsal branch of palmar digital artery

Terminal arch of palmar digital artery

Solear canal

Radial solear branch of circumflex marginal artery

Circumflex marginal artery

Materialise
innovators you can count on

• **Figure 7.4 (B)** Frontal view of Mimics modeled computed tomography (CT) data of arteries and bones after infusion of the median artery of the left forelimb with the contrast medium barium sulfate (normal cadaver specimen). The distal phalanx is shown in sagittal section without its lateral half. The terminal arch of the medial and lateral palmar digital arteries is visible, deep within the solear canal of the distal phalanx. The arterial branches that radiate from the terminal arch exit through foramina in the parietal cortex of the distal phalanx. The proximal parietal branches of the terminal arch arborize in the proximal sublamellar dermis, sending branches to both the proximal lamellar dermis and the coronary dermis. Arteries from the coronal circumflex artery anastomose with branches of the proximal parietal branches of the terminal arch, supplying blood to the coronary growth zone of the proximal hoof wall. The distal parietal branches of the terminal arch exit the distal phalanx and unite to form the circumflex marginal artery. From the circumflex marginal artery, radial solear branches curl inward under the distal margin of the distal phalanx and supply the solear dermis. Mimics model by Simon Collins.

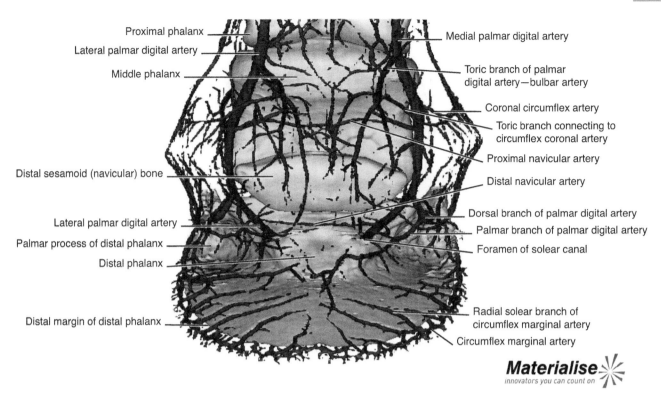

Proximal phalanx

Lateral palmar digital artery

Middle phalanx

Distal sesamoid (navicular) bone

Lateral palmar digital artery

Palmar process of distal phalanx

Distal phalanx

Distal margin of distal phalanx

Medial palmar digital artery

Toric branch of palmar digital artery—bulbar artery

Coronal circumflex artery

Toric branch connecting to circumflex coronal artery

Proximal navicular artery

Distal navicular artery

Dorsal branch of palmar digital artery

Palmar branch of palmar digital artery

Foramen of solear canal

Radial solear branch of circumflex marginal artery

Circumflex marginal artery

Materialise
innovators you can count on

● **Figure 7.5** Palmar view of Mimics modeled computed tomography (CT) data of arteries and bones after infusion of the median artery of the left forelimb with the contrast medium barium sulfate (normal cadaver specimen). This figure shows the medial and lateral palmar digital arteries entering the paired foramina of the distal phalanx to form the terminal arch within the solear canal of the distal phalanx. Level with the proximal border of the ungular cartilage and directed backward and down is the toric branch of the palmar digital artery. This supplies the digital cushion (the pulvinus) and the dermis of the heels and frog. There is also a connecting branch that unites the toric with the coronal circumflex artery, another example of anastomoses ensuring continuity of arterial blood supply within the foot. Above and below the distal sesamoid (navicular) bone are the proximal and distal navicular arteries, anastomosing arteries that cross between the medial and lateral palmar digital arteries. The proximal navicular artery passes above the distal sesamoid (navicular) bone in the fascia of the "T-ligament," thus bridging the medial and lateral palmar digital arteries. Numerous distally directed branches of the proximal navicular artery pass over the dorsal aspect of the collateral sesamoidean ligament and enter the proximal border of the distal sesamoid through nutrient foramina. The distal navicular artery passes through the distal sesamoid impar ligament and gives off a series of ascending axial vessels, which enter the distal border of the distal sesamoid (navicular) bone dorsal to the foramina of the synovial invaginations of the distal interphalangeal joint (DIPJ) capsule. From the circumflex marginal artery, radial solear branches pass inward (axially), under the distal margin of the distal phalanx to supply the solear dermis. The radial solear arteries finally anastomose with the axial cuneal artery not completely filled in this specimen. Mimics model by Simon Collins.

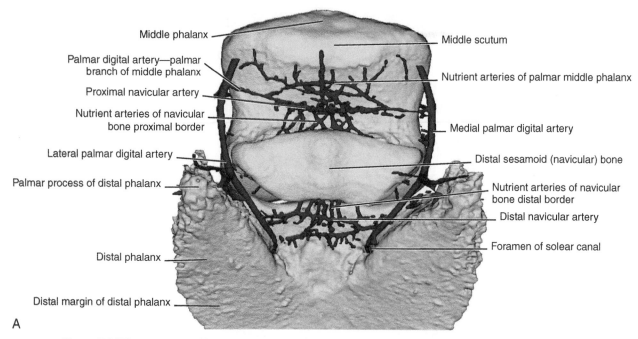

A

• **Figure 7.6 (A)** Palmar view of Mimics modeled computed tomography (CT) data of arteries and bones after infusion of the median artery of the left forelimb with the contrast medium barium sulfate (normal cadaver specimen). The palmar branch of the middle phalanx anastomoses with its opposite member, uniting the medial and lateral palmar digital arteries. Anastomoses deep to the flexor tendons give rise to nutrient vessels that ascend into the proximal palmar border of the middle phalanx immediately distad to the middle scutum. An additional more distad anastomosis of the palmar branch of the middle phalanx forms the proximal navicular artery passing above the distal sesamoid (navicular) bone in the fascia of the "T-ligament." Numerous distally directed branches of the proximal navicular artery pass over the dorsal aspect of the collateral sesamoidean ligament and enter the proximal border of the distal sesamoid through nutrient foramina. The distal navicular artery passes through the distal sesamoid impar ligament and gives off a series of ascending axial vessels, which enter the distal border of the distal sesamoid (navicular) bone dorsal to the foramina of the synovial invaginations of the distal interphalangeal joint (DIPJ) capsule. Mimics model by Simon Collins.

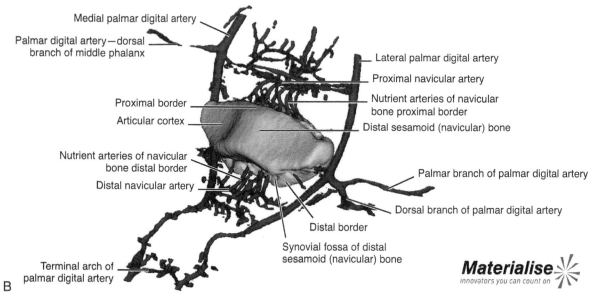

B

• **Figure 7.6 (B)** Oblique medial-lateral view of Mimics modeled computed tomography (CT) data of the arteries associated with the distal sesamoid (navicular). The palmar branch of the middle phalanx anastomoses with its opposite member, uniting the medial and lateral palmar digital arteries. The palmar branch of the middle phalanx anastomoses to form the proximal navicular artery passing above the distal sesamoid (navicular) bone in the fascia of the "T-ligament." Numerous distally directed branches of the proximal navicular artery pass over the dorsal aspect of the collateral sesamoidean ligament and enter the proximal border of the distal sesamoid through nutrient foramina. The curve in shape of the distally directed branches of the proximal navicular artery is due to the vessels conforming to the dorsal border of the distal sesamoidean collateral ligament, which is round in cross-section. The distal navicular artery passes through the distal sesamoid impar ligament and gives off a series of ascending axial vessels, which enter the distal border of the distal sesamoid (navicular) bone dorsal to the foramina of the synovial invaginations of the distal interphalangeal joint (DIPJ) capsule. Mimics model by Simon Collins.

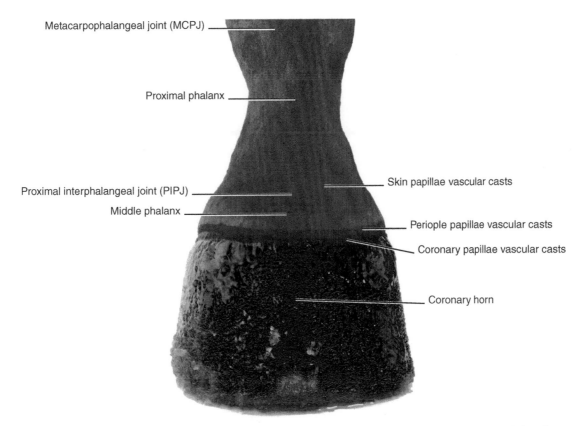

Metacarpophalangeal joint (MCPJ)

Proximal phalanx

Proximal interphalangeal joint (PIPJ)

Middle phalanx

Skin papillae vascular casts

Periople papillae vascular casts

Coronary papillae vascular casts

Coronary horn

• **Figure 7.7** Photograph of horse foot with the vascular system injected with red-colored, polymerized methyl methacrylate (MMA). The specimen has been partially corroded in alkali to remove the skin, hoof periople, and some proximal coronary horn. The outer surface of the hoof capsule has also been corroded, but the bulk of the hoof epidermis remains. Corrosion reveals vascular casts of skin papillae and the elongated tapering papillae of the perioplic and coronary dermis. The size difference between perioplic and coronary papillae can be discerned, and together they form a circular band between the skin and the proximal border of the hoof. Overall, the vascular cast resembles a distal limb showing the shape of the fetlock, pastern, and coronet.

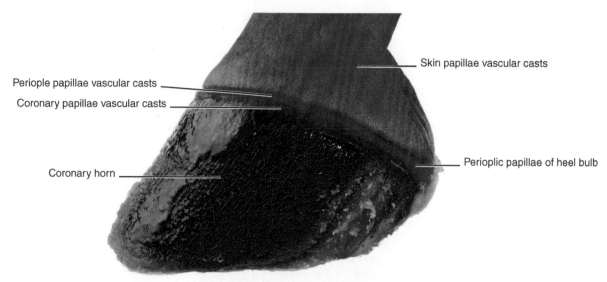

Skin papillae vascular casts

Periople papillae vascular casts

Coronary papillae vascular casts

Perioplic papillae of heel bulb

Coronary horn

• **Figure 7.8** Photograph of horse foot with the vascular system injected with red-colored, polymerized methyl methacrylate (MMA). The specimen has been partially corroded in alkali to remove the skin, hoof periople, and some proximal coronary horn; the bulk of the hoof epidermis remains. Vascular casts of skin papillae and the thin, tapering papillae of the periople and coronary band are visible. The size difference between perioplic and coronary papillae can be discerned, and together they form a border between the skin and the proximal hoof wall. In concert with the periople itself, the zone of perioplic papillae increases in size toward the heel bulbs.

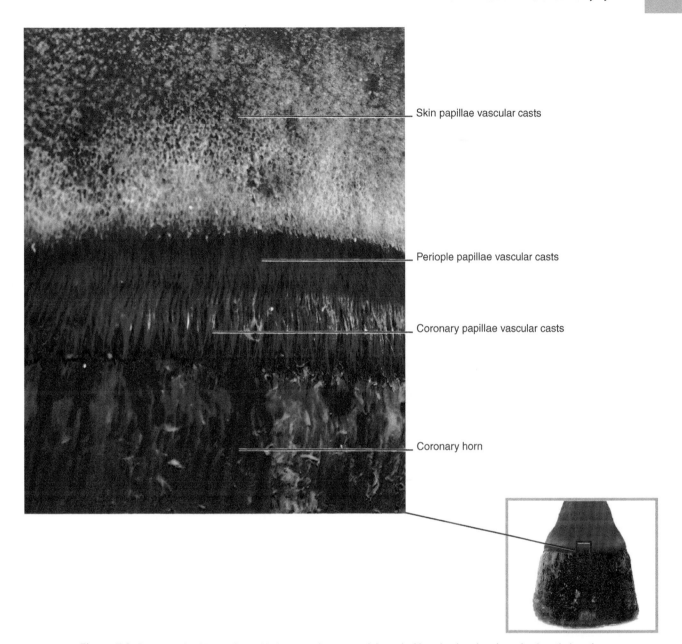

Skin papillae vascular casts

Periople papillae vascular casts

Coronary papillae vascular casts

Coronary horn

• **Figure 7.9** Photograph of horse foot with the vascular system injected with red-colored, polymerized methyl methacrylate (MMA). The specimen has been partially corroded in alkali to remove the skin, hoof periople, and some proximal coronary horn. The outer surface of the hoof capsule has also been corroded, but the bulk of the hoof epidermis remains. Corrosion exposes vascular casts of skin papillae and the elongated, tapering papillae of the perioplic and coronary dermis. There is a size difference and a boundary between the perioplic and coronary papillae. The inset shows the provenance of the specimen.

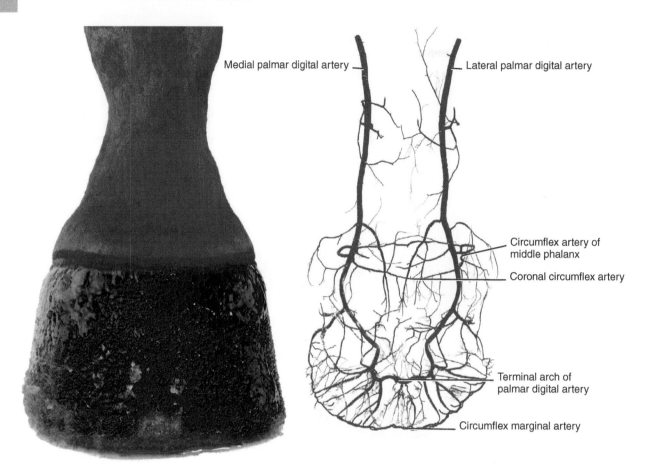

● **Figure 7.10** Photograph of horse foot vascular cast partially corroded in alkali to remove the skin and periople. After full corrosion, the cast on the right was dissected and capillaries, veins, and small arteries removed, leaving only the major arteries. The difference in the volume of blood in the arterial system and the blood in the capillaries and veins is large. The high-pressure arterial system delivers blood to the finest capillaries, ensuring the requirements of every cell, in all tissues, are met.

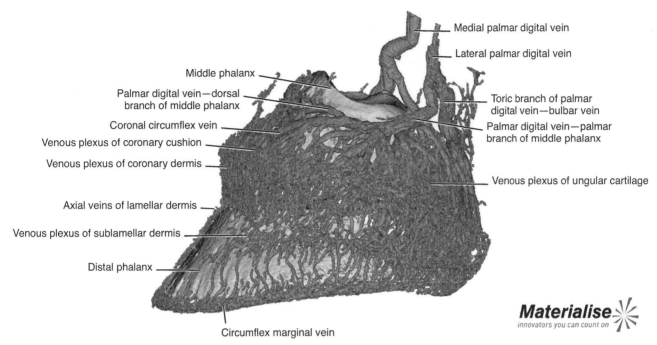

Medial palmar digital vein

Lateral palmar digital vein

Middle phalanx

Palmar digital vein—dorsal branch of middle phalanx

Coronal circumflex vein

Venous plexus of coronary cushion

Venous plexus of coronary dermis

Axial veins of lamellar dermis

Venous plexus of sublamellar dermis

Distal phalanx

Toric branch of palmar digital vein—bulbar vein

Palmar digital vein—palmar branch of middle phalanx

Venous plexus of ungular cartilage

Circumflex marginal vein

Materialise
innovators you can count on

● **Figure 7.11** Lateral view of Mimics modeled computed tomography (CT) data of veins and bones after infusion of the palmar digital vein of the left forelimb with barium sulfate (normal cadaver specimen). The venous plexus of the sublamellar dermis covers the parietal surface of the distal phalanx. The sublamellar plexus is a single layer distally but becomes two overlapping layers proximally. Axial veins of the lamellar dermis drain directly into the sublamellar plexus. The sublamellar and solear plexi unite distally to form the circumflex marginal vein that extends around the entire distal margin of the foot. In the palmar foot, the circumflex marginal vein connects directly to the plexi of the ungular cartilages. Proximally, the sublamellar plexus unites with the venous plexi of the coronary dermis and the coronary subcutis (coronary cushion). The two circumflex vessels of the coronary dermis and subcutis unite as the dorsal branch of the middle phalanx and feed into the medial and lateral palmar digital veins. In this way, a circumferential venous portal is created around the middle phalanx leading to the palmar digital veins. On the abaxial and axial surfaces of the ungular cartilages are the respective superficial and deep plexi of the ungular cartilages that unite with the palmar digital veins and the toric branch of the palmar digital vein. Mimics model by Simon Collins.

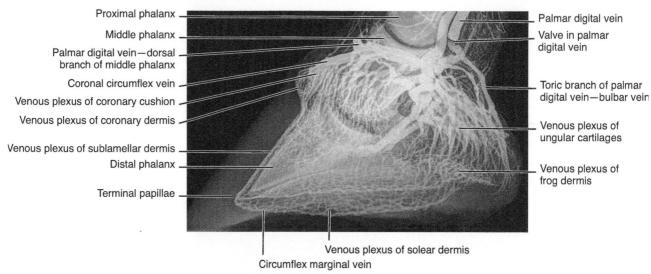

Proximal phalanx

Middle phalanx

Palmar digital vein—dorsal
branch of middle phalanx

Coronal circumflex vein

Venous plexus of coronary cushion

Venous plexus of coronary dermis

Venous plexus of sublamellar dermis

Distal phalanx

Terminal papillae

Palmar digital vein

Valve in palmar
digital vein

Toric branch of palmar
digital vein—bulbar vein

Venous plexus of
ungular cartilages

Venous plexus of
frog dermis

Venous plexus of solear dermis

Circumflex marginal vein

• **Figure 7.12** Lateromedial, contrast enhanced, radiographic image of veins and bones after infusion of the palmar digital vein of the left forelimb with barium sulfate (normal cadaver specimen). The venous plexus of the sublamellar dermis consists of the proximodistally oriented veins covering the parietal surface of the distal phalanx. The sublamellar and solear plexi unite distally to form the circumflex marginal vein that extends around the entire distal margin of the distal phalanx connecting, in the palmar foot, with the plexi of the ungular cartilages. Proximally, the sublamellar plexus unites with the venous plexi of the coronary dermis and the coronary subcutis (coronary cushion). The two circumflex vessels of the coronary dermis and subcutis unite as the dorsal branch of the middle phalanx and feed into the medial and lateral palmar digital veins. In this way, a circumferential venous portal is created around the middle phalanx leading to the palmar digital veins. On the abaxial and axial surfaces of the ungular cartilages are the respective superficial and deep plexi of the ungular cartilages that unite with the palmar digital veins and the toric branch of the palmar digital vein.

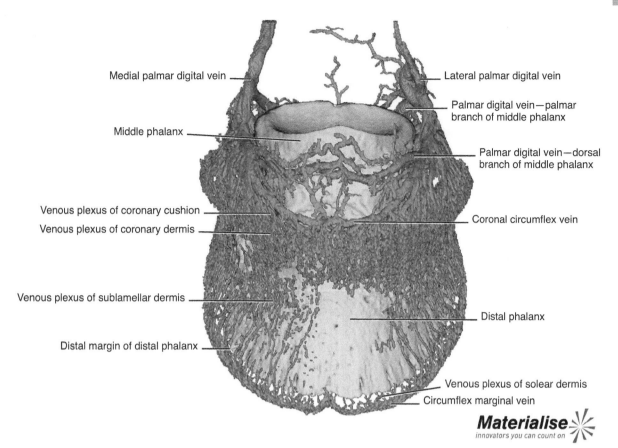

Medial palmar digital vein

Middle phalanx

Venous plexus of coronary cushion

Venous plexus of coronary dermis

Venous plexus of sublamellar dermis

Distal margin of distal phalanx

Lateral palmar digital vein

Palmar digital vein—palmar branch of middle phalanx

Palmar digital vein—dorsal branch of middle phalanx

Coronal circumflex vein

Distal phalanx

Venous plexus of solear dermis

Circumflex marginal vein

Materialise
innovators you can count on

● **Figure 7.13** Frontal view of Mimics modeled computed tomography (CT) data of veins and bones after infusion of the palmar digital vein of the left forelimb with barium sulfate (normal cadaver specimen). The model is reduced in complexity to aid comprehension of the key elements. The model shows the circumflex arrangement of the coronary plexi and the dorsal branch of the middle phalanx. Abaxial to the common digital extensor tendon, the coronal circumflex vein drains the venous plexi of the dorsal coronary dermis and the coronary subcutis (coronary cushion). They join the dorsal branch of the middle phalanx and feed into the medial and lateral palmar digital veins. The medial and lateral branches of the dorsal branch of the middle phalanx unite beneath the axial surface of the common digital extensor tendon. **The venous plexus of the sublamellar dermis covers the parietal surface of the distal phalanx (reduced in this model).** The sublamellar and solear plexus unites distally to form the circumflex marginal vein that extends around the entire distal margin of the foot. Proximally, the sublamellar plexus drains into the venous plexi of the coronary dermis and coronary subcutis. Mimics model by Simon Collins.

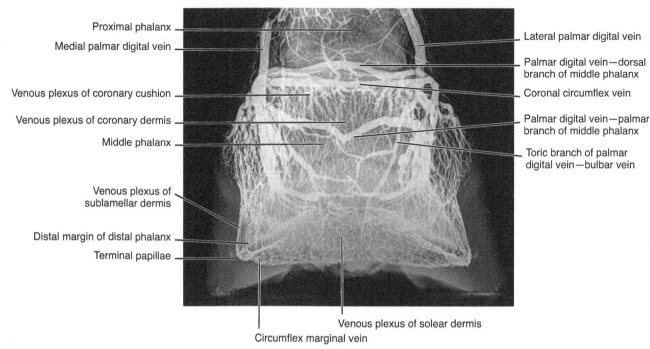

Proximal phalanx
Medial palmar digital vein
Venous plexus of coronary cushion
Venous plexus of coronary dermis
Middle phalanx
Venous plexus of sublamellar dermis
Distal margin of distal phalanx
Terminal papillae

Lateral palmar digital vein
Palmar digital vein—dorsal branch of middle phalanx
Coronal circumflex vein
Palmar digital vein—palmar branch of middle phalanx
Toric branch of palmar digital vein—bulbar vein

Venous plexus of solear dermis
Circumflex marginal vein

• **Figure 7.14** Dorsopalmar radiographic image of veins and bones after infusion of the palmar digital vein of the left forelimb with barium sulfate (normal cadaver specimen). Note circumflex arrangement of the coronary plexi and the dorsal branch of the middle phalanx. Abaxial to the common digital extensor tendon the coronal circumflex vein drains the venous plexi of the dorsal coronary dermis and the coronary subcutis (coronary cushion). They join the dorsal branch of the middle phalanx and feed into the medial and lateral palmar digital veins. The medial and lateral branches of the dorsal branch of the middle phalanx unite beneath the axial surface of the common digital extensor tendon. The venous plexus of the sublamellar dermis covers the parietal surface of the distal phalanx and drains proximally into the venous plexi of the coronary dermis and coronary subcutis. The sublamellar and solear plexus unite distally to form the circumflex marginal vein that extends around the entire distal margin of the foot. Note the reticular network of the venous plexus of the solear dermis.

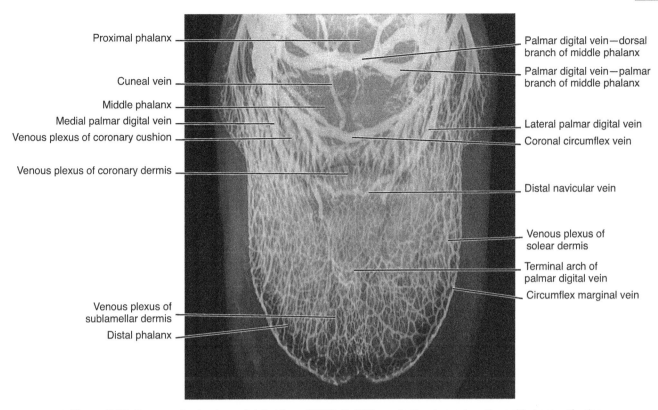

Proximal phalanx

Cuneal vein

Middle phalanx

Medial palmar digital vein

Venous plexus of coronary cushion

Venous plexus of coronary dermis

Venous plexus of sublamellar dermis

Distal phalanx

Palmar digital vein—dorsal branch of middle phalanx

Palmar digital vein—palmar branch of middle phalanx

Lateral palmar digital vein

Coronal circumflex vein

Distal navicular vein

Venous plexus of solear dermis

Terminal arch of palmar digital vein

Circumflex marginal vein

• **Figure 7.15** Dorsoproximal-palmarodistal oblique (D45Pr-PaDiO), contrast enhanced, radiographic image of veins and bones after infusion of the palmar digital vein of the left forelimb with barium sulfate (normal cadaver specimen). Note the circumflex arrangement of the coronary plexi and the dorsal branch of the middle phalanx. Abaxial to the common digital extensor tendon the coronal circumflex vein drains the venous plexi of the dorsal coronary dermis and the coronary subcutis (coronary cushion). They join the dorsal branch of the middle phalanx and feed into the medial and lateral palmar digital veins. The coronal circumflex vein joins the medial and lateral branches of the dorsal branch of the middle phalanx to unite beneath the axial surface of the common digital extensor tendon. The venous plexus of the sublamellar dermis covers the parietal surface of the distal phalanx and drains proximally into the venous plexi of the coronary dermis and coronary subcutis. The sublamellar and solear plexus unite distally to form the circumflex marginal vein that extends around the entire distal margin of the foot. Note the reticular network of the venous plexus of the solear dermis. The sublamellar veins and solear plexus are superimposed in this projection; the proxiodistally oriented vessels are sublamellar veins, and the reticular pattern outlines the solear plexus.

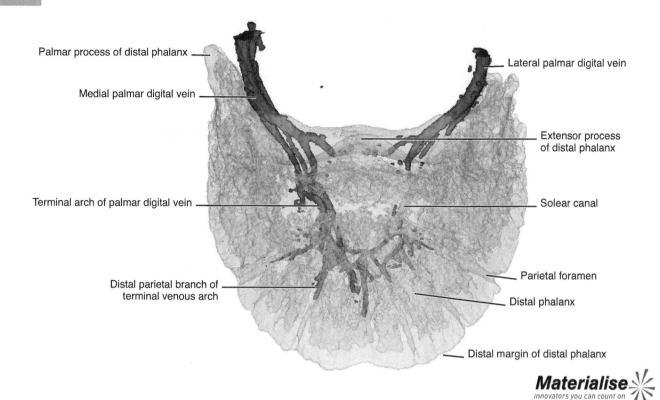

Palmar process of distal phalanx

Medial palmar digital vein

Terminal arch of palmar digital vein

Distal parietal branch of
terminal venous arch

Lateral palmar digital vein

Extensor process
of distal phalanx

Solear canal

Parietal foramen

Distal phalanx

Distal margin of distal phalanx

Materialise
innovators you can count on

● **Figure 7.16** Transparent solear view of Mimics-modeled computed tomography (CT) data of the veins of the distal phalanx after infusion of the palmar digital vein of the left forelimb with barium sulfate (normal cadaver specimen). The solear canal of the distal phalanx contains two or more anastomosing veins, the terminal arch of the palmar digital vein, which surround the terminal arch of the palmar digital artery. It is thought that venules emanating from deep within the distal phalanx feed into these venous vessels within the solear canal. Branches of the palmar digital vein terminal arch enter the distal and proximal parietal foramina and extend along their length, accompanying their arterial counterparts. However, retrograde venography fails to entirely fill the veins in the parietal foramina, perhaps because they are compressed by the adjoining parietal arteries or subdivide into venules too small to fill with barium sulfate. Mimics model by Simon Collins.

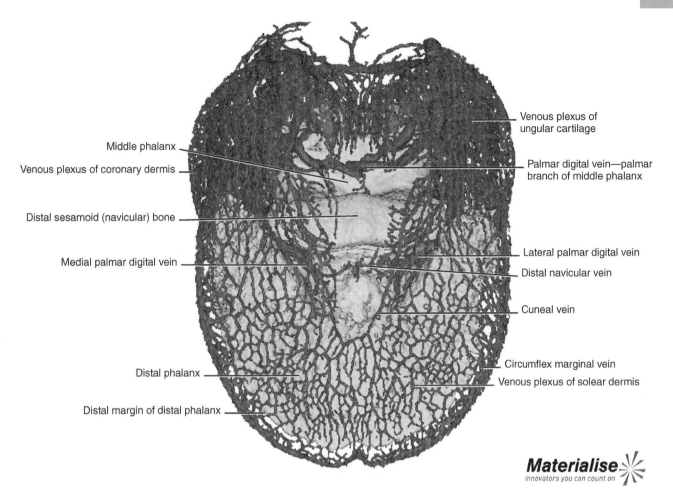

Middle phalanx

Venous plexus of coronary dermis

Distal sesamoid (navicular) bone

Medial palmar digital vein

Distal phalanx

Distal margin of distal phalanx

Venous plexus of
ungular cartilage

Palmar digital vein—palmar
branch of middle phalanx

Lateral palmar digital vein

Distal navicular vein

Cuneal vein

Circumflex marginal vein

Venous plexus of solear dermis

Materialise
innovators you can count on

• **Figure 7.17** Solear view of Mimics-modeled computed tomography (CT) data of veins and bones after infusion of the palmar digital vein of the left forelimb with barium sulfate (normal cadaver specimen). The model shows the reticular network of the venous plexus of the solear dermis. The solear plexus unites with the distal sublamellar plexus to form the circumflex marginal vein that extends around the entire distal margin of the foot. Mimics model by Simon Collins.

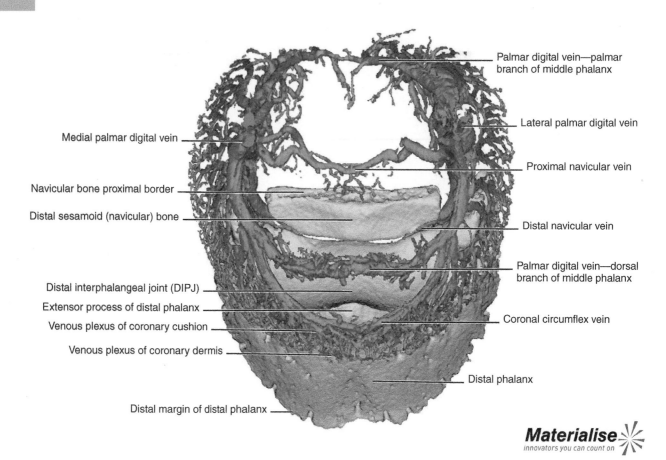

Palmar digital vein—palmar branch of middle phalanx

Lateral palmar digital vein

Medial palmar digital vein

Proximal navicular vein

Navicular bone proximal border

Distal sesamoid (navicular) bone

Distal navicular vein

Palmar digital vein—dorsal branch of middle phalanx

Distal interphalangeal joint (DIPJ)

Extensor process of distal phalanx

Coronal circumflex vein

Venous plexus of coronary cushion

Venous plexus of coronary dermis

Distal phalanx

Distal margin of distal phalanx

Figure 7.18 Skyline view of Mimics-modeled computed tomography (CT) data of veins and bones after infusion of the palmar digital vein of the left forelimb with barium sulfate (normal cadaver specimen). The model is reduced in complexity to aid comprehension of the key elements. The model shows the circumflex arrangement of the coronary plexi and the dorsal branch of the middle phalanx. Dorsally (abaxial to the common digital extensor tendon) the coronal circumflex vein drains the venous plexi of the dorsal coronary dermis and the coronary subcutis (coronary cushion). They join the dorsal branch of the middle phalanx and feed into the medial and lateral palmar digital veins. The medial and lateral branches of the dorsal branch of the middle phalanx unite beneath the axial surface of the common digital extensor tendon. The distal navicular vein receives several venules from the distal margin of the distal sesamoid (navicular bone) and drains directly into the medial and lateral palmar digital vein. Similarly, the proximal navicular vein receives venules from the proximal border of the bone and joins the medial and lateral palmar digital veins via the palmar branch of the middle phalanx. Mimics model by Simon Collins.

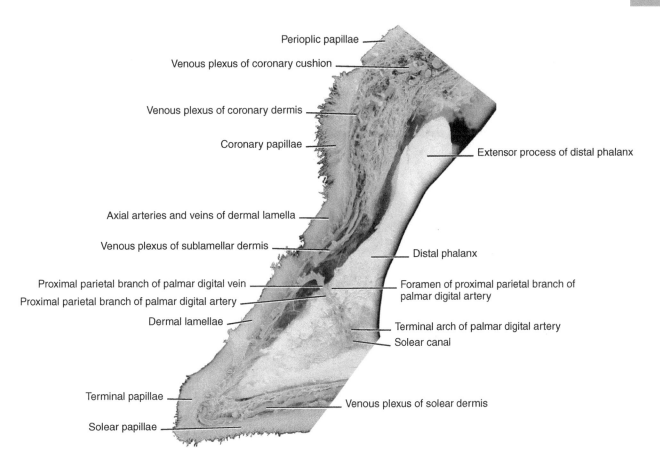

Perioplic papillae

Venous plexus of coronary cushion

Venous plexus of coronary dermis

Coronary papillae

Extensor process of distal phalanx

Axial arteries and veins of dermal lamella

Venous plexus of sublamellar dermis

Distal phalanx

Proximal parietal branch of palmar digital vein

Proximal parietal branch of palmar digital artery

Foramen of proximal parietal branch of palmar digital artery

Dermal lamellae

Terminal arch of palmar digital artery

Solear canal

Terminal papillae

Venous plexus of solear dermis

Solear papillae

• **Figure 7.19** Macro photograph of a partially macerated, dorsal sagittal section of a normal Australian Stockhorse foot. The blood vessels were previously perfused with liquid polyurethane (pigmented blue), which has polymerized, resulting in a vascular cast. Maceration of the specimen in 10% sodium hydroxide for 2 days has removed all tissues except bone. The specimen is remarkable in showing the extent of the large venous plexi in the coronary, sublamellar, and solear dermis. The large venous plexus of the coronary subcutis (coronary cushion) is a feature familiar to radiologists performing foot venograms where these veins are particularly prominent.

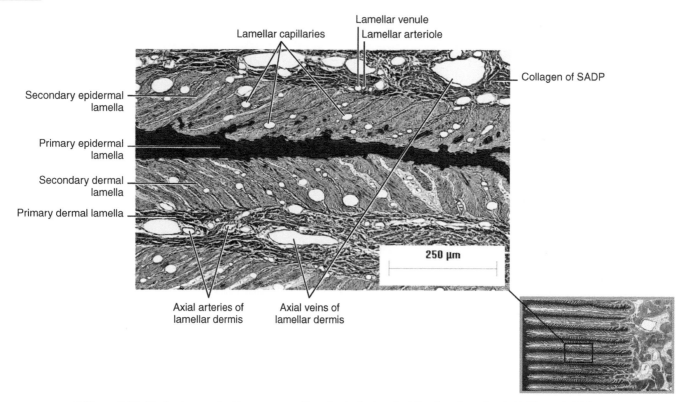

Figure 7.20 Photomicrograph of transverse section of a single dorsal midline lamella stained with Masson's trichrome (blue collagen and red epidermis). The specimen has been perfused with heparinized normal saline followed by 10% neutral buffered formalin fixation. Blood vessels are dilated to their maximum extent, and in particular lamellar capillaries are obvious; there are capillaries within virtually every secondary dermal lamella but none in the primary dermal lamella. The vessels adjacent to the secondary epidermal lamellar tips are venules and arterioles. In the primary lamellar dermis the veins are still laterally compressed despite pressure perfusion. They range in size from 70 to 180 μm. Arteries are smaller in diameter (around 12 μm in diameter) and dilation after fixation perfusion has made their thick, smooth muscle walls less apparent. The box in the inset shows the provenance of the section.

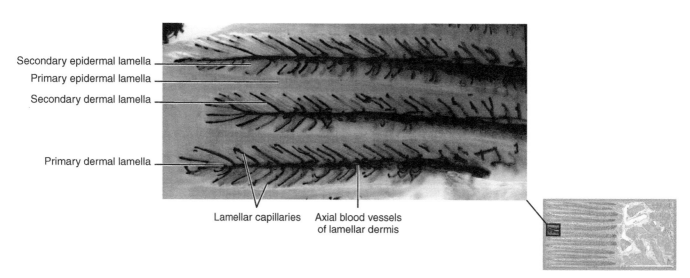

Figure 7.21 Macro photograph of an unstained, 2 mm–thick transverse section of dorsal midline lamellae perfused with India Ink in gelatin. All blood vessels, including the finest capillaries, contain India ink and appear black. The specimen is backlit, and because loops of capillaries are superimposed in the vertical plane, they highlight the capillaries in each secondary dermal lamella (SDL). Capillaries are present in the majority of SDLs. The vessels in the primary dermal lamellae are axial arteries and arterioles, (which deliver blood to the capillaries), and venules and axial veins, (which return blood to the sublamellar venous plexus). The box in the inset shows the provenance of the section.

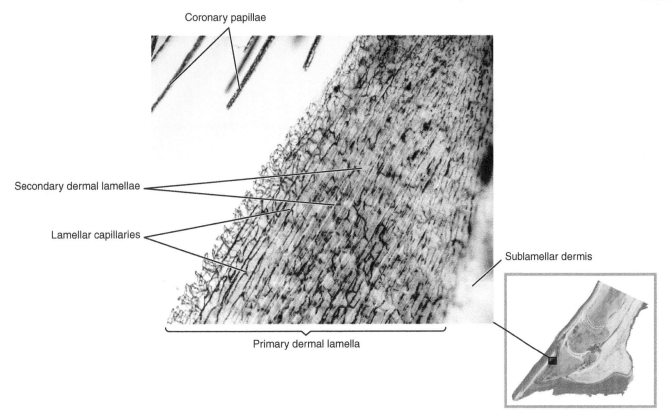

Coronary papillae

Secondary dermal lamellae

Lamellar capillaries

Sublamellar dermis

Primary dermal lamella

● **Figure 7.22** Macro photograph of an unstained, single dermal lamella, perfused with India ink in gelatin. All blood vessels, including the finest capillaries, contain India Ink and appear black. The specimen was lightly fixed in formalin and then macerated in 10% sodium hydroxide. The alkali has removed all hoof and epidermal lamellae, sparing the fixed dermal tissues, which have a white appearance. The axial arteries and veins are obscured deep in the opaque primary dermal lamella (PDL). The secondary dermal lamellae (SDLs) are the white parallel ridges running proximodistally on the surface of the PDL. The majority of the SDLs have black capillaries forming loops arising from arterioles deep in the PDL. The box in the inset shows the provenance of the section.

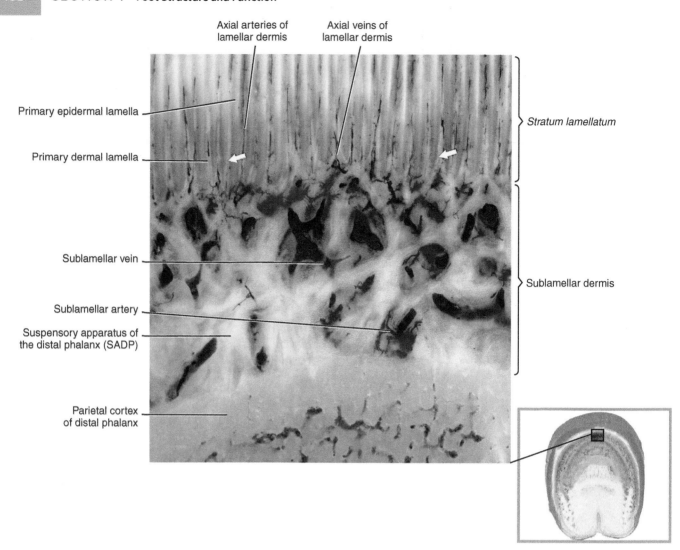

Axial arteries of
lamellar dermis

Axial veins of
lamellar dermis

Primary epidermal lamella

Primary dermal lamella

Sublamellar vein

Sublamellar artery

Suspensory apparatus of
the distal phalanx (SADP)

Parietal cortex
of distal phalanx

Stratum lamellatum

Sublamellar dermis

• **Figure 7.23** Macro photograph of an unstained, transverse section of dorsal midline lamellae with blood vessels previously perfused with liquid methyl methacrylate (MMA). The MMA has polymerized, resulting in a vascular cast. The arterial system contains red-pigmented MMA and the venous system blue. The viscosity of the MMA mixtures was deliberately kept high so that only major vessels were perfused. The keratinized axes of primary epidermal lamellae are whitish in color and between them, in complementary parallel rows, are primary dermal lamellae (PDLs). Within PDLs are axial lamellar arteries and veins sectioned obliquely along their length, so only portions remain. The white-colored collagen bundles of the suspensory apparatus of the distal phalanx (SADP) criss-cross the sublamellar dermis, forming a reticular network (*Stratum reticulare*). The thickest collagen bundles are embedded in the parietal cortex of the distal phalanx. Close to the lamellae (*stratum lamellatum*) small SADP branches enter the PDLs (*arrowed*), where ultimately the finest filaments of the SADP attach to the lamellar basement membrane. The inset shows the provenance of the specimen.

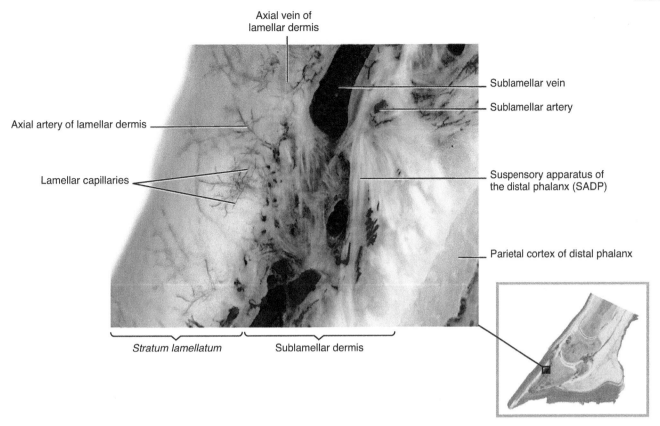

Axial vein of
lamellar dermis

Sublamellar vein

Sublamellar artery

Axial artery of lamellar dermis

Suspensory apparatus of
the distal phalanx (SADP)

Lamellar capillaries

Parietal cortex of distal phalanx

Stratum lamellatum   Sublamellar dermis

• **Figure 7.24** Macro photograph of an unstained, sagittal section of dorsal midline lamellae with blood vessels previously perfused with liquid methyl methacrylate (MMA). The MMA has polymerized, resulting in a vascular cast. The *Stratum medium* of the hoof wall has been removed. The arterial system contains red-pigmented MMA and the venous system blue. The viscosity of the MMA mixtures was deliberately kept high so that only major vessels were perfused. Nevertheless, a few larger capillaries did partially fill from the arteriolar (red) side. The white collagen bundles of the SADP are highlighted against the large, dark-blue veins of the sublamellar venous plexus. In this proximal lamellar region (see inset), the suspensory apparatus of the distal phalanx (SADP) is oriented near vertically. Sublamellar arteries and veins are located in the spaces between the collagen bundles of the SADP. Small axial lamellar arteries branch from the sublamellar arteries and enter the primary dermal lamellae at the same oblique angle as the collagen bundles of the SADP. Arterioles branching from the axial arteries give rise to capillaries that change orientation and run parallel to the secondary epidermal lamellae. In other words, they align parallel to the hoof wall and the dorsal surface of the distal phalanx. The axial veins are aligned similarly to the axial arteries and drain to the large sublamellar venous plexus. The box in the inset shows the provenance of the specimen.

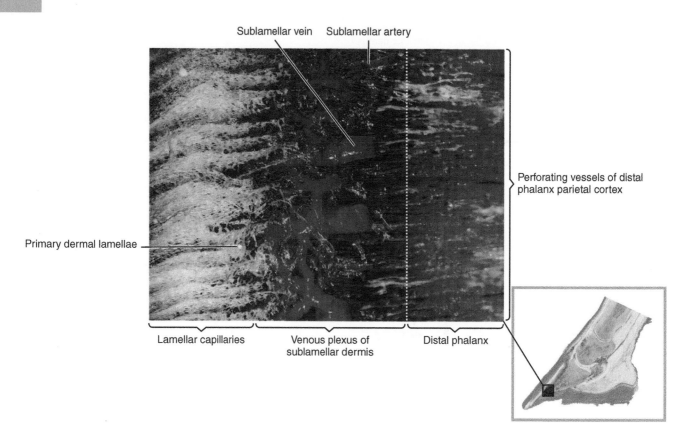

Sublamellar vein   Sublamellar artery

Perforating vessels of distal phalanx parietal cortex

Primary dermal lamellae

Lamellar capillaries   Venous plexus of   Distal phalanx
                        sublamellar dermis

• Figure 7.25 Macro photograph of a transverse section of dorsal midline, lamellar, sublamellar, and transcortical blood vessels containing red, polymerized methyl methacrylate (MMA). The specimen was macerated in 10% sodium hydroxide to remove epidermis, dermis, and bone. There are several vascular casts of lamellae in parallel rows; the capillaries of the lamellae are so fine that they appear translucent and white. Deep to the lamellae are the large, sublamellar collecting veins that drain into the prominent sublamellar venous plexus; note the multiple anastomoses between the veins of the plexus. The sublamellar plexus drains blood proximad to the coronary plexus and ultimately to the palmar digital veins. The dotted line shows the boundary between bone and dermis. Dissolving the bony cortex of the distal phalanx has revealed the extent of the transcortical vasculature, showing that it consists of numerous small arteries and veins. Some of the transcortical veins join the sublamellar venous plexus, creating the possibility that blood can either drain or enter the distal phalanx under certain circumstances (e.g., peaks of hydraulic pressure). The transcortical arteries are branches of the parietal arteries, themselves branches of the terminal arch of the palmar digital arteries. They supply blood to the lamellar arterioles and capillaries. The box in the inset shows the provenance of the specimen.

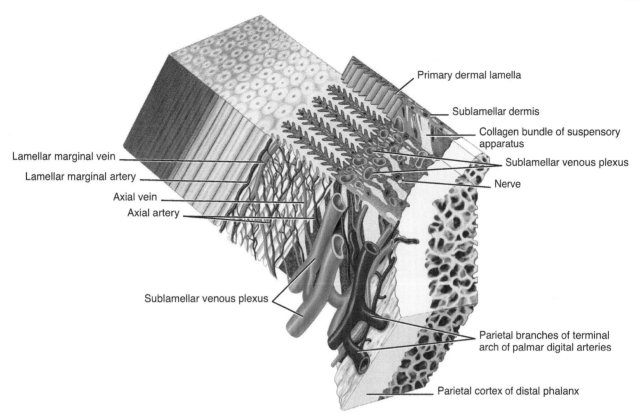

Primary dermal lamella

Sublamellar dermis

Collagen bundle of suspensory apparatus

Sublamellar venous plexus

Nerve

Lamellar marginal vein

Lamellar marginal artery

Axial vein

Axial artery

Sublamellar venous plexus

Parietal branches of terminal arch of palmar digital arteries

Parietal cortex of distal phalanx

• **Figure 7.26** Anatomic diagram showing the relationship between the dorsal midwall blood vessels and the suspensory apparatus of the distal phalanx (SADP). The collagen bundles of the SADP are oriented at 70° to the horizontal at this mid–hoof wall site. The numerous large diameter veins of the sublamellar plexus are oriented proximodistally (parallel to the parietal cortex of the distal phalanx) and are surrounded by the SADP collagen bundles. The axial lamellar arteries branch from sublamellar arteries and run parallel to the SADP collagen bundles in the primary dermal lamella (i.e., at 70° to the horizontal). The axial arteries freely anastomose and form peripheral loops joining to form the marginal lamellar artery. Likewise, axial veins run beside the arteries and drain to the sublamellar venous plexus, which in turn returns blood proximally to the large veins in the coronary dermis and coronary subcutis. Illustration designed by the author.

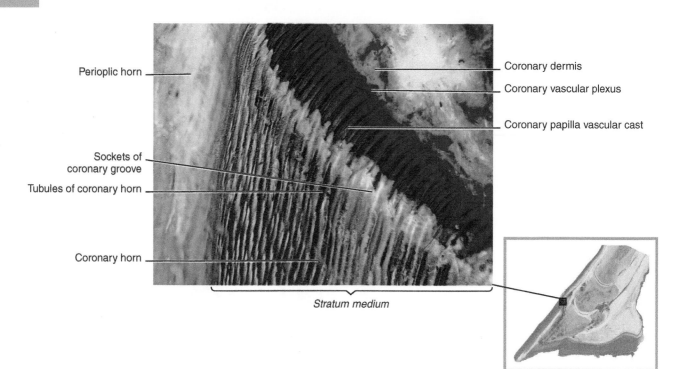

Perioplic horn

Coronary dermis

Coronary vascular plexus

Coronary papilla vascular cast

Sockets of coronary groove

Tubules of coronary horn

Coronary horn

Stratum medium

• **Figure 7.27** Macro photograph of an unstained, sagittal section of dorsal midline, proximal coronet with blood vessels containing red-colored, polymerized methyl methacrylate (MMA). The specimen was lightly macerated in warm saline for 24 hours to loosen dermal–epidermal attachments. The coronary dermis was teased from the proximal hoof wall to show the bases of numerous coronary papillae. Each dermal papilla fits into its own socket in the coronary groove of the hoof wall, and in turn, via its blood supply, nurtures the proximal coronary epidermal basal cells responsible for the production of new tubular hoof wall. There is one papilla per tubule. The majority of the visible vessels in the papillae and the plexus above are venules and veins. The elements of papillary anatomy are repeated wherever tubular horn is produced. The inset shows the provenance of the specimen.

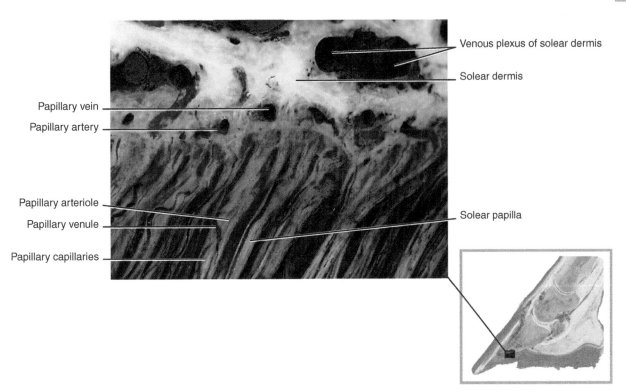

Venous plexus of solear dermis

Solear dermis

Papillary vein

Papillary artery

Papillary arteriole

Papillary venule

Solear papilla

Papillary capillaries

● **Figure 7.28** Macro photograph of an unstained, sagittal section of dorsal midline, solear dermis with blood vessels containing red (arteries) and blue (veins) polymerized, methyl methacrylate (MMA). The specimen was lightly macerated in warm saline for 24 hours to loosen dermal–epidermal attachments. The solear dermis was teased from the sole horn (now absent) to show the numerous solear papillae. At the base of each papilla is a nutrient artery from which an arteriole branches and enters the papilla. Capillaries branch from this central papillary arteriole as it spirals down the center of the papillae to its tip. The central venule entwines around the central arteriole, receiving capillaries from the venous side of the capillary bed. The central venule drains venous blood into the large papillary vein that in turn joins the extensive venous plexus of the sole. Fine capillaries form a sheath around the central arteriole and venule; a few are filled with red MMA. The whitish appearance of the papillae is due to collagenous connective tissue that is continuous with the connective tissue of the solear dermis. The box in the inset shows the provenance of the specimen.

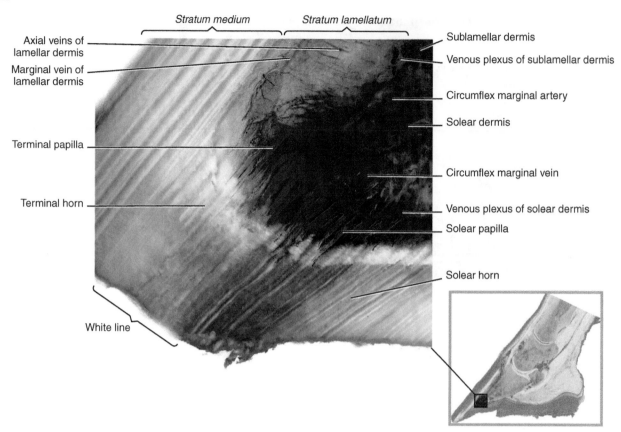

• **Figure 7.29** Macro photograph of an unstained, sagittal section of dorsal midline, hoof wall, lamellar, sole junction (white line) with blood vessels containing red polymerized, methyl methacrylate (MMA). The specimen was lightly macerated in warm saline for 24 hours to loosen dermal–epidermal attachments. The solear and distal lamellar dermis was teased from the sole and terminal (white line) horn to show the terminal and solear papillae. The terminal papillae are the largest papillae of the hoof integument and nurture the tubular horn production of the white line. Terminal papillae form the distal border of the lamellar dermis and merge with the solear papillae. The inset shows the provenance of the specimen.

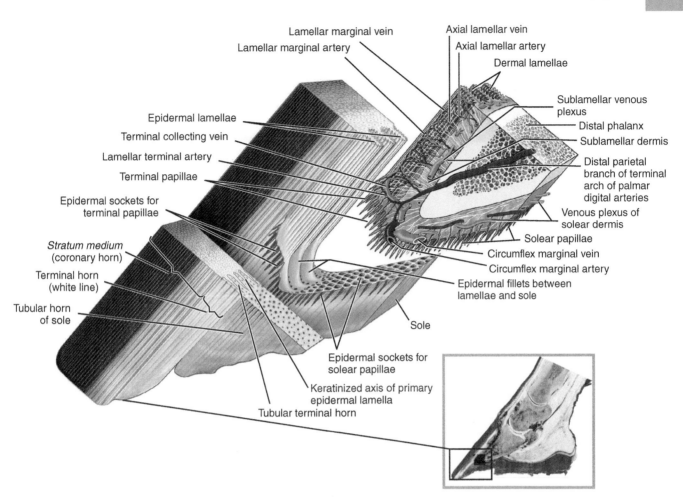

Lamellar marginal vein
Lamellar marginal artery
Axial lamellar vein
Axial lamellar artery
Dermal lamellae

Epidermal lamellae
Terminal collecting vein
Lamellar terminal artery
Terminal papillae
Epidermal sockets for terminal papillae
Stratum medium (coronary horn)
Terminal horn (white line)
Tubular horn of sole

Sublamellar venous plexus
Distal phalanx
Sublamellar dermis
Distal parietal branch of terminal arch of palmar digital arteries
Venous plexus of solear dermis
Solear papillae
Circumflex marginal vein
Circumflex marginal artery
Epidermal fillets between lamellae and sole

Sole

Epidermal sockets for solear papillae
Keratinized axis of primary epidermal lamella
Tubular terminal horn

• **Figure 7.30** Diagram of the terminal papillae, sole papillae and lamellae at the junction of the hoof wall, white line and sole. The terminal papillae are the largest papillae of the hoof integument and nurture the tubular horn production of the white line. The lamellar epidermis proximal to the terminal horn production region is nonproliferative. However, the epidermis lining the sockets of the terminal papillae and the epidermis around them is highly proliferative and forms the terminal horn of the white line. The corner formed between the epidermal wall and the sole is filled with a stress-reducing fillet. The fillets align with each epidermal lamella and distribute stresses over a broader area, making the angle between wall and sole more durable and capable of bearing larger loads. Terminal horn production joins the 10-month-old wall that has grown down from the coronary band to the adjacent two- to three-month-old sole. The inset shows the provenance of the specimen. (Illustration designed by the author.)

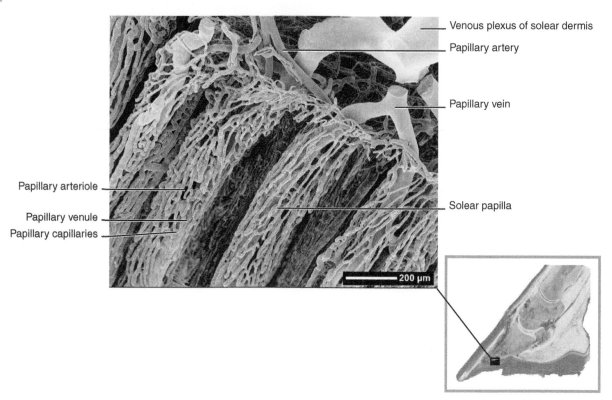

Venous plexus of solear dermis

Papillary artery

Papillary vein

Solear papilla

Papillary arteriole

Papillary venule

Papillary capillaries

200 µm

● **Figure 7.31** Scanning electron micrograph of dorsal midline methyl methacrylate vascular cast of solear papillae. The blood delivered to each solear papilla nurtures a single sole horn tubule. The basal cells of the intertubular horn between tubular horn is also supplied by a network of capillaries. At the base of each papilla is a nutrient papillary artery from which a papillary arteriole arises and enters the papilla. Capillaries branch from this central papillary arteriole and form a capillary sheath around the central vessels. The central venule entwines around the central arteriole, receiving capillaries from the venous side of the capillary bed. The central venule drains venous blood into the large papillary vein that in turn joins the extensive venous plexus of the sole. The inset shows the provenance of the specimen.

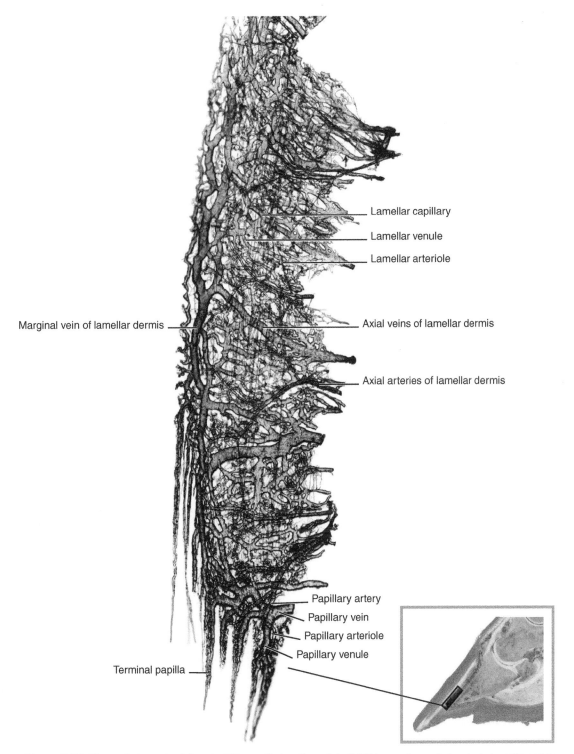

Lamellar capillary

Lamellar venule

Lamellar arteriole

Marginal vein of lamellar dermis

Axial veins of lamellar dermis

Axial arteries of lamellar dermis

Papillary artery

Papillary vein

Papillary arteriole

Papillary venule

Terminal papilla

• **Figure 7.32** Macro photograph of dorsal midline methyl methacrylate (MMA) vascular cast of a single lamella and its **terminal papillae.** The cast was made by pressure-injecting liquid MMA into the median artery just palmar to the carpus. Arterially delivered MMA reached the distal lamellae and toe and entered the axial arteries (colored red). Arterioles branching from the axial arteries supply numerous lamellar capillaries oriented proximodistally in parallel rows in secondary dermal lamellae. The fine parallel lines running from top to bottom of the cast are lamellar capillaries. The relatively large lamellar venules and axial veins filled last (colored blue). The volume of blood in venules and veins far exceeds the volume in arterioles and axial arteries. Axial arteries and veins alternate with each other the entire proximodistal length of the lamella. The inset shows the provenance of the specimen.

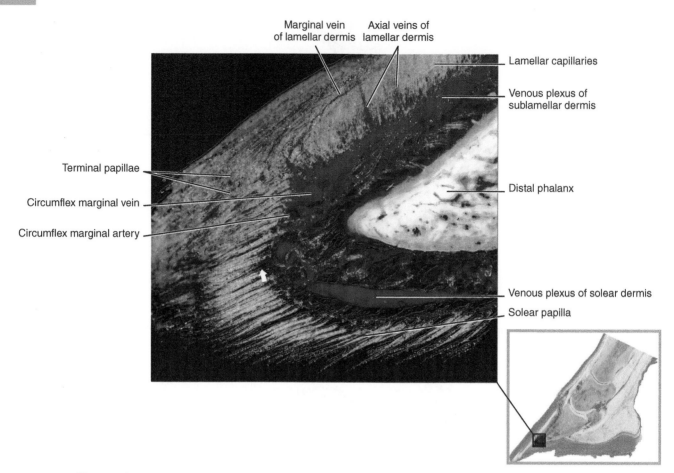

• **Figure 7.33** Macro photograph of a sagittal section of dorsal midline, lamellar sole junction with blood vessels containing red polymerized, methyl methacrylate (MMA). The specimen was partially macerated in 10% sodium hydroxide to remove epidermis and photographed before the margin of the distal phalanx was dissolved. Some residual black pigmented solear epidermis remains (arrow) There are several vascular casts of lamellae in parallel rows; their marginal veins outline their abaxial, most peripheral, borders. Projecting from the distal border of each lamella are the vascular casts of five to seven terminal papillae. These blend with the more palmar solear papillae. Draining the papillary and lamellar circulations are the large solear and sublamellar venous plexi. The inset shows the provenance of the specimen.

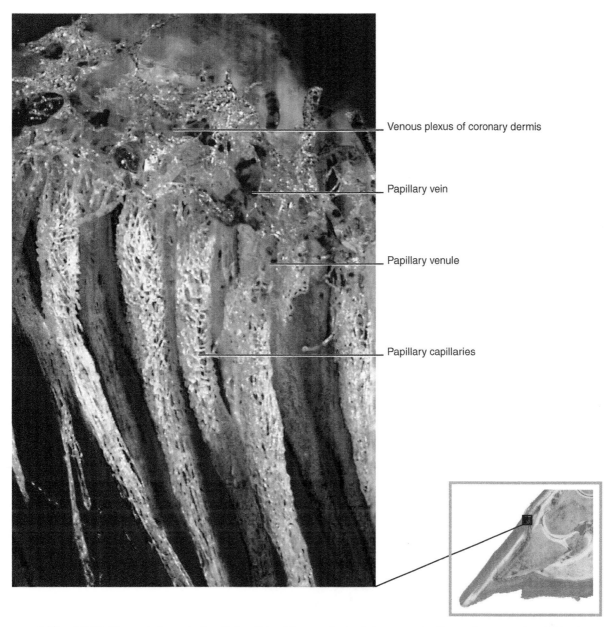

Venous plexus of coronary dermis

Papillary vein

Papillary venule

Papillary capillaries

• **Figure 7.34** Macro photograph of methyl methacrylate vascular cast of coronary papillae and coronary dermis blood vessels. Arteries in the coronary dermis branch to supply each papilla with an arteriole. The papillary arteriole runs the entire length of the papilla, giving off branches from which numerous capillaries arise. In this photograph, taken with bright white light, the specimen was air dried and the transparent capillaries are highly reflective. They form a whitish sheath around the central arteriole and venule. The central venule entwines around the central arteriole, receiving capillaries from the venous side of the capillary bed. The central venule drains venous blood into the large papillary vein that in turn joins the extensive coronary venous plexus. The inset shows the provenance of the specimen.

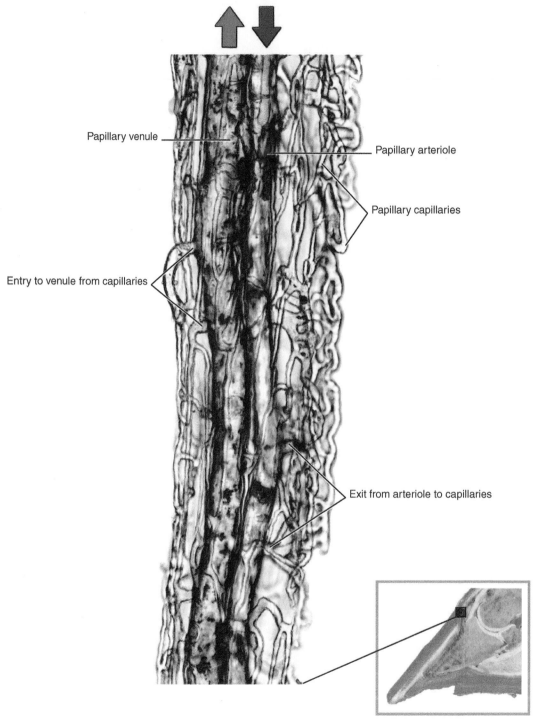

Papillary venule

Papillary arteriole

Papillary capillaries

Entry to venule from capillaries

Exit from arteriole to capillaries

• **Figure 7.35** Macro photograph of methyl methacrylate vascular corrosion cast of a single coronary papilla. The arrows show the direction of blood flow (red = arteriole inflow; blue = venule outflow). The papillary arteriole and venule run the entire length of the papilla, giving off short branches that connect to and from the capillary bed. The capillaries line the periphery of the papilla close to the proliferating epidermal basal cells of the hoof wall tubule. There are multiple exit points, to the capillary bed, along the length of the arteriole and, likewise, multiple entry points from the capillary bed to the venule. The inset shows the provenance of the specimen.

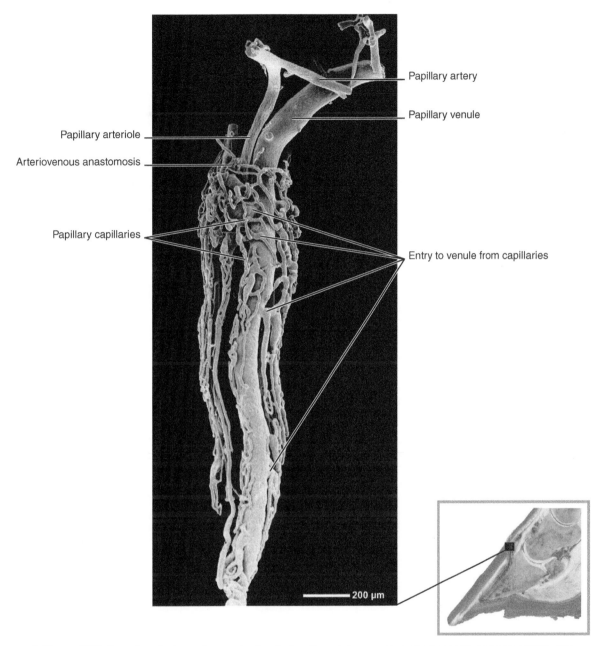

Papillary artery

Papillary venule

Papillary arteriole

Arteriovenous anastomosis

Papillary capillaries

Entry to venule from capillaries

200 µm

• **Figure 7.36** Scanning electron micrograph of methyl methacrylate vascular cast of a single coronary papilla. The papillary arteriole and venule run the entire length of the papilla, giving off short branches that connect to and from the capillary bed. In this preparation the papillary arteriole is obscured behind the papillary venule. There are multiple entry points from the capillary bed to the venule. The inset shows the provenance of the specimen.

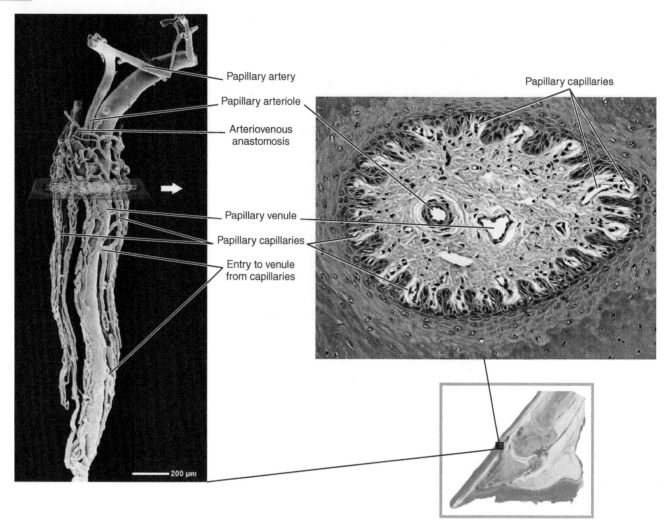

Papillary artery

Papillary arteriole

Arteriovenous
anastomosis

Papillary venule

Papillary capillaries

Entry to venule
from capillaries

200 µm

Papillary capillaries

Figure 7.37 Scanning electron micrograph of methyl methacrylate vascular corrosion cast of a single coronary papilla and photomicrograph of transverse section of a coronary papilla stained with haematoxylin and eosin. The arteriole and venule of the papilla run the entire length of the papilla, giving off short branches that connect to and from the capillary bed. The transverse section photomicrograph shows a papilla surrounded by a freshly synthesized coronary hoof wall tubule. The coronary arteriole has a thick muscular wall compared with the larger, relatively thin-walled venule. At the level of the section (shown superimposed on the vascular cast) epidermal basal cells are proliferating at a high rate to manufacture new tubular horn that keratinizes centrifugally. In the dermis between the epidermal ridges that line the inner surface of the tubule socket are numerous capillaries in very close proximity to the coronary epidermal basal cells. The inset shows the provenance of the specimens.

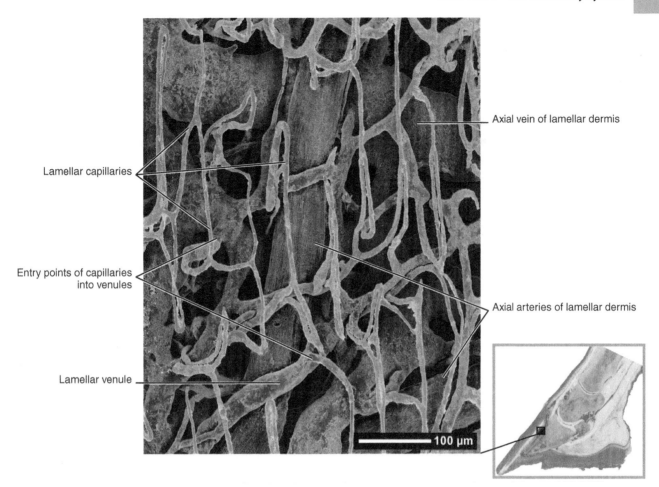

Axial vein of lamellar dermis

Lamellar capillaries

Entry points of capillaries into venules

Axial arteries of lamellar dermis

Lamellar venule

100 µm

● **Figure 7.38** Scanning electron micrograph of methyl methacrylate vascular cast of lamellar microcirculation. The cast of the axial lamellar artery (colored red) is circular in profile and identified by the surface impressions of its longitudinally oriented endothelial cells. Veins are identified by circular pavement-like, endothelial cell impressions. Numerous capillaries branch from arterioles obscured beneath the dense venous network. The capillaries loop upward toward the viewer and are arranged in parallel rows. In life the capillaries are within rows of proximodistal oriented secondary dermal lamellae. The space between the capillary rows is occupied by secondary epidermal lamellae. The capillary loops arise from arterioles and terminate with venules. There are numerous points of entry of capillaries into venules. The inset shows the provenance of the specimen.

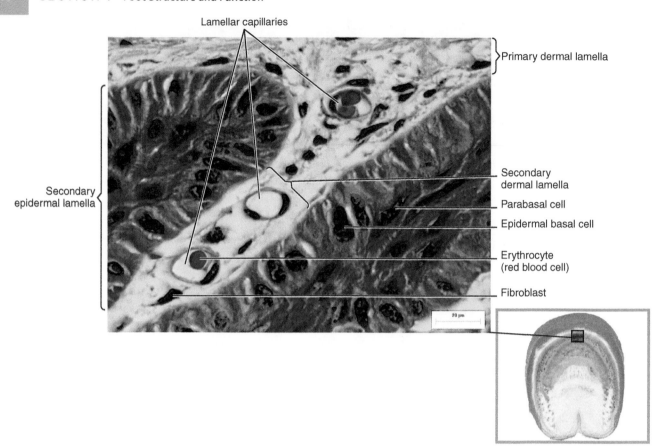

Lamellar capillaries

Primary dermal lamella

Secondary epidermal lamella

Secondary dermal lamella

Parabasal cell

Epidermal basal cell

Erythrocyte (red blood cell)

Fibroblast

20 µm

Figure 7.39 Photomicrograph of normal secondary epidermal and dermal lamellae. Within the connective tissue of the secondary dermal lamella are three capillaries, two of which contain erythrocytes (red blood cells). Numerous fibroblasts within the secondary and primary dermal lamellae maintain the extracellular matrix; the lamellar basement membrane is not visible in this haematoxylin and eosin stained section. The distance between capillary wall and epidermal basal cell is less than the diameter of a red blood cell. This small distance ensures efficient delivery of glucose and other nutrients to the epidermal basal cell. (Capillary diameter [mean ± s.e] = 15.41 ± 0.75 µm; mean erythrocyte diameter = 8.23 ± 0.17 µm; mean distance to nearest epidermal basal cell = 4.51 ± 0.74 µm.) The inset shows the provenance of the specimen.

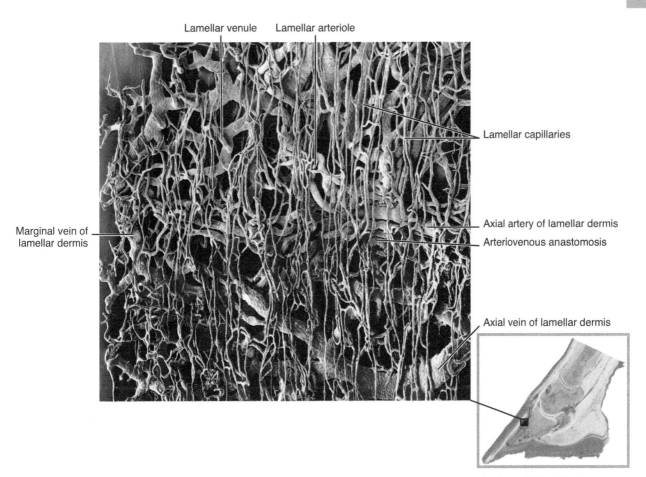

Lamellar venule   Lamellar arteriole

Lamellar capillaries

Axial artery of lamellar dermis

Arteriovenous anastomosis

Marginal vein of
lamellar dermis

Axial vein of lamellar dermis

● **Figure 7.40** Scanning electron micrograph of methyl methacrylate vascular corrosion cast of a single dermal lamella. The cast of the axial lamellar artery (colored red) is identified by the surface impressions of its longitudinally oriented endothelial cells. Veins (colored blue) are identified by circular, pavement-like endothelial cell impressions. In life the axial arteries and veins are within the primary dermal lamella and capillaries within the secondary lamellae. The numerous capillaries arise from arterioles that have branched from branches of the axial lamellar artery. The capillaries (uncolored) loop upward toward the viewer and are arranged in parallel rows that, in life, are within rows of proximodistal oriented secondary dermal lamellae. The spaces between the capillary rows is occupied by secondary epidermal lamellae. Capillaries are the smallest blood vessels in the circulation, and the lamellar capillary network delivers the nutrients essential for epidermal basal cell metabolism. The capillary loops converge into venules that join the larger veins draining to the sublamellar plexus. Arteriovenous anastomoses (colored yellow) connect artery to vein, enabling blood to bypass the capillary bed should the need arise. The inset shows the provenance of the specimen.

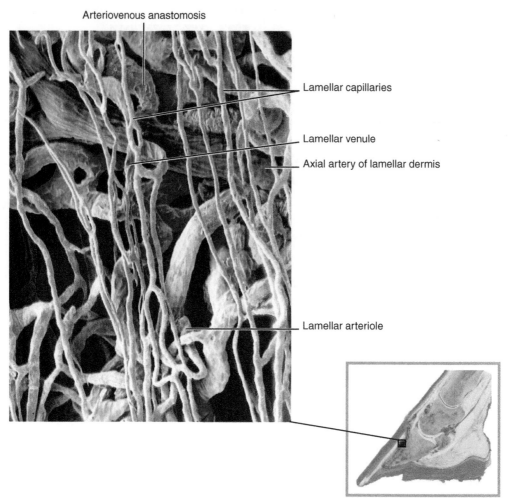

Arteriovenous anastomosis

Lamellar capillaries

Lamellar venule

Axial artery of lamellar dermis

Lamellar arteriole

• **Figure 7.41** Scanning electron micrograph of methyl methacrylate vascular corrosion cast of an axial lamellar artery (colored red) and surrounding lamellar veins (colored blue). An arteriole arising from a branch of the axial artery gives rise to a tuft of capillaries (uncolored). The capillaries are arranged in rows that align, in life, with secondary dermal lamellae. The capillary loops that arise from the arteriole converge into a venule that in turn merges into a larger vein. Arteriovenous anastomoses (colored yellow) connect artery to vein. The base of the arteriolar cast is undercut, denoting the presence of a muscular sphincter in the wall of the vessel at this location. The inset shows the provenance of the specimen.

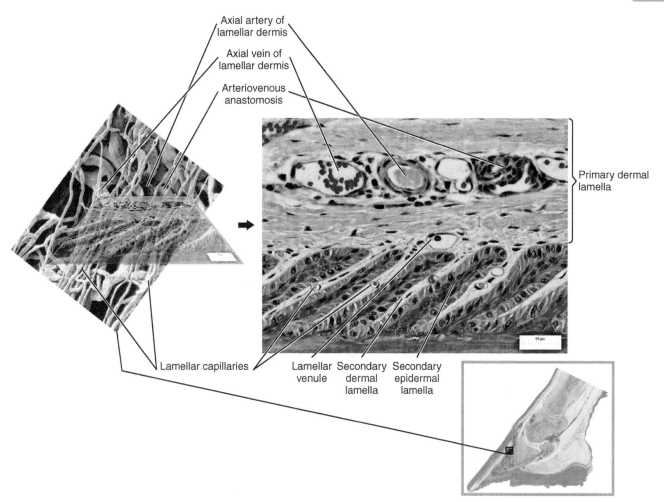

Axial artery of
lamellar dermis

Axial vein of
lamellar dermis

Arteriovenous
anastomosis

Primary dermal
lamella

Lamellar capillaries

Lamellar
venule

Secondary
dermal
lamella

Secondary
epidermal
lamella

• **Figure 7.42** Scanning electron micrograph of methyl methacrylate vascular corrosion cast of lamellar blood vessels (as in Figure 7-41). To aid conceptual understanding, the vascular cast scanning electron micrograph has been aligned with a light photomicrograph sectioned transversely (TS) through the same region. Within the primary dermal lamella is an axial artery and vein. The artery has a thick muscular wall typical of high-pressure delivery vessels, and the adjacent thin-walled vein contains numerous red blood cells (erythrocytes). Numerous capillaries are present within secondary dermal lamellae (SDLs). The arteriovenous anastomosis (AVA) also has a thick muscular wall and prominent endothelial cells; the connection between artery and vein that is not evident in the two-dimensional section is explained by the three-dimensional vascular cast. The cast shows the AVA clearly connected to both the artery and vein above and below the plane of transverse section. The rows of capillaries in the vascular cast have their TS equivalent in the capillaries within consecutive rows of SDLs. The inset shows the provenance of the specimen. Bar = 50 μm (0.05 mm).

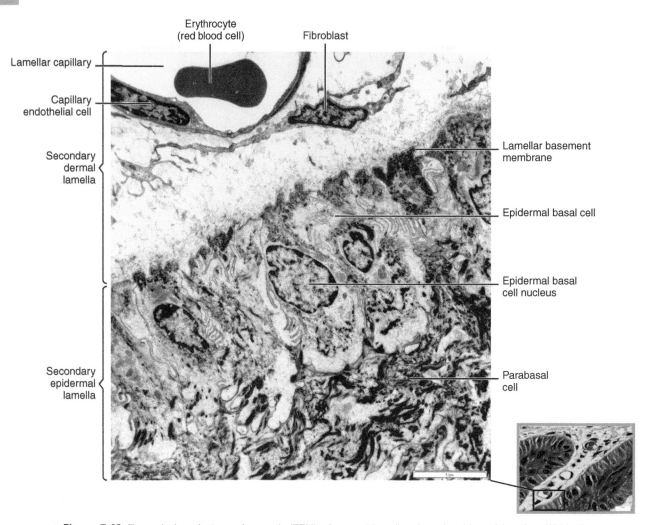

Erythrocyte
(red blood cell)

Fibroblast

Lamellar capillary

Capillary
endothelial cell

Secondary
dermal
lamella

Secondary
epidermal
lamella

Lamellar basement
membrane

Epidermal basal cell

Epidermal basal
cell nucleus

Parabasal
cell

• **Figure 7.43** Transmission electron micrograph (TEM) of normal lamellar dermal–epidermal junction. Within the connective tissue of the secondary dermal lamella is a capillary containing a single erythrocyte (red blood cell). The vascular endothelial cell forms the thin wall of the capillary through which nutrients and gases diffuse from the capillary lumen to the extracellular fluid outside. This maintains a concentration gradient whereby the epidermal basal cell can sequester nutrients, especially glucose, within its cytoplasm. The distance between capillary wall and epidermal basal cell is approximately 10 μm, less than the diameter of the red blood cell. This small distance ensures efficient delivery of glucose and other nutrients to the epidermal basal cell. Fibroblasts within the secondary dermal lamella maintain the extracellular matrix; the lamellar basement membrane is just visible at this magnification. The inset shows the provenance of the specimen. Bar = 5 μm (0.005 mm).

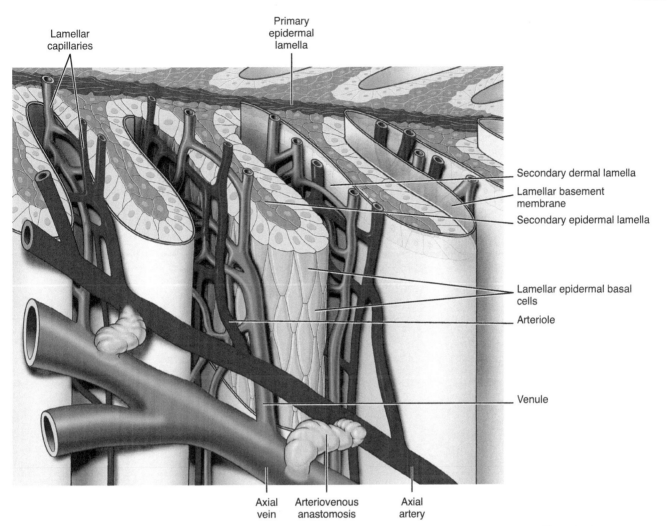

Lamellar
capillaries

Primary
epidermal
lamella

Secondary dermal lamella

Lamellar basement
membrane

Secondary epidermal lamella

Lamellar epidermal basal
cells

Arteriole

Venule

Axial   Arteriovenous   Axial
vein   anastomosis   artery

● **Figure 7.44** Diagram of the lamellar microcirculation. The epidermal lamellae are well served by a capillary circulation; every secondary dermal lamella (SDL) has capillaries delivering essential nutrients (mainly glucose) to the target
tissue, the adjacent epidermal basal cells. Lamellar capillaries are within 5 to 7 μm (the diameter of one red blood cell)
of all faces of the secondary epidermal lamellae (SELs) and are virtually absent from the primary dermal lamellae
(PDLs) and the sublamellar dermis. Arterioles branch from the lamellar axial arteries in the PDL and transition into the
smallest unit of the circulation the capillary (shaded red in the diagram). The capillaries exiting the SDLs (shaded blue)
merge with thin-walled venules that in turn join the axial veins in the PDL. Capillaries have small diameters and thin
endothelial cell walls, and this allows molecules inside the capillary lumen to rapidly diffuse to the interstitial fluid just
outside the vessel. Most gases and inorganic ions pass through the capillary wall in less than 2 milliseconds. The direct
connections between arteries and veins are arterio-venous anastomoses or AV shunts. They are under the control of
the nervous system and, by opening and closing, facilitate heat transfer through the hoof wall and thus thermoregulation. The inset shows the provenance of the specimen. (Illustration designed by the author.)

References

1. Bell, D. R. (2013). The microcirculation and the lymphatic system. In R. A. Rhoades & D. R. Bell (Eds.), *Medical physiology: Principles for clinical medicine* (4th ed.). Philadelphia, PA: Lippincott Williams & Wilkins.

2. Bragulla, H., & Hirschberg, R. M. (2003). Horse hooves and bird feathers: Two model systems for studying the structure and development of highly adapted integumentary accessory organs – The role of the dermo-epidermal interface for the micro-architecture of complex epidermal structures. *Journal of Experimental Zoology Part B: Molecular and Developmental Evolution, 298B*, 140–151.

3. Lanovaz, J. L., Clayton, H. M., & Watson, L. G. (1998). In vitro attenuation of impact shock in equine digits. *Equine Veterinary Journal (Suppl.)*, (26), 96–102.

4. Molyneux, G. S., Haller, C. J., Mogg, K., & Pollitt, C. C. (1994). The structure, innervation and location of arteriovenous anastomoses in the equine foot. *Equine Veterinary Journal, 26*, 305–312.

5. Nordstrom, C. H. (2010). Cerebral energy metabolism and microdialysis in neurocritical care. *Childs Nervous System, 26*, 465–472.

6. Pass, M. A., Pollitt, S., & Pollitt, C. C. (1998). Decreased glucose metabolism causes separation of hoof lamellae in vitro: A trigger for laminitis? *Equine Veterinary Journal (Suppl.)*, (26), 133–138.

7. Pawlak, E., Wang, L., Johnson, P. J., Nuovo, G., Taye, A., Belknap, J. K., et al. (2012). Distribution and processing of a disintegrin and metalloproteinase with thrombospondin motifs-4, aggrecan, versican, and hyaluronan in equine digital laminae. *American Journal of Veterinary Research, 73*, 1035–1046.

8. Ratzlaff, M. H., Shindell, R. M., & Debowes, R. M. (1985). Changes in digital venous pressures of horses moving at the walk and trot. *American Journal of Veterinary Research, 46*, 1545–1549.

9. Wattle, O., & Pollitt, C. C. (2004). Lamellar metabolism. *Clinical Techniques in Equine Practice, 3*, 22–33.

10. Weber, J. M., Dobson, G. P., Parkhouse, W. S., Wheeldon, D., Harman, J. C., Snow, D. H., et al. (1987). Cardiac output and oxygen consumption in exercising Thoroughbred horses. *American Journal of Physiology, 253*, R890–R895.

LAMELLAR HISTOLOGY

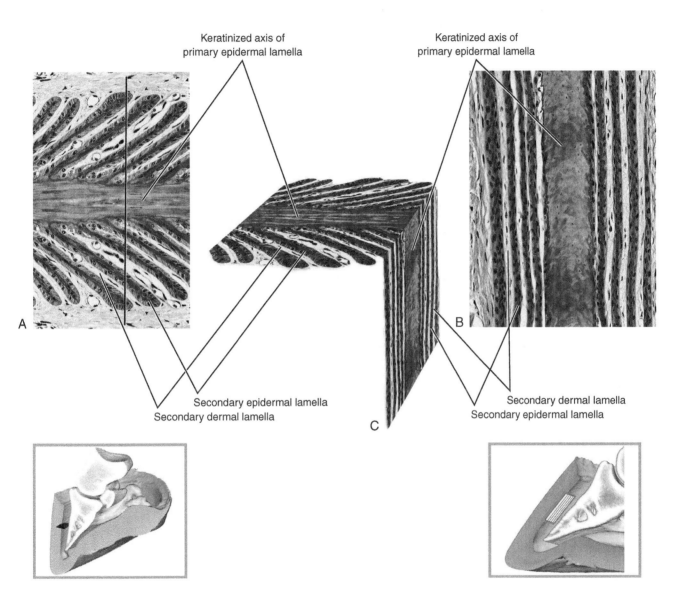

Keratinized axis of
primary epidermal lamella

Keratinized axis of
primary epidermal lamella

Secondary epidermal lamella
Secondary dermal lamella

Secondary dermal lamella
Secondary epidermal lamella

A

B

C

● **Figure 8.1** A transverse compared with a dorsal section of normal midwall lamellae. The transverse (**A**) is the traditional plane of section and is prepared from bandsaw cuts made perpendicular to the dorsal hoof wall. The dorsal plane of section is parallel to the hoof wall and gives a less familiar, but instructive, longitudinal view of the lamellae. The line in **A** transects three to four lamellae on either side of the keratinized axis of the primary epidermal lamella (PEL). A dorsal lamellar section (**B**) through the line also shows three to four lamellae, but now the profiles are longitudinal. The composite in **C** explains the relationship between the two planes of section. The dorsal section shows that the lamellar epidermal basal cells are fusiform in shape with the long axis of their nuclei and cytoskeleton aligned proximodistally along lines of stress. The insets show the provenance planes of the sections. (Stain = haematoxylin and eosin.)

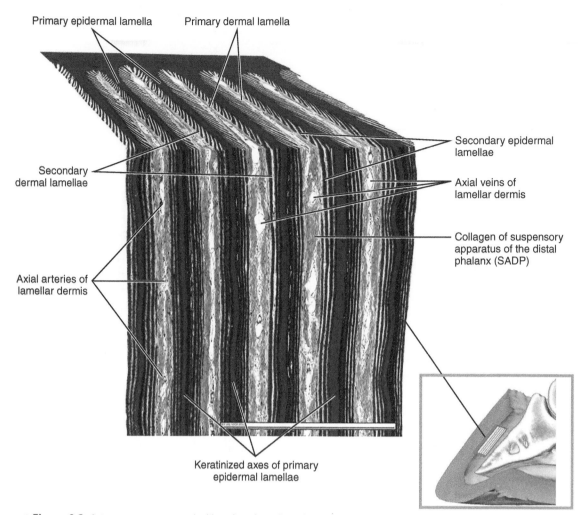

Primary epidermal lamella   Primary dermal lamella

Secondary epidermal
lamellae

Axial veins of
lamellar dermis

Collagen of suspensory
apparatus of the distal
phalanx (SADP)

Secondary
dermal lamellae

Axial arteries of
lamellar dermis

Keratinized axes of primary
epidermal lamellae

● **Figure 8.2** A transverse compared with a dorsal section of normal midwall lamellae from the toe of a normal horse foot stained with Masson's trichrome. Connective tissue is stained blue and epidermis red. The dorsal plane of section is midlamellar, and the lamellae are arranged in parallel, proximodistal rows. There are approximately 4 lamellae per millimeter. On either side of each keratinized primary epidermal lamellar axis are three to four secondary epidermal lamellae with interdigitating dermal lamellae. There is an axial artery every 3 mm in each primary dermal lamella with laterally compressed veins in between. Note the proximodistal orientation of the linear collagen bundles of the suspensory apparatus of the distal phalanx, an alignment parallel to load-bearing lines of stress. The box in the inset shows the provenance of the specimen. (Bar = 1000 μm [1 mm]).

TRANSVERSE HISTOLOGY

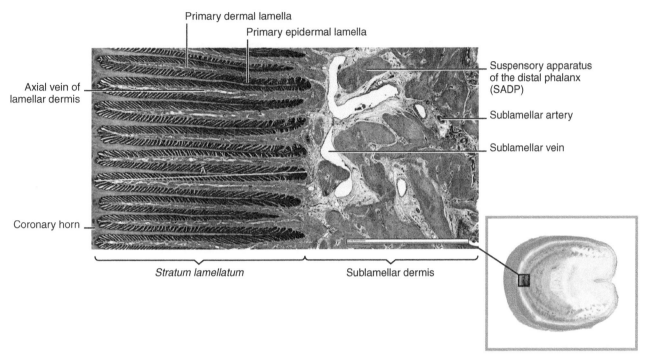

Primary dermal lamella

Primary epidermal lamella

Axial vein of lamellar dermis

Suspensory apparatus of the distal phalanx (SADP)

Sublamellar artery

Sublamellar vein

Coronary horn

Stratum lamellatum

Sublamellar dermis

● **Figure 8.3** Low-magnification photomicrograph of transverse section of dorsal, midwall lamellae (*stratum lamellatum*) and the sublamellar dermis from a normal horse front foot, stained with haematoxylin and eosin (H&E). The term *stratum lamellatum* defines both the dermal and epidermal lamellae. There are nine primary epidermal lamellae (PELs) inter-digitating with nine primary dermal lamellae (PDLs). The mean length (line A) of a PEL is 3335 ± 194 μm.[1] Each PEL has a cornified axis wider at its base where it merges with the coronary horn of the *stratum medium* (the hoof wall proper). There are no cell nuclei in the PEL cornified axis (or the coronary horn of the *stratum medium*), so this eosinophilic tissue stains light pink. In contrast, the living cells of the secondary epidermal lamellae are rich in baso-philic nuclei, and the tissue stains dark blue. The sublamellar dermis consists of bundles of dense collagen sectioned transversely. The bundles of collagen are the main component of the suspensory apparatus of the distal phalanx. PDLs also consist of bundles of collagenous connective tissue but are smaller in size because they are subbranches of the larger bundles in the sublamellar dermis. In between the bundles of collagen in the sublamellar dermis are prominent arteries and veins serving the relatively high metabolic requirements of lamellar tissue. The box in the inset shows the provenance of the section. (Stain = haematoxylin and eosin. Bar = 2000 μm [2 mm]).

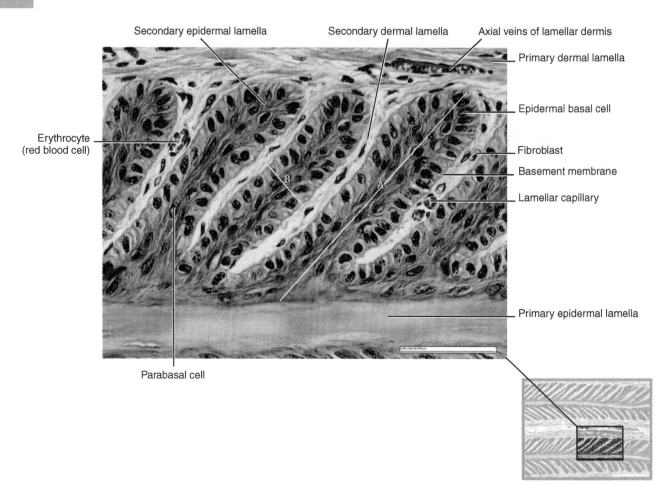

• **Figure 8.4** Medium magnification photomicrograph of transverse section of dorsal, midwall lamellae from a normal horse foot, stained with haematoxylin and eosin (H&E). The eosinophilic, cornified axis of the primary epidermal lamella is devoid of cell nuclei and is stained light pink. In contrast, the living basal and parabasal cells of the secondary epidermal lamellae (SELs) have basophilic nuclei, which stain dark blue. The club-shaped tips of SELs are always rounded and never tapered or pointed. Branches from the bundles of collagenous connective tissue in the primary dermal lamella enter the secondary dermal lamellae (SDLs) and insert as fine collagenous filaments into the lamellar basement membrane (BM), penetrating to the farthest extremities of the SDL. Most of the nuclei of the epidermal basal cells are oval and situated at the apical pole of the cell; the pole farthest from the BM. The long axis of the basal cell nucleus is oriented at right angles to the BM. The median width (line B) of an SEL is 25 µm (range 21.5 to 28.5 µm), and the median length (line A) is 142 µm (range 107 to 173 µm).[1] The box in the inset shows the provenance of the section. (Stain = haematoxylin and eosin. Bar = 50 µm [0.05 mm]).

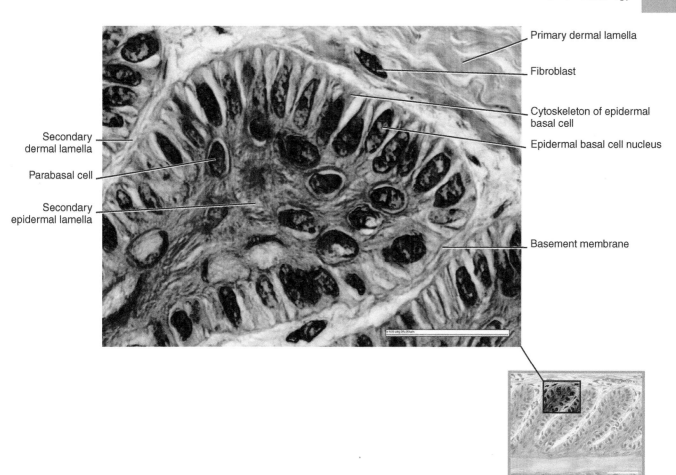

Primary dermal lamella

Fibroblast

Cytoskeleton of epidermal basal cell

Epidermal basal cell nucleus

Secondary dermal lamella

Parabasal cell

Secondary epidermal lamella

Basement membrane

● **Figure 8.5** High-magnification photomicrograph of transverse section of dorsal, midwall secondary epidermal lamella (SEL) from a normal horse foot, stained with haematoxylin and eosin. The living basal cells of the SEL have basophilic nuclei (dark blue) oriented with their long axes at 90° to the basement membrane (BM). The tip of the SEL in transverse section is typically club-shaped and never tapered or pointed. In secondary dermal lamellae (SDLs) fine connective tissue filaments merge into the lamellar basement membrane (BM). The pink-staining cytoskeleton of the epidermal basal cell suspends the oval nuclei at the apical pole of the cell. The cytoplasm of parabasal cells contains more keratin intermediate filaments and is thus more eosinophilic (dark red). The box in the inset shows the provenance of the section. (Stain = haematoxylin and eosin. Bar = 25 μm [0.025 mm]).

Secondary dermal lamella   Secondary epidermal lamella   Basement membrane

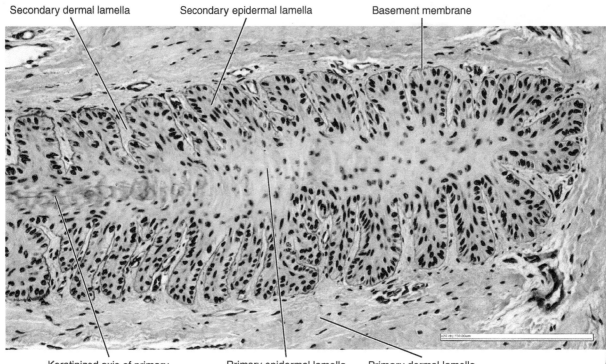

Keratinized axis of primary
epidermal lamella

Primary epidermal lamella

Primary dermal lamella

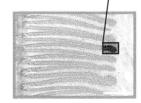

● **Figure 8.6** Photomicrograph of transverse section of dorsal, midwall secondary epidermal lamellar tip from a normal horse foot, stained with periodic acid Schiff (PAS). The glycoprotein-rich lamellar basement membrane (BM) has stained dark magenta, clearly outlining the perimeter of the secondary epidermal lamellae. The keratinized axis of the primary epidermal lamella has also stained magenta, marking the extent of this relatively rigid component of the lamella. The remainder of the lamellar tip is flexible and tends to separate from its basement membrane during acute laminitis. The box in the inset shows the provenance of the section. (Stain = periodic acid Schiff. Bar = 150 μm [0.15 mm]).

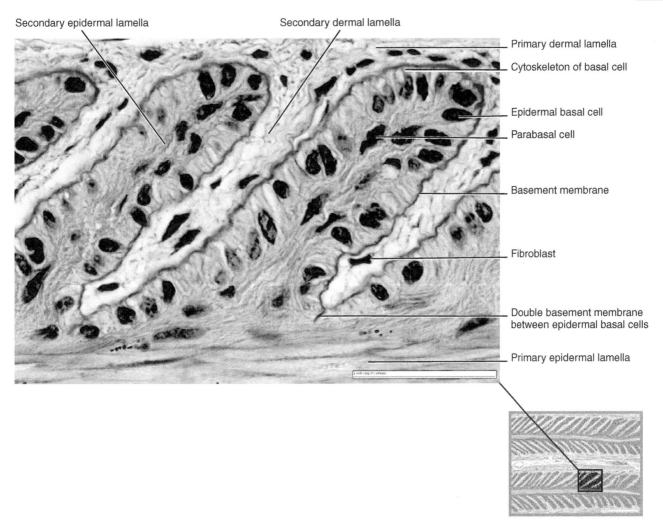

Secondary epidermal lamella

Secondary dermal lamella

Primary dermal lamella

Cytoskeleton of basal cell

Epidermal basal cell

Parabasal cell

Basement membrane

Fibroblast

Double basement membrane
between epidermal basal cells

Primary epidermal lamella

• **Figure 8.7** High-magnification photomicrograph of transverse section of dorsal, midwall secondary epidermal lamella (SEL) from a normal horse foot, stained with periodic acid Schiff (PAS). Notably, the glycoprotein-rich lamellar basement membrane (BM) has stained dark magenta, clearly outlining the perimeter of each secondary epidermal lamella. The BM appears tightly adherent to the basal border of the epidermal basal cells. A double BM inserts between two basal cells at the base of adjacent SELs. The living basal cells of the SEL have basophilic nuclei (dark blue) oriented with their long axes at 90° to the BM. The tip of the SEL is typically club-shaped and never tapered or pointed. The box in the inset shows the provenance of the section. (Stain = periodic acid Schiff. Bar = 25 μm [0.025 mm]).

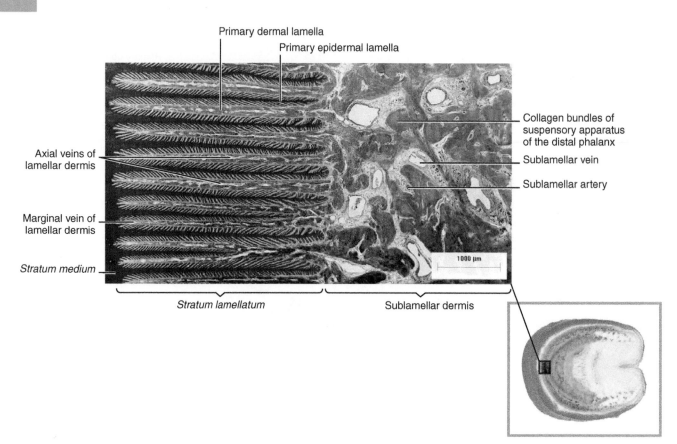

Primary dermal lamella

Primary epidermal lamella

Collagen bundles of suspensory apparatus of the distal phalanx

Sublamellar vein

Sublamellar artery

Axial veins of lamellar dermis

Marginal vein of lamellar dermis

Stratum medium

1000 µm

Stratum lamellatum

Sublamellar dermis

● **Figure 8.8** Low magnification photomicrograph of transverse section of dorsal, midwall lamellae (*stratum lamellatum*) and the connective tissue of the sublamellar dermis from a normal horse front foot, stained with Masson's trichrome (MTC) a connective tissue stain. Stained with MTC, the collagen of the sublamellar and lamellar dermis is blue and epidermal structures (the *stratum medium* of the inner hoof wall and the primary and secondary epidermal lamellae) are red. In this transverse plane of section the collagen bundles of the suspensory apparatus of the distal phalanx are cut obliquely across their long axis and are thus ovoid and rounded in shape. In the loose connective tissue between the collagen bundles are several large-diameter, thin-walled sublamellar veins, approximately 450 µm in diameter. Adjacent to the veins but much smaller in diameter (15 µm) are thick-walled arteries. In the primary lamellar dermis the veins are also cut obliquely across their long axis and resemble long, thin ribbons. The box in the inset shows the provenance of the section. (Stain = Masson's trichrome. Bar = 1000 µm [1 mm]).

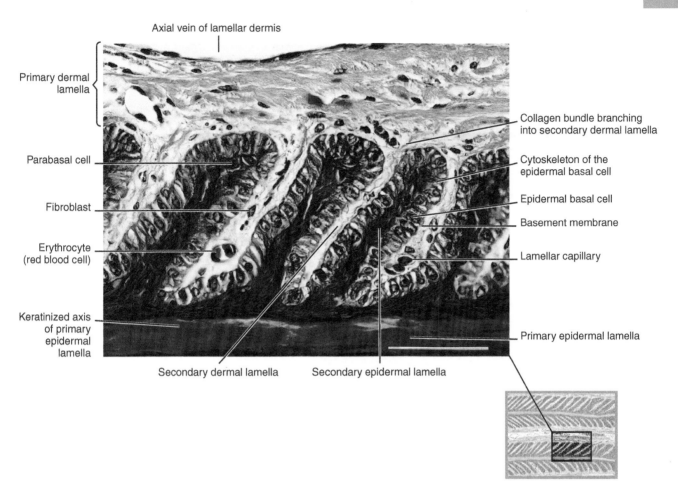

Axial vein of lamellar dermis

Primary dermal lamella

Parabasal cell

Fibroblast

Erythrocyte (red blood cell)

Keratinized axis of primary epidermal lamella

Collagen bundle branching into secondary dermal lamella

Cytoskeleton of the epidermal basal cell

Epidermal basal cell

Basement membrane

Lamellar capillary

Primary epidermal lamella

Secondary dermal lamella   Secondary epidermal lamella

• **Figure 8.9** Medium magnification photomicrograph of transverse section of dorsal, midwall lamellae, stained with Masson's trichrome (MTC), a connective tissue stain. Stained with MTC, the collagen of the primary and secondary dermal lamellae is blue and the primary and secondary epidermal lamellae (SELs) are red. Blue-staining collagen bundles of the suspensory apparatus of the distal phalanx (SADP) are cut transversely across their long axes in the primary dermal lamella. Axial arteries and veins accompany branching collagen bundles of the SADP into the primary dermal lamella. The box in the inset shows the provenance of the section. (Stain = Masson's trichrome. Bar = 50 μm [0.05 mm]).

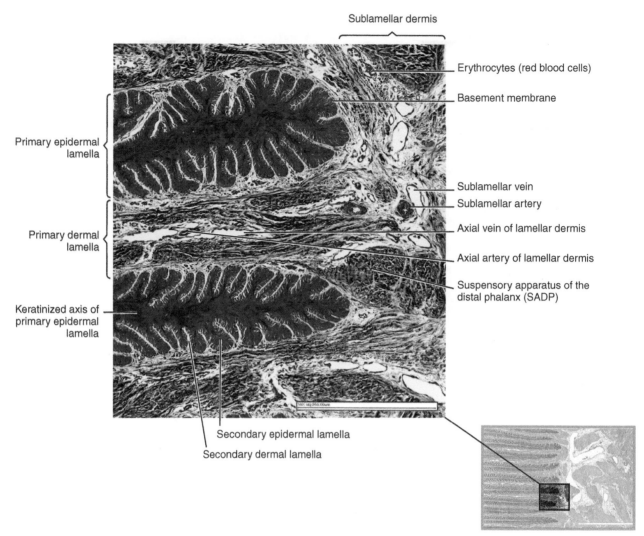

Sublamellar dermis

Erythrocytes (red blood cells)

Basement membrane

Primary epidermal lamella

Sublamellar vein

Sublamellar artery

Axial vein of lamellar dermis

Primary dermal lamella

Axial artery of lamellar dermis

Suspensory apparatus of the distal phalanx (SADP)

Keratinized axis of primary epidermal lamella

Secondary epidermal lamella

Secondary dermal lamella

• **Figure 8.10** Medium magnification photomicrograph of transverse section of dorsal, midwall lamellae, stained with Masson's trichrome (MTC), a connective tissue stain. Stained with MTC, the collagen of the sublamellar dermis, the primary and secondary dermal lamellae are blue and the primary and secondary epidermal lamellae (SELs) are red. Ovoid, blue-staining collagen bundles of the suspensory apparatus of the distal phalanx (SADP), cut transversely across their long axes, dominate the sublamellar dermis. Between the collagen bundles are the numerous arteries and veins of the sublamellar dermis, also cut across their long axes. Axial arteries and veins accompany branching collagen bundles into the primary dermal lamellae. The box in the inset shows the provenance of the section. (Stain = Masson's trichrome. Bar = 250 μm [0.25 mm]).

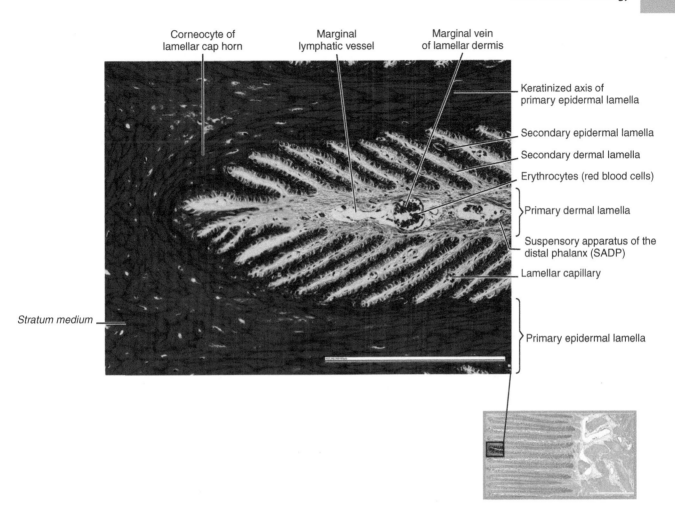

Corneocyte of lamellar cap horn

Marginal lymphatic vessel

Marginal vein of lamellar dermis

Keratinized axis of primary epidermal lamella

Secondary epidermal lamella

Secondary dermal lamella

Erythrocytes (red blood cells)

Primary dermal lamella

Suspensory apparatus of the distal phalanx (SADP)

Lamellar capillary

Primary epidermal lamella

Stratum medium

• **Figure 8.11** Medium magnification photomicrograph of transverse section of dorsal, midwall lamellae, stained with Masson's trichrome (MTC), a connective tissue stain. Stained with MTC, the collagen of the sublamellar dermis, the primary and secondary dermal lamellae are blue and the primary and secondary epidermal lamellae (SELs) are red. The region shows the most peripheral (abaxial) lamellae between the bases of two primary epidermal lamellae at the abaxial tip of a primary dermal lamella. The blue-staining collagen bundles of the suspensory apparatus of the distal phalanx (SADP) are less dense and are at their farthest distance from the distal phalanx virtually attaching directly to the stratum medium of the hoof wall. The density of blood vessels in this region appears the same as elsewhere in the lamellar circulation despite the vessels being as far as they can be from the terminal arch of the palmar digital arteries. The marginal vein of the lamellar venous system connects the distal terminal papillary collecting vein to the coronary dermal venous plexus. Likewise, a major lymphatic vessel, always adjacent to the marginal vein, drains lymphatic fluid from distal lamellar and papillary tissues to collecting ducts in the coronary band. The box in the inset shows the provenance of the section. (Stain = Masson's trichrome stain. Bar = 250 µm [0.25 mm]).

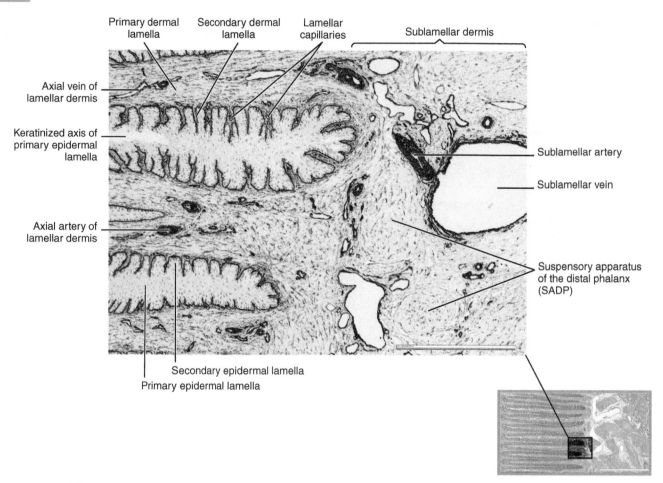

Primary dermal lamella
Secondary dermal lamella
Lamellar capillaries
Sublamellar dermis

Axial vein of lamellar dermis

Keratinized axis of primary epidermal lamella

Sublamellar artery

Sublamellar vein

Axial artery of lamellar dermis

Suspensory apparatus of the distal phalanx (SADP)

Secondary epidermal lamella
Primary epidermal lamella

• **Figure 8.12** Dorsal section of midwall lamellae from the toe of a normal horse foot immunostained for the basement membrane protein collagen IV. Collagen IV is exclusively a basement membrane (BM) protein that forms a sheetlike mesh, the structural framework of the lamina densa of the basement membrane. It interacts with other molecules that influence cell adhesion, migration, and differentiation. Loss of lamellar collagen IV occurs early in the development of laminitis.[2] Basement membranes (BMs) underlie both epidermal cells and vascular endothelial cells; thus the BMs of the lamellae, as well as all the blood vessels in this transverse section, show dark brown positive immunostaining. The box in the inset shows the provenance of the specimen. (Bar = 500 μm [0.50 mm]).

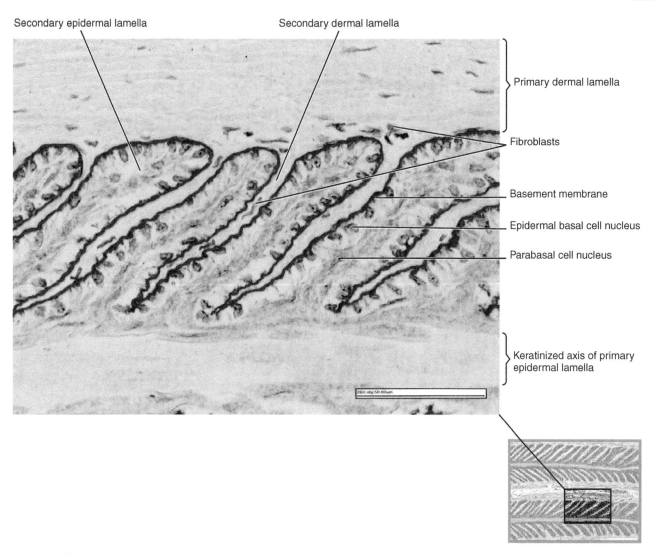

Secondary epidermal lamella   Secondary dermal lamella

Primary dermal lamella

Fibroblasts

Basement membrane

Epidermal basal cell nucleus

Parabasal cell nucleus

Keratinized axis of primary epidermal lamella

• **Figure 8.13** Transverse section of midwall lamellae from the toe of a normal horse foot immunostained for the basement membrane protein laminin 332. Laminin 332 is the anchoring filament protein that links basal cell hemidesmosomes to the lamina densa of the basement membrane (BM). Laminin 332 is unique to dermal–epithelial junctions, so there is no immunostaining of vascular BMs. The dark-brown positive immunostaining of the BM at the lamellar dermal-epidermal interface clearly differentiates secondary epidermal lamellae from dermal lamellae. The box in the inset shows the provenance of the specimen. (Bar = 50 μm [0.05 mm]).

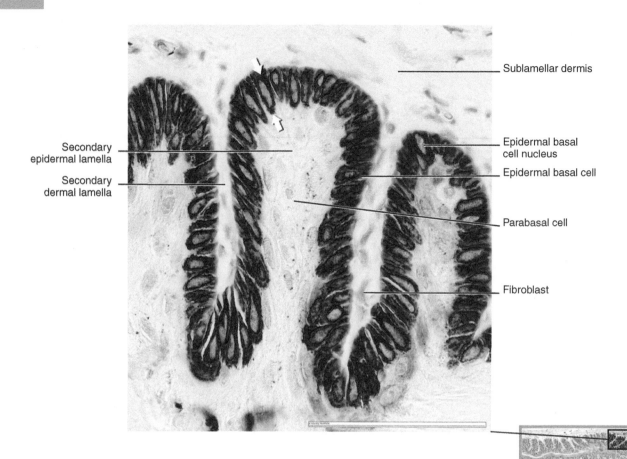

Secondary epidermal lamella

Secondary dermal lamella

Sublamellar dermis

Epidermal basal cell nucleus

Epidermal basal cell

Parabasal cell

Fibroblast

•Figure 8.14 Photomicrograph of transverse section of dorsal, midwall lamellae from a normal horse foot, immunostained for cytokeratin 14 (K14). Cytokeratin is an intermediate filament (10 nm diameter) and the major element of the lamellar epidermal basal cell (LEBC) cytoskeleton (in addition to actin). There are two attachment plaques associated with cytokeratin: the hemidesmosomes at the basal border and desmosomes at the lateral and apical walls of the LEBC. The brown positive immunostaining (*arrows*) shows cytokeratin localized to these attachment plaques at all borders of the LEBCs. Unlike actin, cytokeratin connects to the nucleus, forming a multifilament cradle in the cytoplasm of the cell. The box in the inset shows the provenance of the specimen. (Bar = 50 μm [0.05 mm]).

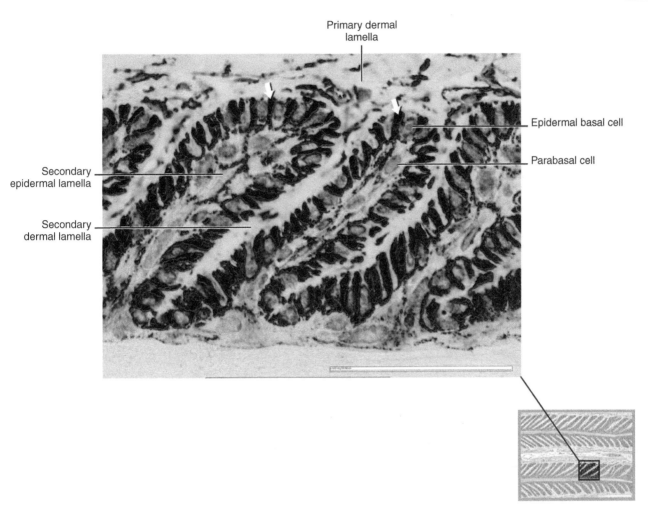

Primary dermal
lamella

Epidermal basal cell

Parabasal cell

Secondary
epidermal lamella

Secondary
dermal lamella

• **Figure 8.15** Photomicrograph of transverse section of dorsal, midwall lamellae from a normal horse foot, immuno-stained for actin. Actin is a microfilament (7 nm diameter) and major element of the lamellar epidermal basal cell (LEBC) cytoskeleton (in addition to keratin intermediate filaments). The attachment plaque associated with actin is the adherens junction (AJ) and multiple AJs form zones of attachment (zona adherens) between adjacent cells thus joining them together. The dark-brown positive immunostaining (*arrows*) shows actin localized to the AJs in the lateral borders of LEBCs. It is conspicuously absent at the basal LEBC border, which lacks adherens junctions. The cell boundaries of adjacent secondary epidermal lamellar (SEL) parabasal cells show punctate actin staining, suggesting the partici-pation of actin in the numerous desmosomes that connect parabasal cells to one another. The actin cytoskeleton network is confined to the periphery of the LEBC cytoplasm and does not connect to the nucleus. The box in the inset shows the provenance of the specimen. (Bar = 50 μm [0.05 mm]).

DORSAL HISTOLOGY

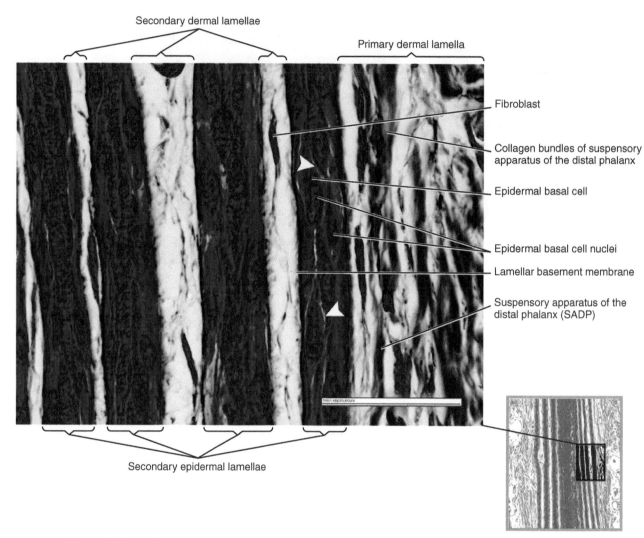

Secondary dermal lamellae

Primary dermal lamella

Fibroblast

Collagen bundles of suspensory apparatus of the distal phalanx

Epidermal basal cell

Epidermal basal cell nuclei

Lamellar basement membrane

Suspensory apparatus of the distal phalanx (SADP)

Secondary epidermal lamellae

• **Figure 8.16** Dorsal section of midwall lamellae from the toe of a normal horse foot stained with Masson's trichrome. Connective tissue is stained blue and epidermis red. Note the proximodistal orientation of the linear collagen bundles of the suspensory apparatus of the distal phalanx; an alignment parallel to load-bearing lines of stress. Also aligned proximodistally are the fusiform, lamellar epidermal basal cells. The cells appear joined head to tail where their tapered ends overlap (*arrowheads*). The box in the inset shows the provenance of the specimen. (Bar = 25 μm [0.025 mm]).

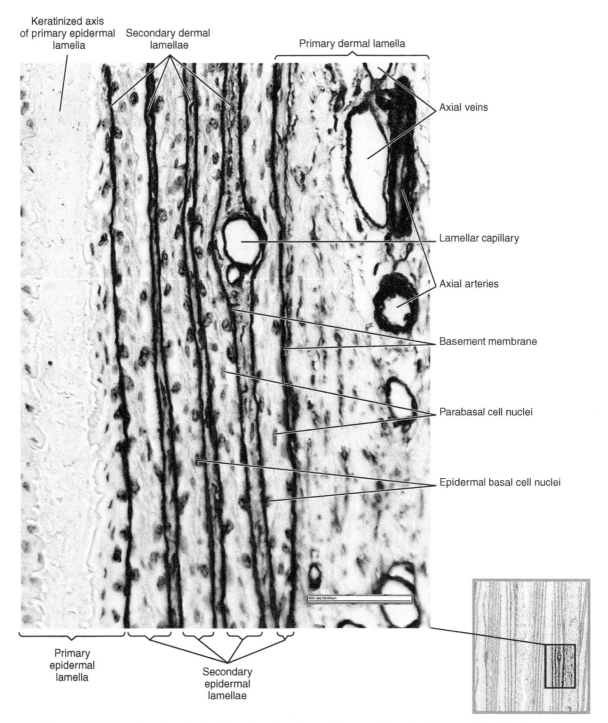

Keratinized axis
of primary epidermal
lamella

Secondary dermal
lamellae

Primary dermal lamella

Axial veins

Lamellar capillary

Axial arteries

Basement membrane

Parabasal cell nuclei

Epidermal basal cell nuclei

Primary
epidermal
lamella

Secondary
epidermal
lamellae

• **Figure 8.17** Dorsal section of midwall lamellae from the toe of a normal horse foot immunostained for the basement membrane protein type IV collagen. Basement membranes (BMs) underlie both epidermal cells and vascular endothelial cells. The BMs of all the blood vessels (lamellar capillaries, axial arteries, and veins) in this dorsal section show dark-brown positive immunostaining. Notably, the positive immunostaining of the BM at the lamellar dermal-epidermal junction clearly differentiates secondary epidermal from dermal lamellae. Within the secondary dermal lamellae, collagen fibrils from the extremities of the suspensory apparatus of the distal phalanx insert onto the entire surface area of the lamellar basement membrane. Most of the epidermal cell nuclei are oval in shape, with their long axes oriented proximodistally. The box in the inset shows the provenance of the specimen. (Bar = 50 μm [0.05 mm]).

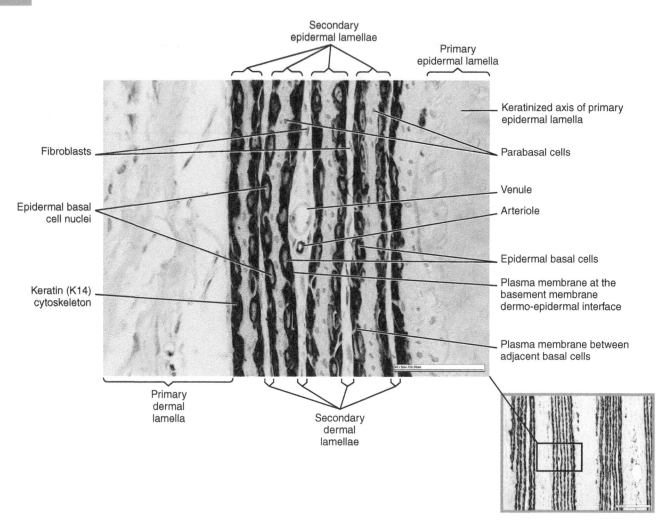

Secondary
epidermal lamellae

Primary
epidermal lamella

Keratinized axis of primary
epidermal lamella

Fibroblasts

Parabasal cells

Venule

Arteriole

Epidermal basal
cell nuclei

Epidermal basal cells

Plasma membrane at the
basement membrane
dermo-epidermal interface

Keratin (K14)
cytoskeleton

Plasma membrane between
adjacent basal cells

Primary
dermal
lamella

Secondary
dermal
lamellae

• **Figure 8.18** Dorsal section of midwall lamellae from the toe of a normal horse foot immunostained for cytokeratin 14 (K14). Brown, positive immunostaining is present only in the cytoplasm of lamellar epidermal basal cells (compare with the transverse section in figure 8.14). The dorsal lamellar section shows the fusiform shape of epidermal basal cells joined end-to-end at their tapering proximal and dorsal borders. Cross-branching cytokeratin 14 intermediate filaments are pan-cytoplasmic and cradle the nucleus by attaching to the nuclear envelope. Keratin intermediate filaments attach to all the inner walls of the epidermal basal cell, via hemidesmosomes at the basal plasma membrane and via desmosomes between the plasma membranes adjoining basal and parabasal cells. Thus all the lamellar epidermal cells are firmly linked to each other by their cytoskeletons and adhesion plaques, providing the lamellae with the structural integrity needed to withstand the peaks of mechanical loading that the horse foot encounters. The box in the inset shows the provenance of the specimen. (Bar = 100 μm [0.1 mm]).

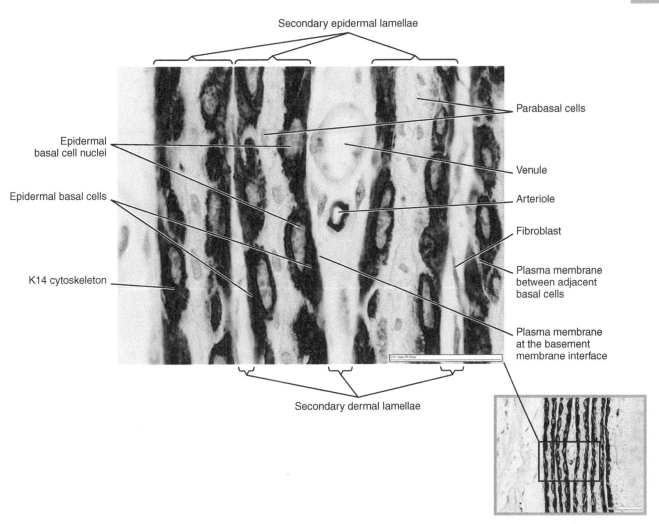

Secondary epidermal lamellae

Parabasal cells

Epidermal
basal cell nuclei

Venule

Epidermal basal cells

Arteriole

Fibroblast

K14 cytoskeleton

Plasma membrane
between adjacent
basal cells

Plasma membrane
at the basement
membrane interface

Secondary dermal lamellae

• **Figure 8.19** Dorsal section of midwall lamellae from the toe of a normal horse foot immunostained for cytokeratin 14 (K14). Brown, positive immunostaining is present only in the cytoplasm of lamellar epidermal basal cells (compare with the transverse section in figure 8.14). The dorsal lamellar section shows the fusiform shape of epidermal basal cells joined end-to-end at their tapering proximal and dorsal borders. Cross-branching cytokeratin 14 intermediate filaments are pan-cytoplasmic and cradle the nucleus by attaching to the nuclear envelope. Keratin intermediate filaments attach to all the inner walls of epidermal basal cells, via hemidesmosomes at the basal plasma membrane and via desmosomes between the plasma membranes adjoining basal and parabasal cells. Thus all the lamellar epidermal cells are firmly linked to each other by their cytoskeletons and adhesion plaques, providing the lamellae with the structural integrity needed to withstand the peaks of mechanical loading that the horse foot encounters. The box in the inset shows the provenance of the specimen. (Bar = 50 μm [0.05 mm]).

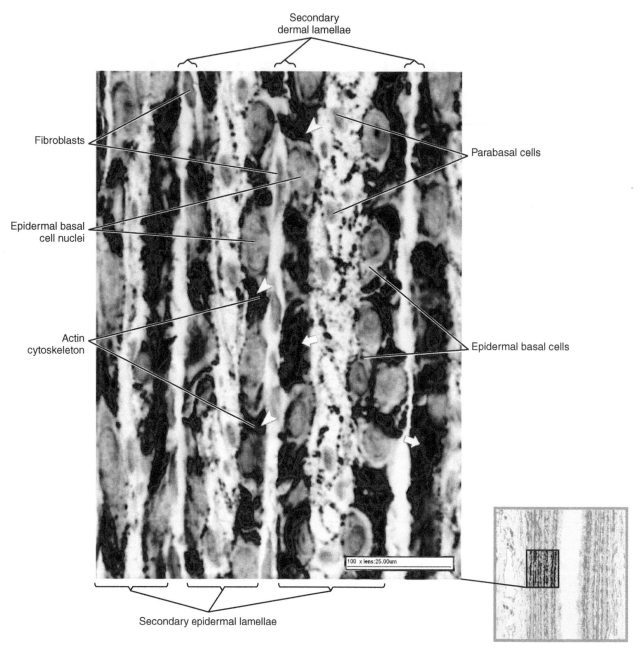

● Figure 8.20 Photomicrograph of dorsal section of dorsal, midwall lamellae from a normal horse foot, immunostained for actin. The dorsal lamellar section shows the fusiform shape of epidermal basal cells joined by actin-rich, zona adherens at their proximal, distal, and lateral borders. The section plane passes through the center of some cells and close to the lateral wall of others. Where the center of the epidermal basal cells is sectioned, the proximal and distal borders of adjoining cells show positive (dark brown) actin immunostaining (*arrowheads*). Where the section is close to a lateral wall, the location of multiple adherens junctions, the entire cell shows positive actin immunostaining (*arrows*). Basal cell borders facing a secondary dermal lamella show no actin immunostaining as the basal plasma membrane lacks adherens junctions. The cell boundaries of adjacent secondary epidermal lamellar parabasal cells show punctate actin staining, suggesting localization of actin to the numerous desmosomes that connect parabasal cells to one another. The actin cytoskeleton network is confined to the periphery of the lamellar epidermal basal cell cytoplasm and does not connect to the nucleus. The box in the inset shows the provenance of the specimen. (Bar = 25 μm [0.025 mm]).

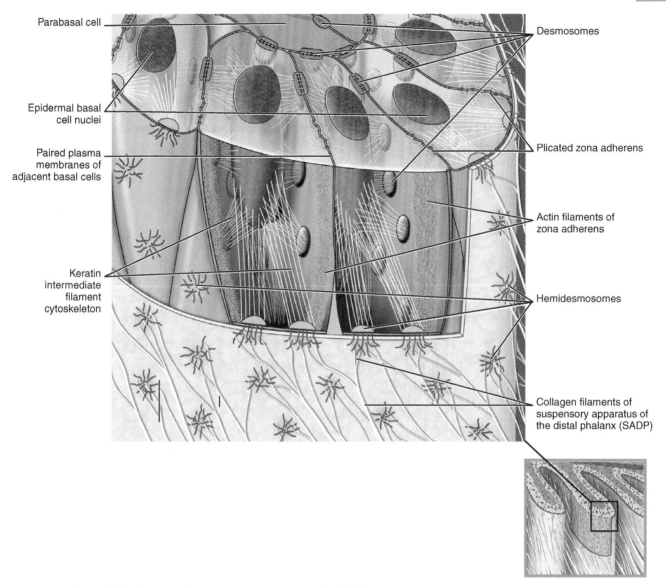

Parabasal cell

Epidermal basal cell nuclei

Paired plasma membranes of adjacent basal cells

Keratin intermediate filament cytoskeleton

Desmosomes

Plicated zona adherens

Actin filaments of zona adherens

Hemidesmosomes

Collagen filaments of suspensory apparatus of the distal phalanx (SADP)

• **Figure 8.21** Diagram of lamellar epidermal basal cells (LEBCs) and their cytoskeleton. As an integral part of the suspensory apparatus of the distal phalanx (SADP), the LEBC must remain not only attached to its adjacent basement membrane but also to neighboring LEBCs and the parabasal cells in the core of the secondary epidermal lamella (SEL). Attachment to the lamellar basement membrane is achieved with attachment plaques called *hemidesmosomes*. Attachment to neighboring cells is achieved with attachment plaques called desmosomes. Uniting hemidesmosomes and desmosomes to the cell nucleus is the dense filamentous keratin intermediate filament cytoskeleton (colored white in the diagram). The cytoskeleton also maintains the shape and rigidity of LEBCs, as well as being a conduit of information between nuclei and the extracellular milieu. The actin cytoskeleton (colored green in the diagram) does not connect to the nucleus but is associated with the plicated, actin-rich *zona adherens* that encircles the basilateral and apical walls of each cell. Actin filaments are contractile and elastic and enable the SEL to return to its original state after loading. (Illustration designed by the author).

References

1. de Laat, M. A., van Eps, A. W., McGowan, C. M., Sillence, M. N., & Pollitt, C. C. (2011). Equine laminitis: Comparative histopathology 48 hours after experimental induction with insulin or alimentary oligofructose in Standardbred horses. *Journal of Comparative Pathology, 145,* 399–409.

2. Visser, M. B., & Pollitt, C. C. (2011). The timeline of lamellar basement membrane changes during equine laminitis development. *Equine Veterinary Journal, 43,* 471–477.

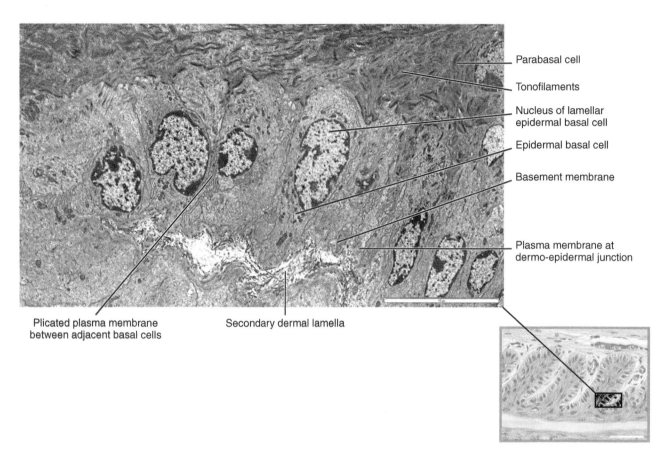

Parabasal cell

Tonofilaments

Nucleus of lamellar epidermal basal cell

Epidermal basal cell

Basement membrane

Plasma membrane at dermo-epidermal junction

Plicated plasma membrane between adjacent basal cells

Secondary dermal lamella

• **Figure 9.1** Transmission electron microscopic (TEM) image of normal lamellar epidermal basal cells (LEBCs) surrounding the tip of a secondary dermal lamella in transverse section. There are at least seven nucleated LEBCs arranged side by side attached to the basement membrane. Note the heavily plicated (folded), paired plasma membranes between adjacent LEBCs. The plicated zones are rich in filamentous actin and accommodate deformation and stretching of the LEBCs during mechanical loading. Collagen bundles at the tip of the secondary dermal lamella insert into the basement membrane, thus contributing in the suspension of the distal phalanx. At this magnification the lamina densa of the basement membrane is just visible as a gray line bordering the dermal side of the LEBC plasma membrane. The LEBC nuclei are oval, and their long axes are perpendicular to the basement membrane. (Bar = 10 nm.) The box in the inset shows the provenance of the specimen.

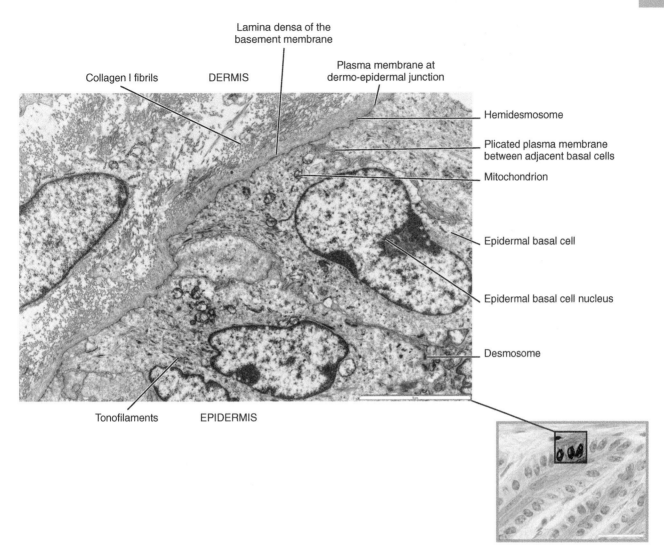

Lamina densa of the
basement membrane

Plasma membrane at
dermo-epidermal junction

Collagen I fibrils   DERMIS

Hemidesmosome

Plicated plasma membrane
between adjacent basal cells

Mitochondrion

Epidermal basal cell

Epidermal basal cell nucleus

Desmosome

Tonofilaments   EPIDERMIS

● **Figure 9.2** Transmission electron microscopic (TEM) image of normal lamellar epidermal basal cells (LEBCs) and their dermal junction in transverse section. The dermis is upper left, and the epidermis is lower right. At this magnification the lamina densa of the basement membrane is just visible as a gray line bordering the dermal side of the LEBC plasma membrane. Cytoskeletal tonofilaments converge on numerous electron dense hemidesmosomes embedded in the LEBC plasma membrane. The long axis of the oval LEBC nuclei is perpendicular to the basement membrane. In the dermis the numerous small dots are collagen bundles, cut transversely. (Bar = 5 nm.) The box in the inset shows the provenance of the specimen.

Parabasal cell   Desmosome   Epidermal basal cell   Mitochondrion

Hemidesmosome

Fibroblast

Nucleus of lamellar
epidermal basal cell

Lamina densa of
basement membrane

Plasma membrane at
dermo-epidermal junction

Collagen type I fibrils

Tonofilaments   Plicated plasma membrane between
adjacent basal cells

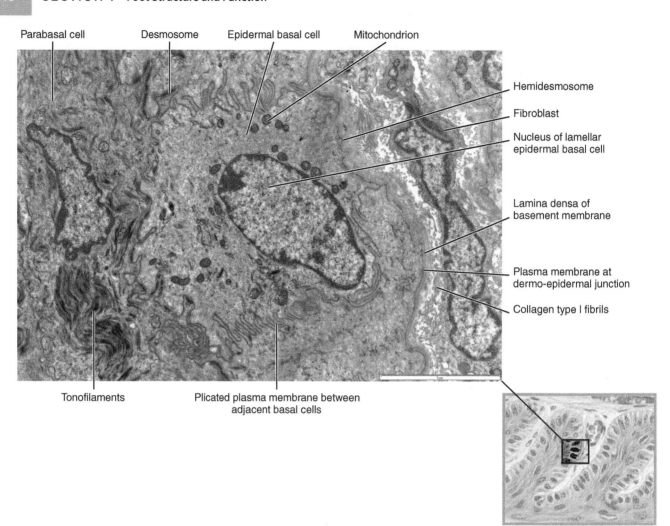

• **Figure 9.3** Transmission electron microscopic (TEM) image of immersion fixed normal lamellar epidermal basal cells (LEBCs) in transverse section. The nucleated parabasal cell on the left is packed with wavy, dark-staining, keratin tonofilaments and is attached to adjacent LEBCs by numerous electron dense desmosomes. The lamellar basement membrane demarcates the lamellar dermal–epidermal junction, and numerous hemidesmosomes attach the LEBC plasma membrane to the lamina densa of the basement membrane. The plasma membranes between adjacent LEBCs are remarkably plicated, forming multiple interdigitations between cells. The plasma membranes in the plicated zones are tightly apposed, moderately electron dense, and surrounded by fine filamentous material, presumably F-actin. The plicated membranes appear to be a zone of near continuous adherens junctions, part of the actin-rich *zona adherens* that encircles the basilateral and apical walls of each cell. (Bar = 10 nm.) The box in the inset shows the provenance of the specimen.

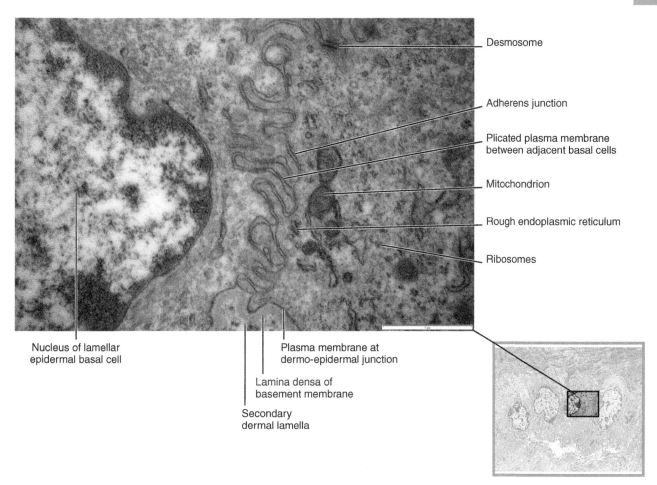

Desmosome

Adherens junction

Plicated plasma membrane
between adjacent basal cells

Mitochondrion

Rough endoplasmic reticulum

Ribosomes

Nucleus of lamellar
epidermal basal cell

Plasma membrane at
dermo-epidermal junction

Lamina densa of
basement membrane

Secondary
dermal lamella

● **Figure 9.4** Transmission electron microscopic (TEM) image of two normal immersion-fixed lamellar epidermal basal cells (LEBCs) in transverse section. Resembling tram tracks, the parallel plasma membranes of the two adjacent cells are plicated, forming multiple interdigitations between the cells. The plasma membranes in the plicated zones are tightly apposed, moderately electron dense, and surrounded by fine filamentous material, presumably F-actin. In the cytoplasm beside the plicated zone are numerous ribosomes, mitochondria, and rough endoplasmic reticulum, suggesting a region of protein translation and production. The plicated membranes appear to be a zone of near continuous adherens junctions, part of the actin-rich *zona adherens* that encircles the basilateral and apical walls of each cell. (Bar = 1 μm.) The box in the inset shows the provenance of the specimen.

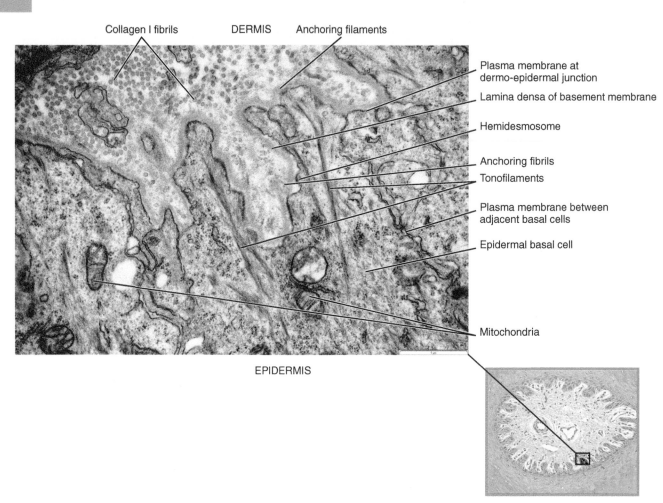

Collagen I fibrils   DERMIS   Anchoring filaments

Plasma membrane at
dermo-epidermal junction

Lamina densa of basement membrane

Hemidesmosome

Anchoring fibrils

Tonofilaments

Plasma membrane between
adjacent basal cells

Epidermal basal cell

Mitochondria

EPIDERMIS

• **Figure 9.5** Transmission electron micrograph of dermal–epidermal junction between proximal *stratum medium* (coronary horn), epidermal basal cells, and adjacent dermis of coronary papilla in transverse section. The basal cell layer encircles the coronary papilla and is folded into short pegs, which indent the surface of the papilla. This increases the surface area of attachment between papillae and the epidermal sockets of the proximal hoof wall. Prominent cytokeratin (K14) tonofilaments of the cytoskeleton attach to hemidesmosomes at the dermal–epidermal junction. Anchoring fibrils (type collagen VII) on the dermal side of the lamina densa of the basement membrane attach to the type collagen I fibrils of the suspensory apparatus of the distal phalanx. The basal cells associated with coronary papillae proliferate throughout the life of the horse, adding new cells, destined for cornification, to the hoof wall tubules of the *stratum medium*. (Bar = 1 nm.) The box in the inset shows the provenance of the specimen.

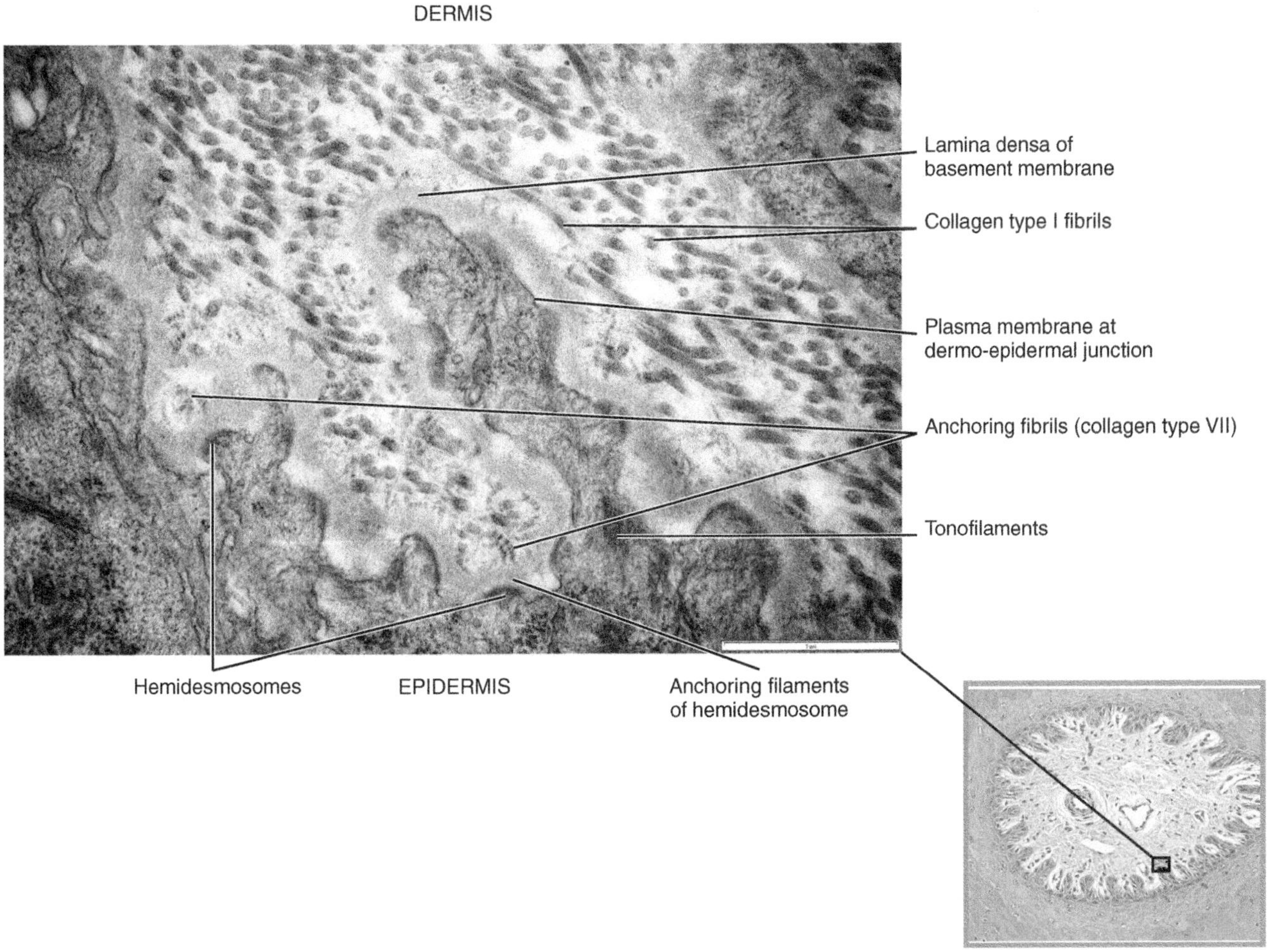

DERMIS

Lamina densa of
basement membrane

Collagen type I fibrils

Plasma membrane at
dermo-epidermal junction

Anchoring fibrils (collagen type VII)

Tonofilaments

Hemidesmosomes   EPIDERMIS   Anchoring filaments
of hemidesmosome

● **Figure 9.6** Transmission electron micrograph of dermal–epidermal junction between proximal *stratum medium* (coronary horn), epidermal basal cells, and adjacent dermis of coronary papilla in transverse section. Tonofilaments of the basal cell cytoskeleton attach to hemidesmosomes at the dermal–epidermal junction. Anchoring fibrils (type VII collagen) on the dermal side of the *lamina densa* of the basement membrane integrate strongly with the type collagen I fibrils of the suspensory apparatus of the distal phalanx. Anchoring fibrils are characterized by their hooked shape and the specific type VII collagen banding pattern. Type I collagen fibrils with circular profiles are sectioned transversely; others, sectioned lengthwise, show the banding pattern typical of type I collagen. (Bar = 1 nm.) The box in the inset shows the provenance of the specimen.

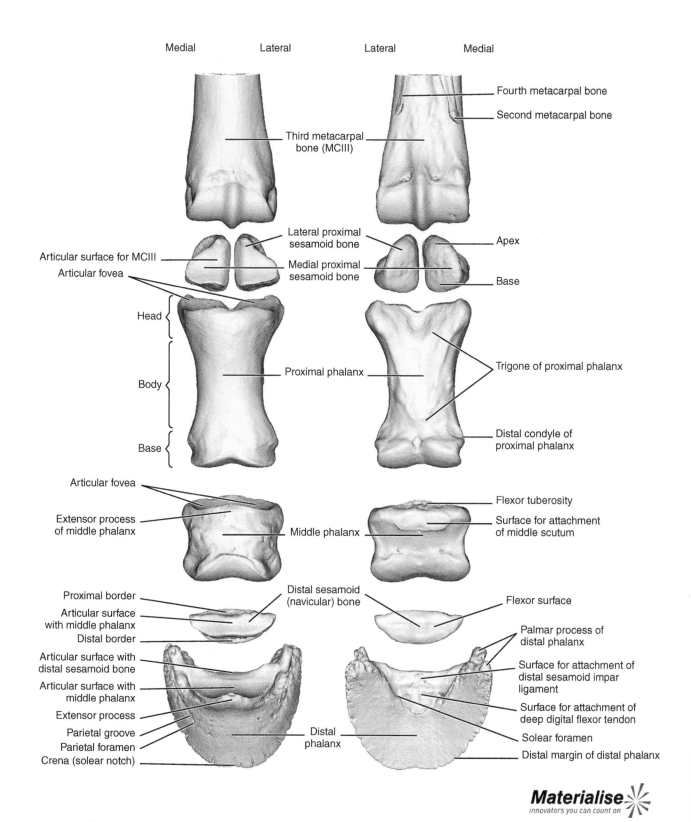

Medial   Lateral   Lateral   Medial

Fourth metacarpal bone

Second metacarpal bone

Third metacarpal bone (MCIII)

Lateral proximal sesamoid bone

Apex

Articular surface for MCIII

Articular fovea

Medial proximal sesamoid bone

Base

Head

Proximal phalanx

Trigone of proximal phalanx

Body

Base

Distal condyle of proximal phalanx

Articular fovea

Flexor tuberosity

Extensor process of middle phalanx

Surface for attachment of middle scutum

Middle phalanx

Proximal border

Distal sesamoid (navicular) bone

Flexor surface

Articular surface with middle phalanx

Distal border

Palmar process of distal phalanx

Articular surface with distal sesamoid bone

Surface for attachment of distal sesamoid impar ligament

Articular surface with middle phalanx

Surface for attachment of deep digital flexor tendon

Extensor process

Parietal groove

Parietal foramen

Distal phalanx

Solear foramen

Crena (solear notch)

Distal margin of distal phalanx

Materialise
innovators you can count on

• **Figure 10.1** Mimics models of the bones of the distal left forelimb of the normal Standardbred stallion described in Chapter 6. The dorsal aspect is on the left and the palmar aspect is on the right. This is an exploded view of the phalangeal, sesamoidean, and metacarpal bones.

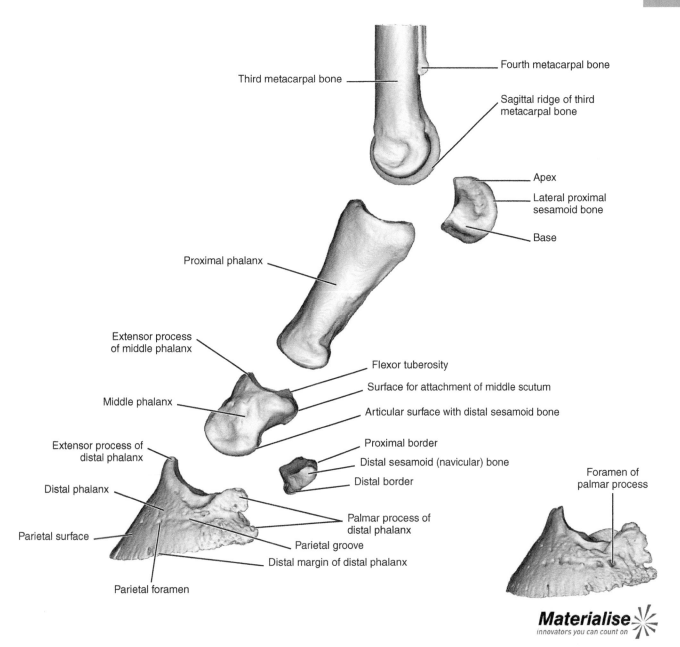

Third metacarpal bone

Fourth metacarpal bone

Sagittal ridge of third metacarpal bone

Apex

Lateral proximal sesamoid bone

Base

Proximal phalanx

Extensor process of middle phalanx

Flexor tuberosity

Surface for attachment of middle scutum

Articular surface with distal sesamoid bone

Middle phalanx

Proximal border

Distal sesamoid (navicular) bone

Distal border

Extensor process of distal phalanx

Distal phalanx

Foramen of palmar process

Parietal surface

Palmar process of distal phalanx

Parietal groove

Distal margin of distal phalanx

Parietal foramen

Materialise
innovators you can count on

• **Figure 10.2** Mimics models of the bones of the distal left forelimb of the normal Standardbred stallion described in Chapter 6 (lateromedial aspect). This is an exploded lateral view of phalangeal, sesamoidean, and metacarpal bones. The foramen of the palmar process is absent in the distal phalanx but present in the specimen on the right.

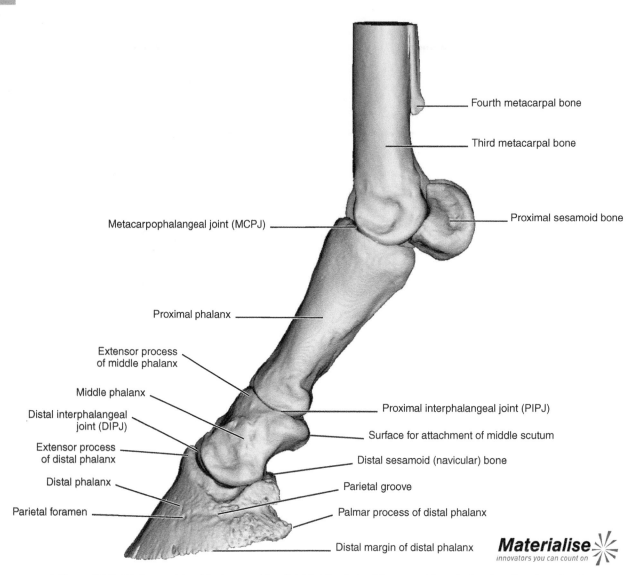

Fourth metacarpal bone

Third metacarpal bone

Proximal sesamoid bone

Metacarpophalangeal joint (MCPJ)

Proximal phalanx

Extensor process
of middle phalanx

Middle phalanx

Distal interphalangeal
joint (DIPJ)

Extensor process
of distal phalanx

Distal phalanx

Parietal foramen

Proximal interphalangeal joint (PIPJ)

Surface for attachment of middle scutum

Distal sesamoid (navicular) bone

Parietal groove

Palmar process of distal phalanx

Distal margin of distal phalanx

Materialise
innovators you can count on

● **Figure 10.3** Mimics models of the bones of the distal left forelimb of the normal Standardbred stallion described in Chapter 6 (lateromedial aspect). The foot is in the resting stance position.

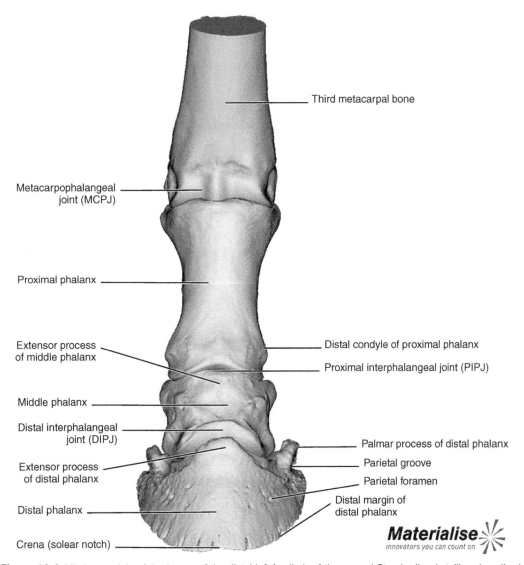

Third metacarpal bone

Metacarpophalangeal
joint (MCPJ)

Proximal phalanx

Extensor process
of middle phalanx

Distal condyle of proximal phalanx

Proximal interphalangeal joint (PIPJ)

Middle phalanx

Distal interphalangeal
joint (DIPJ)

Palmar process of distal phalanx

Parietal groove

Parietal foramen

Extensor process
of distal phalanx

Distal margin of
distal phalanx

Distal phalanx

Crena (solear notch)

Materialise
innovators you can count on

• **Figure 10.4** Mimics models of the bones of the distal left forelimb of the normal Standardbred stallion described in Chapter 6 (dorsal aspect). The foot is in the resting stance position.

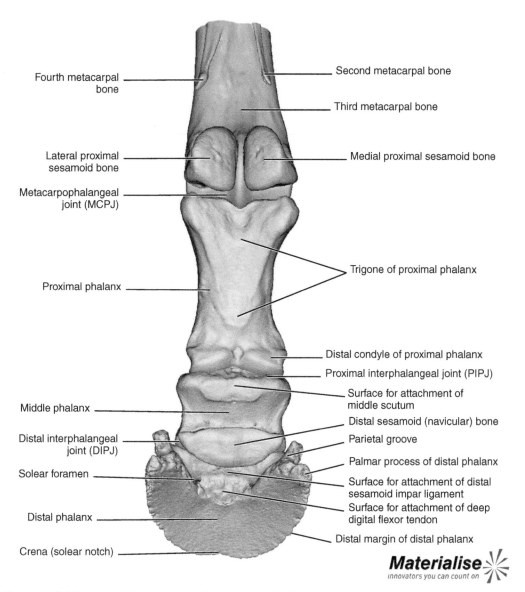

Fourth metacarpal bone

Second metacarpal bone

Third metacarpal bone

Lateral proximal sesamoid bone

Medial proximal sesamoid bone

Metacarpophalangeal joint (MCPJ)

Proximal phalanx

Trigone of proximal phalanx

Distal condyle of proximal phalanx

Proximal interphalangeal joint (PIPJ)

Surface for attachment of middle scutum

Middle phalanx

Distal sesamoid (navicular) bone

Distal interphalangeal joint (DIPJ)

Parietal groove

Palmar process of distal phalanx

Solear foramen

Surface for attachment of distal sesamoid impar ligament

Surface for attachment of deep digital flexor tendon

Distal phalanx

Distal margin of distal phalanx

Crena (solear notch)

Materialise
innovators you can count on

• **Figure 10.5** Mimics models of the bones of the distal left forelimb of the normal Standardbred stallion described in Chapter 6 (palmar aspect). The foot is in the resting stance position.

Large foramina for distal parietal
branches of the terminal arch

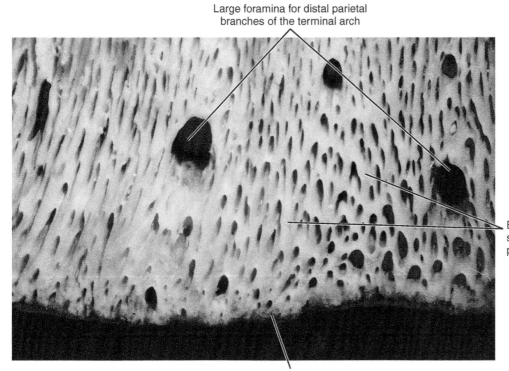

Bone ridges for insertion of
suspensory apparatus of distal
phalanx (SADP)

Distal margin of
distal phalanx

• Figure 10.6 Dorsal parietal cortex and distal margin of the distal phalanx. Numerous foramina perforate the dorsal surface of the distal phalanx. Between the foramina are ridges of cortical bone: the insertion sites for collagen bundles of the suspensory apparatus of the distal phalanx. The larger foramina are visible on radiographs and are conduits for the larger parietal branches of the terminal arch of the paired digital arteries and veins. Small arteries and veins pass through the lesser foramina, and all form the vascular bed of the sublamellar dermis. The entire dorsal lamellar blood supply passes through the foramina in the parietal cortex of the distal phalanx.

Articular surface

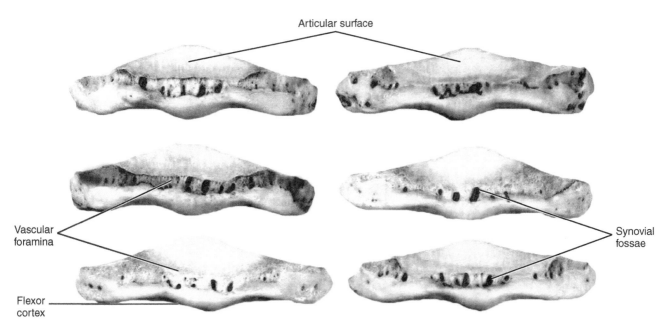

Vascular
foramina

Synovial
fossae

Flexor
cortex

• Figure 10.7 Six navicular bones standing on their proximal borders, showing the variability in size and number of the synovial fossae that characterize the distal border. Between the synovial fossae are numerous foramina through which branches of the distal navicular artery enter to supply the distal half of the navicular bone. These structures are integrated among the collagen bundles of the distal sesamoidean impar ligament (DSIL) that insert on the distal border. The pink shaded area shows the area of insertion of the DSIL.

Articular surfaces

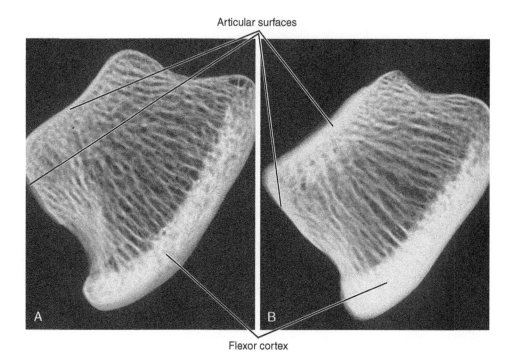

Flexor cortex

Figure 10.8 Radiographic images of distal sesamoid bone sections. Bone is a living tissue and during life is constantly remodeling in response to the biomechanical forces it encounters. New bone is laid down to reinforce the sites of greatest stress. A navicular bone section from an untrained two-year-old racehorse is shown in **A**. The flexor cortex has to withstand the greatest stress and is thus the densest part of the bone. The calcified trabeculae in the center of the bone are a loose network of supporting struts. The section **B** is taken from a mature, working Thoroughbred. The distal two thirds of the flexor surface is densely calcified and is thicker than in the young horse. The trabeculae have lost their meshlike appearance and are organized, along lines of stress, into stronger columns and struts. In addition, the two surfaces, which relate to the distal interphalangeal joint (DIPJ), have been reinforced. These adaptive changes take months to occur, and excessive loading of the flexor surface and failure to remodel are important factors in the development of navicular disease.

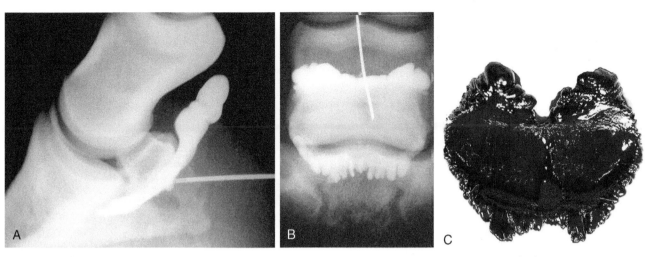

• **Figure 10.9** Lateromedial (**A**) and dorsoproximal palmarodistal oblique (**B**) radiographic images of a foot with 5 ml of radiopaque contrast medium injected into the navicular bursa and (C) an acrylic cast of the navicular bursa. Note the proximal and distal extent of the bursa as it conforms to the shape of the palmar pouch of the distal interphalangeal joint (DIPJ) and the collateral sesamoidean ligament. The irregular distal border of the bursa (**B** and **C**) conforms to the arrangement of the collagen bundles in the distal sesamoiden impar ligament, which insert on the distal phalanx proximad to the DDFT. The center of the acrylic cast of the bursa (C) is imprinted with the shape of the distal sesamoid bone.

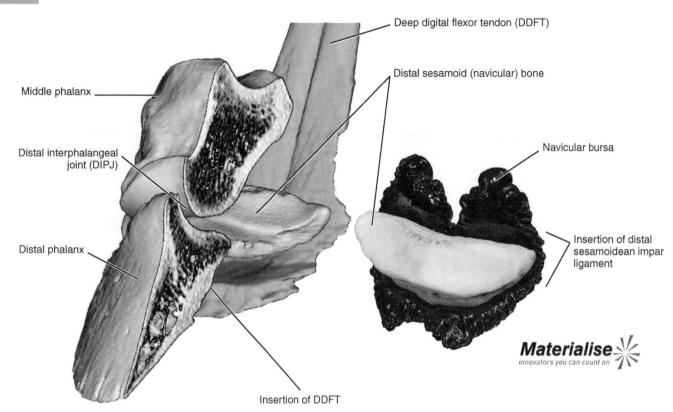

● **Figure 10.10** Mimics model of the distal interphalangeal joint (DIPJ), distal sesamoid (navicular) bone, the deep digital flexor tendon (DDFT) and an acrylic cast of the navicular bursa. Between the flexor cortex of navicular bone and the DDFT is a lubricated bursa. The acrylic cast of the bursa shows the anatomic relationship between bone and tendon. The irregular distal border of the bursa conforms to the arrangement of the collagen bundles in the distal sesamoiden impar ligament, which insert on the distal phalanx proximad to the DDFT.

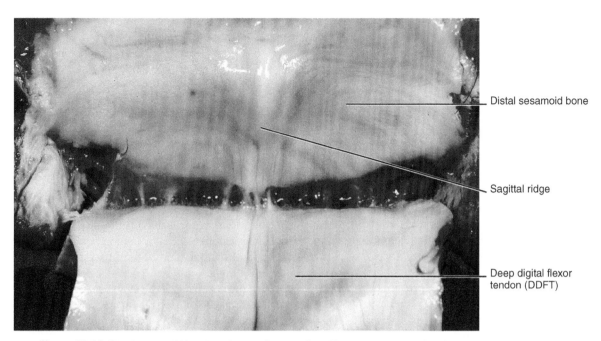

Distal sesamoid bone

Sagittal ridge

Deep digital flexor tendon (DDFT)

● **Figure 10.11** Distal sesamoid (navicular) bone: flexor surface. The navicular bursa has been opened, and the deep digital flexor tendon has been reflected downward to show the smooth, shiny fibrocartilage of the flexor surface of a normal distal sesamoid (navicular) bone. Pathologic degeneration of the flexor surface is associated with navicular disease. Bisecting the bone is the sagittal ridge where, the first lesions of navicular disease often appear.

11 Joints

DISTAL INTERPHALANGEAL JOINT, OR COFFIN JOINT

The distal interphalangeal joint (DIPJ) is a composite joint (a joint composed of three or more skeletal elements) formed by the distal trochlea of the second phalanx, the distal phalanx, and the distal sesamoid (navicular) bone. It has a limited range of lateral and rotational movements but a wide range of flexion and extension. The joint capsule has a small dorsal and a large palmar pouch. The dorsal pouch is beneath the common extensor tendon about 10 to 15 mm proximal to the coronet. The palmar pouch is beneath the deep digital flexor tendon (DDFT) and extends to the upper third of the middle phalanx.

The DIPJ stabilizes the distal sesamoid impar ligament, collateral sesamoidean ligaments, collateral ligaments of the DIPJ, DDFT, and distal digital annular ligament.

When the foot is unbalanced or moving over rough, uneven terrain, the distal phalanx twists and slides, relative to the middle phalanx, increasing the likelihood of DIPJ injury. This limited range of lateral and rotational movement is used diagnostically; trotting in a circle is more painful when the DIPJ is injured.

METACARPOPHALANGEAL, OR FETLOCK JOINT

The metacarpophalangeal joint (MCPJ), or fetlock joint, is frequently injured in athletic horses due to its extreme range of motion and the intense loads to which it is subjected. The risk of injury increases as horses approach their maximum speed and the loaded fetlock joint, in the stance phase of the gallop, shares a peak force 2.6 times its own body weight.[4] The record speed for Quarter Horses racing over 1/4 mile is around 19 meters/second, which is 68.4 kilometers/hour or 42.5 miles/hour (www.aqha.com). The peak vertical forces on the forelimbs compared with the hind limbs are markedly greater, explaining why the forelimbs are more frequently injured.[2]

The MCPJ is formed from the distal end of the large, third metacarpal (McIII) or cannon bone, the proximal end of the first phalanx, and both proximal sesamoid bones. It acts as a hinge joint, flexing and extending with limited lateral movement.

The distal end of McIII is cylinder shaped and is bisected by a prominent sagittal ridge (Fig. 11.8). The ridge fits into a reciprocal groove on the proximal surface of the proximal phalanx. The groove continues palmarly, between the proximal sesamoid bones, in the fibrocartilagenous intersesamoidean ligament that binds together the axial surfaces of the proximal sesamoid bones. The palmar (plantar) surface of the intersesamoidean ligament is also grooved to accommodate the deep flexor tendon.

The MCPJ capsule is attached around the borders of the articular surfaces. The joint has a wide range of motion and thus a joint capsule that extends a long way proximally on both the dorsal and palmar surfaces of McIII. In the dorsal joint capsule, to help cushion the impact of the proximal phalanx against the distal McIII during extreme extension (dorsal flexion of the fetlock), there is a bilobed synovial pad.[3] The palmar pouch of the capsule is located between the distal, palmar aspect of McIII and the suspensory ligament and extends proximally 3 cm above the apices of the proximal sesamoid bones.

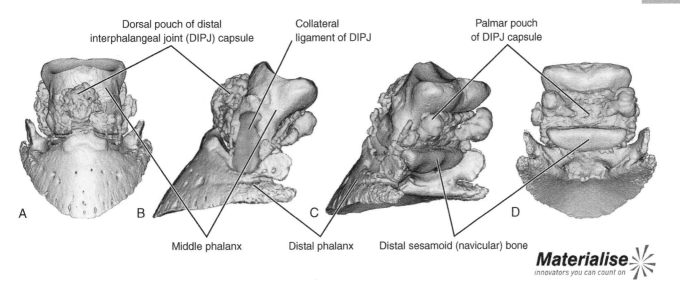

Dorsal pouch of distal interphalangeal joint (DIPJ) capsule

Collateral ligament of DIPJ

Palmar pouch of DIPJ capsule

A   B   C   D

Middle phalanx   Distal phalanx   Distal sesamoid (navicular) bone

Materialise
innovators you can count on

• **Figure 11.1** Mimics modeled computed tomography (CT) data of the distal interphalangeal joint (DIPJ) capsule of a normal adult horse foot. The capsule (*green*) has been infused with a suspension of the contrast agent barium sulfate to create a virtual cast. The joint capsule has a dorsal and a palmar pouch. The dorsal pouch (**A & B**) is beneath the common extensor tendon about 10 to 15 mm above the proximal border of the hoof wall. The palmar pouch (**C & D**) is beneath the distal sesamoid (navicular) bone and the deep digital flexor tendon and extends to the upper third of the middle phalanx. In **B**, the joint capsule is shown beneath the collateral ligament of the DIPJ. Original Mimics model by Simon Collins.

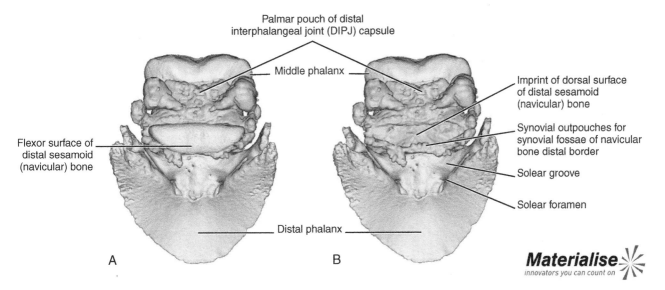

Palmar pouch of distal interphalangeal joint (DIPJ) capsule

Middle phalanx

Imprint of dorsal surface of distal sesamoid (navicular) bone

Synovial outpouches for synovial fossae of navicular bone distal border

Flexor surface of distal sesamoid (navicular) bone

Solear groove

Solear foramen

Distal phalanx

A   B

Materialise
innovators you can count on

• **Figure 11.2** Mimics modeled computed tomography (CT) data of the palmar aspect of the distal phalanx and its distal interphalangeal joint (DIPJ) capsule with and without the distal sesamoid (navicular) bone. The joint capsule (*green*) has been infused with a suspension of the contrast agent barium sulfate, creating a virtual cast. The articular surface of the navicular bone, a component of the DIPJ, is bathed in the same synovial fluid as the articular surfaces of the middle and distal phalanges. The articular surface makes a navicular bone–shaped imprint into the cast of the DIPJ capsule as it wraps around the bone, thus revealing its close association with the joint. Outpouches of the joint capsule project into 3 to 5 fossae in the distal border of the navicular bone; the synovial outpouches are obscured when the navicular bone is in place (**A**) and revealed when it is absent (**B**). The palmar digital nerves associate closely with the palmar pouch and, in time, may be blocked by diffusion of local anesthetic injected into the joint.

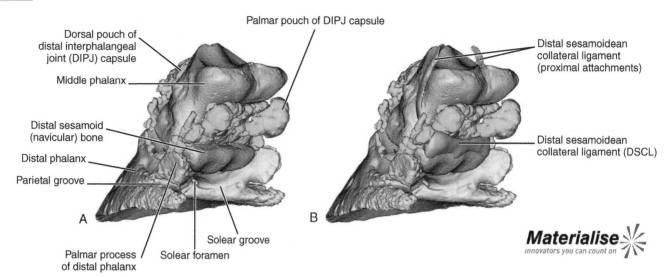

Figure 11.3 Mimics modeled computed tomography (CT) data of the palmar aspect of the distal phalanx and its distal interphalangeal joint (DIPJ) capsule with and without the distal sesamoidean collateral ligament. The joint capsule (*green*) has been infused with a suspension of the contrast agent barium sulfate. The collateral ligament is attached to the proximal border of the navicular bone, and its medial and lateral bands pass proximo-dorsally, enveloped by the palmar pouch, to insert on the distal end of the proximal phalanx. The body of the distal sesamoidean collateral ligament, attached to the proximal border of the navicular bone, makes a complementary imprint into the distal border of the palmar pouch of the DIPJ.

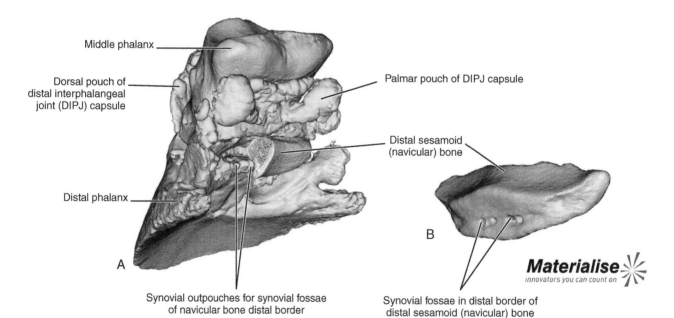

Figure 11.4 Mimics modeled computed tomography (CT) data of the palmar aspect of the distal phalanx and its distal interphalangeal joint (DIPJ) capsule with the distal sesamoid (navicular) bone bisected (**A**). The joint capsule (*green*) has been infused with a suspension of the contrast agent barium sulfate, creating a virtual cast. Outpouches of the joint capsule project into the 3 to 5 fossae in the distal border of the navicular bone (**B**). The distal impar ligament inserts on the distal border of the navicular bone distal to the row of synovial fossae.

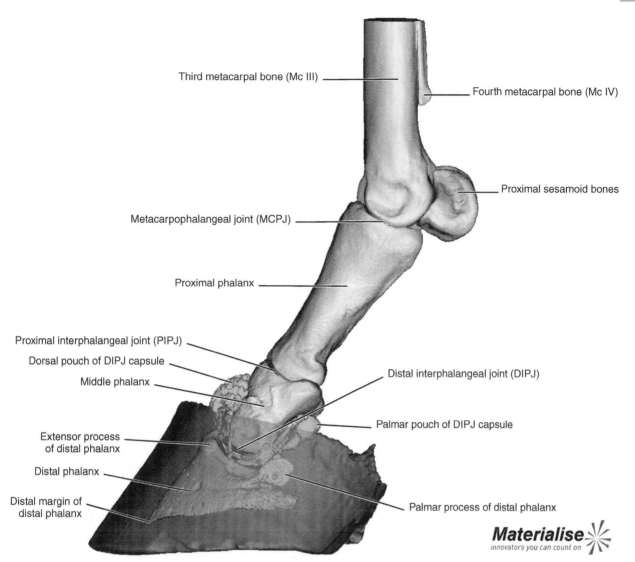

Third metacarpal bone (Mc III)

Fourth metacarpal bone (Mc IV)

Proximal sesamoid bones

Metacarpophalangeal joint (MCPJ)

Proximal phalanx

Proximal interphalangeal joint (PIPJ)

Dorsal pouch of DIPJ capsule

Middle phalanx

Distal interphalangeal joint (DIPJ)

Palmar pouch of DIPJ capsule

Extensor process of distal phalanx

Distal phalanx

Distal margin of distal phalanx

Palmar process of distal phalanx

Materialise
innovators you can count on

• **Figure 11.5** Mimics model of the distal left forelimb of the normal Standardbred stallion described in Chapter 6. The distal interphalangeal joint (DIPJ) capsule (*green*) has been infused with a suspension of the contrast agent barium sulfate, creating a virtual cast. The hoof capsule has been made transparent to show how far the dorsal pouch of the DIPJ extends above the proximal hoof wall. The dorsal pouch is beneath the common digital extensor tendon and extends about 22 mm above the proximal border of the hoof wall. For arthrocentesis of the DIPJ, a hypodermic needle can be consistently placed into the dorsal pouch using the following technique.[1] A horizontally directed 20-gauge, 2.5 to 4 cm needle, on the dorsal midline, 10 mm above the hoof wall margin, is inserted through the common digital extensor tendon into the dorsal pouch.

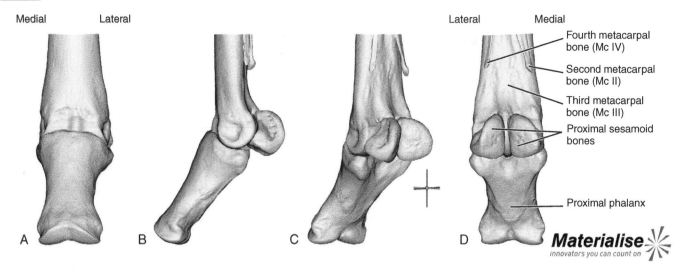

Medial   Lateral   Lateral   Medial

Fourth metacarpal
bone (Mc IV)

Second metacarpal
bone (Mc II)

Third metacarpal
bone (Mc III)

Proximal sesamoid
bones

Proximal phalanx

A   B   C   D

Materialise
innovators you can count on

● **Figure 11.6** Mimics models of the distal left forelimb of the normal Standardbred stallion described in Chapter 6. The metacarpophalangeal joint (MCPJ), or fetlock joint, is formed from the distal end of the large, third metacarpal (McIII), or cannon bone, the proximal end of the first phalanx, and both proximal sesamoid bones. Dorsopalmar, DPa (**A**), lateromedial, LM (**B**), palmarolateral-dorsomedial oblique, Pa45L-DM (**C**), and palmar dorsal, PaD (**D**) aspects.

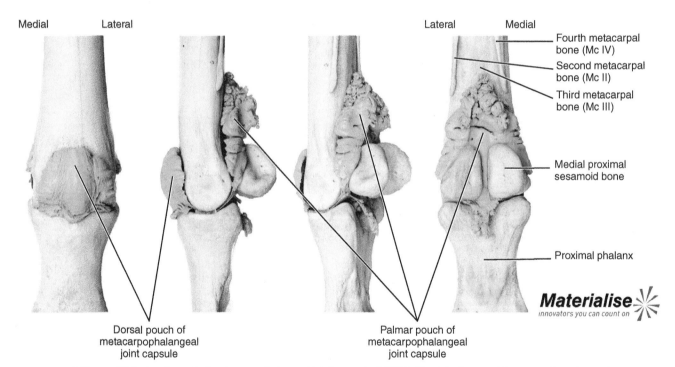

Medial   Lateral   Lateral   Medial

Fourth metacarpal
bone (Mc IV)

Second metacarpal
bone (Mc II)

Third metacarpal
bone (Mc III)

Medial proximal
sesamoid bone

Proximal phalanx

Dorsal pouch of
metacarpophalangeal
joint capsule

Palmar pouch of
metacarpophalangeal
joint capsule

Materialise
innovators you can count on

● **Figure 11.7** Acrylic cast of metacarpophalangeal joint capsule (MCPJ). The joint has a wide range of motion and thus a joint capsule that extends a long way proximally on both the dorsal and palmar surfaces of the third metacarpal bone (McIII). The palmar pouch of the capsule is located between the distal, palmar aspect of McIII and the suspensory ligament and extends proximally 3 cm above the apices of the proximal sesamoid bones. The palmar pouch is relatively easy to access with a hypodermic needle thus simplifying the injection of diagnostic local anesthetic or therapeutic substances.

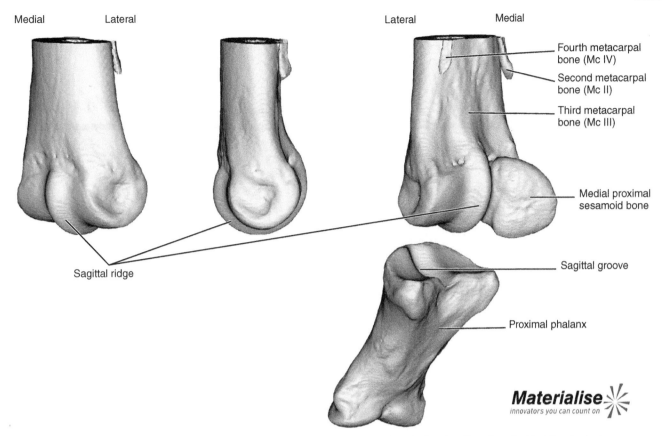

Medial · Lateral · Lateral · Medial

Fourth metacarpal bone (Mc IV)

Second metacarpal bone (Mc II)

Third metacarpal bone (Mc III)

Medial proximal sesamoid bone

Sagittal groove

Proximal phalanx

Sagittal ridge

Materialise
innovators you can count on

• **Figure 11.8** Mimics models of the distal left forelimb of the normal Standardbred stallion described in Chapter 6. A prominent sagittal ridge on the articular surface of the third metacarpal bone (McIII) dovetails into a groove on the proximal articular surface of the proximal phalanx and helps stabilize the joint.

References

1. Bassage, L. H., & Ross, M. W. (2011). Diagnostic analgesia. In M. W. Ross & S. J. Dyson, (Eds.), *Diagnosis and management of lameness in the horse* (pp. 100–135). St Louis, MO: Elsevier.
2. Pfau, T., Witte, T. H., & Wilson, A. M. (2006). Centre of mass movement and mechanical energy fluctuation during gallop locomotion in the Thoroughbred racehorse. *Journal of Experimental Biology, 209*, 3742–3757.
3. Richardson, D. W., & Dyson, S. J. (2011). The metacarpalphalangeal joint. In C. A. Ross & S. J. Dyson (Eds.), *Lameness in the horse; diagnosis and management* (p. 394). St Louis, MO: Elsevier.
4. Witte, T. H., Hirst, C. V., & Wilson, A. M. (2006). Effect of speed on stride parameters in racehorses at gallop in field conditions. *Journal of Experimental Biology, 209*, 4389–4397.

12 Radiography of the Foot

The foot of the horse is a common source of general lameness and the focus of the pathology due to laminitis. Despite the rise of ultrasonography and magnetic resonance imaging, the demand for high-quality diagnostic radiographs of the foot is still important for clinicians in equine practice.[1-3] Portable digital radiography has revolutionized the technology and made obtaining good-quality radiographs of the foot relatively easy. Nevertheless, a sound knowledge of foot anatomy and pathology remains a prerequisite if the images obtained are to be interpreted correctly.

RADIOGRAPHIC TECHNIQUE

The hoof distal phalanx distance (HDPD) never varies in normal horses.[4] If the HDPD increases, laminitis is the likely cause. It is extremely important to know the rate and magnitude of the HDPD increase. Good quality radiographs documenting the shifting status of the distal phalanx within the hoof capsule, supply important diagnostic and prognostic information, and should be a part of the work-up of every laminitis case.

The HDPD can be measured directly from a lateromedial radiograph if radiographic technique has been standardized. The x-ray beam should be a predetermined distance from the film, at a right angle to the sagittal plane of the foot, centered midway between the heel and the toe, and 2 to 3 cm above the bearing surface of the hoof wall. The foot should be clean with the shoe removed, at least for the initial radiographic examination. Excess sole and frog should be pared away with a hoof knife, and any mud and gravel should be removed with a wire brush. Since the beam of most x-ray machines cannot be lowered closer than 10 cm above ground level, the horse should stand with its forefeet on wooden blocks or boxes that are 10 to 15 cm thick. This will allow the x-ray beam to be centered on the foot while the foot is kept parallel to the ground. A radiopaque marker, in the form of a straight metal bar or rod, should be embedded in the edge of the wooden block closest to the X-ray sensor. This creates a horizontal line on the radiograph, against which the angle of the distal phalanx can be calculated. A radiographic marker (such as a screw or tack) can be left in the proximal hoof wall to serve as a reference point for subsequent measurement of downward vertical displacement of the distal phalanx, should this occur. A straight metal marker (a 50 to 70 mm steel rod or a line of barium paste) should be applied to the surface of the dorsal hoof wall in the sagittal plane so that the outer surface of the dorsal hoof wall can be located on the radiograph. For the majority of normal horses in the 400 to 450 kg bodyweight range, the mid-wall HDPD (the distance between the hoof wall marker and the parietal cortex of the distal phalanx) is between 15 to 17mm on calibrated

digital radiographs. The hoof wall and the parietal cortex of the distal phalanx are parallel in the normal horse. The HDPD is also 25% of the length of the distal phalanx palmar cortex measured from the dorsal–distal margin to the articular surface facing the navicular bone.[4]

VENOGRAPHY

Venography was developed in our laboratory in 1991 to determine whether retrograde venous therapy of the equine digit was possible. Radiographs showed that the lack of valves in all veins below the midpastern region enabled near complete retrograde filling with 20 to 25 ml of radiopaque contrast media. In 1992 the technique was shown to Ric Redden, the eminent equine podiatrist of Kentucky, United States, who has since used venography extensively and encouraged its widespread use.[5]

Venography is a relatively simple and practical method for assessing the state of digital circulation in the standing, sedated horse.

Venographic Technique

Performing a venogram requires good radiographic technique and teamwork. To enable subsequent analysis, a radiopaque marker should accurately delineate the surface of the dorsal hoof wall, even if using digital equipment. A narrow strip of barium paste applied to the hoof wall conforms to flares and other wall deformities and is the most accurate method. A 3-mm strip of the lead-impregnated fabric from a discarded lead apron also conforms to the hoof wall and may be used. If the hoof wall is genuinely straight, a fine metal rod will suffice. Satisfactory plain shots should be performed first to ensure that all parameters that may affect radiograph quality are accounted for. The venographic projections of most value are the lateromedial, the horizontal proximal dorsal-distal palmar projections (parallel to the ground) and, if there is time, dorsal 65° proximal–palmarodistal oblique ("upright pedal" or "high coronary") projection. Within a few minutes contrast material diffuses from the digital vessels and blurs the image. Teamwork is essential; everything needs to be ready for rapid action.

The horse should be well sedated with the foot under investigation thoroughly cleaned and nerve blocked at the abaxial sesamoid sites. The lateral side of the pastern should be clipped and prepared as for surgery. An Esmarch's bandage (tourniquet) is applied tightly around the fetlock, starting proximally and progressing distally to distend the digital veins (the opposite of the usual surgical application).

The distended digital vein can be palpated with the gloved finger. The concave curve of the midpastern makes accurate venipuncture placement difficult. A short scalp vein 21G needle set is recommended as the tubing leading from the needle makes syringe attachment easy, especially if an injection site is attached. If the horse moves suddenly, the needle can damage the vein and increase the chance of perivascular injection of contrast medium.

Once free backflow of blood is established and the line is patent and free of air bubbles, the extension tubing is capped with a latex injection site and the wings of the butterfly set are gently taped in place, out of the x-ray beam. Back pressure will dislodge the catheter, so taping is important.

Most 450 kg horses will need 20 to 25 ml of contrast material for the venogram. Employ any of the contrast agents used for myelograms, undiluted (e.g., Iomeron 350 or Omnipaque). The use of two to three smaller 10-ml syringes instead of one large syringe enables greater hydraulic pressure to be exerted and is recommended.

When injection commences, the team must be ready to make radiographs with the x-ray beam focused on the middle of the foot 2 to 3 cm proximad to the bearing border. The horse stands on predesigned boxes or blocks to achieve this. The foot should be made non–weight bearing once during the injection; this encourages filling of dorsal sublamellar vessels. Inject all the contrast agent through the injection site or stop when there is significant back pressure—detectable after the first 15-20 ml. Shoot high- and low-contrast lateral-medial projections first and quickly position the equipment for the horizontal and 65° dorso-palmar shots oblique.

After 5-6 minutes, contrast diffuses from the vessels and subsequent radiographs deteriorate. Release the tourniquet, remove the catheter, and pressure bandage a small gauze pad over the venipuncture site to prevent hematoma formation. Practice on normal horses first. Some believe that venography is therapeutic, but this remains to be properly tested.

Digital Radiography and Venograms

Venograms performed with digital radiographic equipment produce good results with somewhat superior definition and contrast. In lateral-medial radiographs of normal feet the sublamellar veins readily fill with contrast agent, but vessels between lamellae do not. The terminal papillae at the distal ends of the lamellae are visible and form a 'notch' more dorsal than the adjacent distal sublamellar and circumflex vessels. Vessels within the terminal arch of the distal phalanx fill with contrast agent, and these may be veins or arteries or both. Digital arteries also fill with contrast agent and can be recognized midpastern by their "string of beads" appearance. The normally well-filled coronary dermis-coronary cushion venous plexus is a feature of venograms and is visible dorsal to the extensor process of the distal phalanx; it follows the dorsopalmar angle of the coronary band. The ungular cartilage venous plexus combines with the coronary plexus and dominates the radiographic image of the palmar foot.

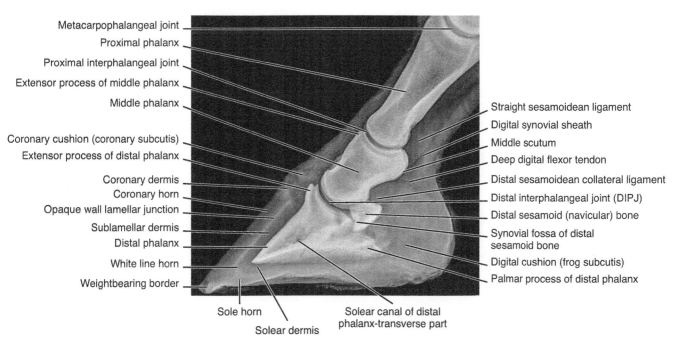

• **Figure 12.1** Radiographic image (latero-medial projection) of a normal adult horse foot. The digital image shows the radiolucent dermis between the distal phalanx and the hoof capsule. Intrusion of the less lucent epidermis into the radiolucent dermis, proximally and distally, characterizes severe, chronic laminitis and is important diagnostically. The radiopaque line marking the junction between the axial *stratum medium* (coronary horn) and the *stratum internum* (epidermal lamellae) is an artifact of the projection but useful in determining the limits of the lamellar and sublamellar dermis. The terminal horn of the white line aligns with the lamellar epidermis, not the coronary horn.

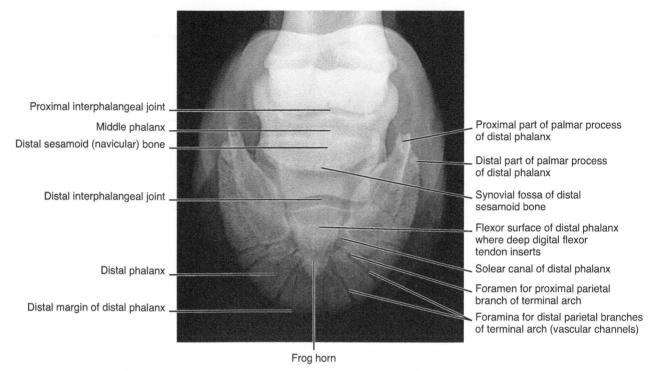

Proximal interphalangeal joint
Middle phalanx
Distal sesamoid (navicular) bone

Distal interphalangeal joint

Distal phalanx

Distal margin of distal phalanx

Proximal part of palmar process of distal phalanx

Distal part of palmar process of distal phalanx

Synovial fossa of distal sesamoid bone

Flexor surface of distal phalanx where deep digital flexor tendon inserts

Solear canal of distal phalanx

Foramen for proximal parietal branch of terminal arch

Foramina for distal parietal branches of terminal arch (vascular channels)

Frog horn

• Figure 12.2 Radiographic image (dorsal 65° proximal–palmarodistal oblique projection) of a normal adult horse foot. Note the intact, sharp boundary of the distal margin of the distal phalanx; lysis and fracture of the distal margin characterize chronic laminitis. The number, shape, and size of the synovial fossae in the distal border of the distal sesamoid (navicular) bone is normal.

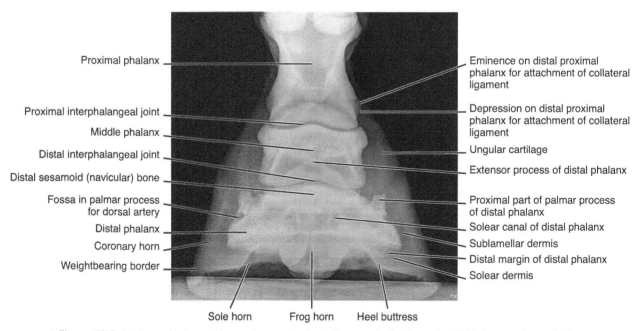

Proximal phalanx

Proximal interphalangeal joint
Middle phalanx
Distal interphalangeal joint
Distal sesamoid (navicular) bone
Fossa in palmar process for dorsal artery
Distal phalanx
Coronary horn
Weightbearing border

Eminence on distal proximal phalanx for attachment of collateral ligament

Depression on distal proximal phalanx for attachment of collateral ligament

Ungular cartilage

Extensor process of distal phalanx

Proximal part of palmar process of distal phalanx

Solear canal of distal phalanx

Sublamellar dermis

Distal margin of distal phalanx

Solear dermis

Sole horn   Frog horn   Heel buttress

• Figure 12.3 Radiographic image (dorsopalmar projection) of a normal adult horse foot. With the x-ray beam horizontal this projection allows assessment of medial-lateral balance and joint space width. Note the ungular cartilages arise from the proximal part of the palmar processes of the distal phalanx. This projection will detect the presence and extent of calcification of the ungular cartilages (sidebone).

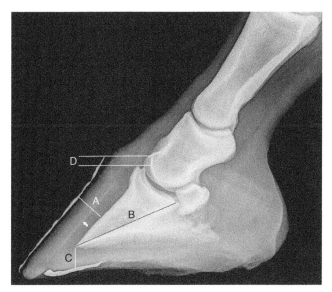

• **Figure 12.4** Radiographic image (lateromedial projection) of the same normal adult horse foot as in Fig. 12.1. The dorsal hoof wall and dorsal sole have been marked with radiopaque barium paste. Note that the convex outer edge of the dorsal wall is radiolucent. Measurement of the distance between the outer hoof wall and the parietal surface of the distal phalanx (*line A*) is more accurate if a radiopaque marker is in place. The distance between the outer hoof wall and the parietal surface of the distal phalanx is notated as the hoof distal phalanx distance (HDPD) in this text. Proximal, middle, and distal HDPD measurements should be obtained; these values should not be significantly different in the normal horse. In the normal horse the HDPD (*line A*) is 25% of line B (the distance between the distal margin of the distal phalanx [DP] and its articulation with the distal sesamoid bone). Radiopaque barium paste on the dorsal sole enables the vertical distance (*line C*) between the DP distal margin and the outer edge of the sole to be measured. The barium paste on the dorsal hoof wall is placed to locate the exact proximal limit of the *stratum medium* (coronary horn), a hard edge beneath the periople. The radiographic image can then be used to measure **D,** the distance between the proximal hoof wall and the extensor process of the DP. Obtaining these measurements is important diagnostically as **A** and **D** increase and **C** decreases as laminitis develops.

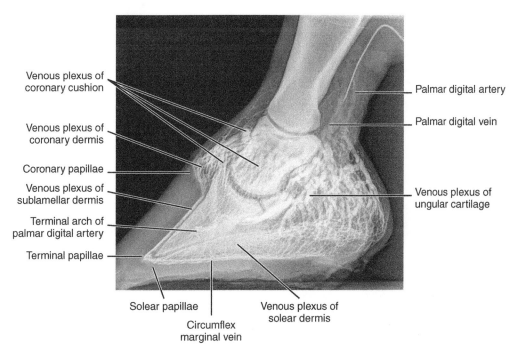

• **Figure 12.5** Lateromedial contrast-enhanced radiographic image of veins after infusion of the palmar digital vein of the left forelimb of a normal adult horse with iodinated contrast medium. Proximally, the sublamellar plexus unites with the venous plexi of the coronary dermis and the coronary subcutis (coronary cushion). Distally, the sublamellar and solear plexi unite to form the circumflex marginal vein that extends around the entire distal margin of the foot, connecting, in the palmar foot, with the plexi of the ungular cartilages. Note the direction of the contrast-filled coronary and terminal papillae; in the normal foot they are aligned (parallel) with the dorsal hoof wall and the parietal surface of the distal phalanx. Also, the distal margin of the distal phalanx is proximad to the terminal papillae and dorsal circumflex marginal vein.

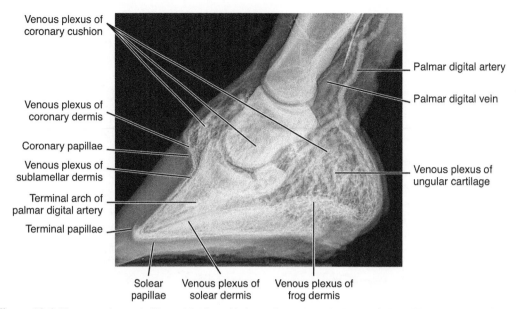

Venous plexus of coronary cushion

Venous plexus of coronary dermis

Coronary papillae

Venous plexus of sublamellar dermis

Terminal arch of palmar digital artery

Terminal papillae

Palmar digital artery

Palmar digital vein

Venous plexus of ungular cartilage

Solear papillae

Venous plexus of solear dermis

Venous plexus of frog dermis

• Figure 12.6 The same foot as in Figure 12-5 but with the radiograph made 3 minutes later. The contrast medium has diffused from the circulation into the surrounding extracellular fluid compartment diffusing parts of the image, especially the papillae. With the tourniquet still in place, contrast medium has backfilled the palmar digital arteries.

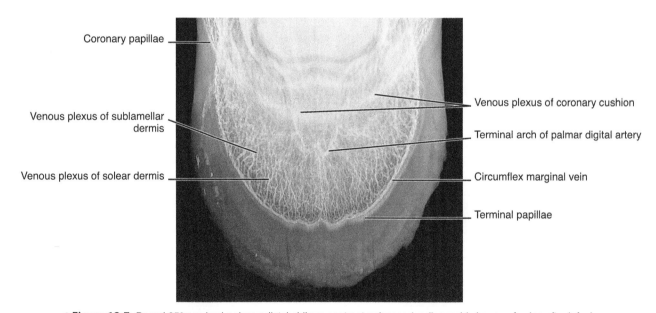

Coronary papillae

Venous plexus of sublamellar dermis

Venous plexus of solear dermis

Venous plexus of coronary cushion

Terminal arch of palmar digital artery

Circumflex marginal vein

Terminal papillae

• Figure 12.7 Dorsal 65° proximal-palmarodistal oblique contrast-enhanced radiographic image of veins after infusion of the palmar digital vein of the left forelimb of a normal adult horse with iodinated contrast medium. The venous plexus of the sublamellar dermis covers the parietal surface of the distal phalanx and drains proximally into the venous plexi of the coronary dermis and coronary subcutis. The coronary vessels form a crescent-shaped band extending medial to lateral in the dorsal coronet. The sublamellar and solear plexi unite distally to form the circumflex marginal vein that extends around the entire distal margin of the foot. Note the reticular network of the venous plexus of the solear dermis. The sublamellar veins and solear plexus are superimposed in this projection; the proximodistally oriented vessels are sublamellar veins, and the reticular pattern is due to the solear plexus. The terminal papillae are aligned dorsoproximally, each one representing the terminal circulation of a single lamella. Contrast medium filling of lamellar vessels is insufficient to be detected by retrograde venography. This projection is important in the investigation of chronic laminitis; dislocation of the distal phalanx obliterates filling of the dorsal solear plexus and the circumflex marginal vein.

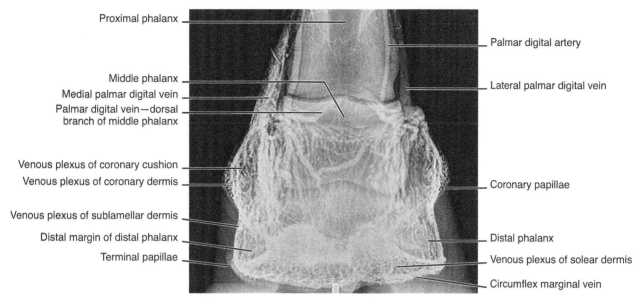

Proximal phalanx

Middle phalanx
Medial palmar digital vein
Palmar digital vein—dorsal
branch of middle phalanx

Venous plexus of coronary cushion
Venous plexus of coronary dermis

Venous plexus of sublamellar dermis
Distal margin of distal phalanx
Terminal papillae

Palmar digital artery

Lateral palmar digital vein

Coronary papillae

Distal phalanx
Venous plexus of solear dermis
Circumflex marginal vein

• **Figure 12.8** Dorsopalmar contrast-enhanced radiographic image of veins after infusion of the palmar digital vein of the left forelimb of a normal adult horse with iodinated contrast medium. The contrast-filled coronary and terminal papillae are aligned (parallel) with the dorsal hoof wall and the parietal surface of the distal phalanx. The sublamellar plexi are also parallel with the medial and lateral hoof walls. Because the plane of the solear plexus is higher at the heels than at the toe, filling of the dorsal (toe) solear plexus and circumflex marginal vein can be inspected using this projection. The dislocation of the distal phalanx associated with chronic laminitis may obliterate filling of the dorsal solear plexus and the circumflex marginal vein.

References

1. Dyson, S. J. (2011). Navicular disease. In M. W. Ross & S. J. Dyson (Eds.), *Diagnosis and management of lameness in the horse* (2nd ed., pp. 324–342). St. Louis, MO: Elsevier.
2. Dyson, S. J. (2011). Radiology and radiography. In M. W. Ross & S. J. Dyson (Eds.), *Diagnosis and management of lameness in the horse* (2nd ed., pp. 168–182). St Louis, MO: Elsevier.
3. Kold, S., & Butler, J. (2003). Radiography of the horse. 2. Foot and pastern. *In Practice, 25,* 208–215.
4. Linford, R.L., OBrien, T.R., Trout, D.R. (1993). Qualitative and morphometric radiographic findings in the distal phalanx and digital soft tissues of sound Thoroughbred racehorses. *American Journal of Veterinary Research.* 54(1) 38-51.
5. Redden, R. F. (2001). A technique for performing digital venography in the standing horse. *Equine Veterinary Education, 13,* 128–134.

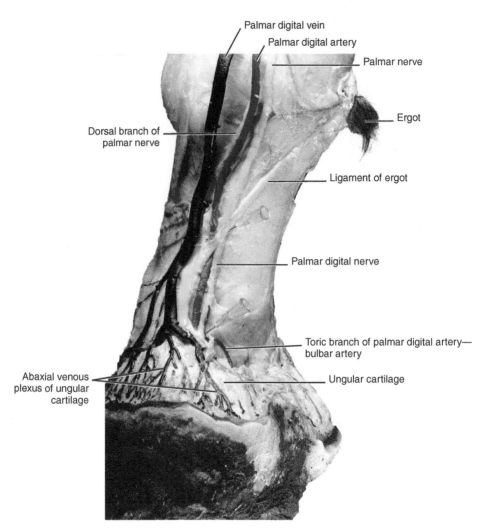

Palmar digital vein
Palmar digital artery
Palmar nerve
Dorsal branch of palmar nerve
Ergot
Ligament of ergot
Palmar digital nerve
Toric branch of palmar digital artery—bulbar artery
Abaxial venous plexus of ungular cartilage
Ungular cartilage

• **Figure 13.1** The palmar digital nerve. Regional anesthesia of the palmar digital nerve is the most common diagnostic procedure performed in practice. In the photograph of the dissection, the palmar digital vein has been injected with blue latex and the palmar digital artery with red latex. The palmar digital nerve is easy to palpate palmar to the artery as it passes under the ligament of ergot in the midpastern region. The needle shows where local anesthetic can be injected to block the palmar digital nerve at the ligament of ergot site. Distally, the nerve can be blocked as it passes axial to the ungular cartilage of the distal phalanx. The pulse of the artery is palpated and the injection made just palmar to it. The needle shows the site. Loss of skin sensation in the midline, between the bulbs of the heels, is assessed and a successful palmar digital nerve block anesthetizes the superficial and deep digital flexor tendons and their sheaths, the distal sesamoid (navicular) bone and its bursa, the solear and palmar third of the distal phalanx, the distal sesamoidean ligaments, the digital cushion, the corium of the frog, and much of the sole, wall, and coronet. Traditionally considered to block only the palmar third of the foot, in practice around 70-80% of the foot is desensitized.[1] Figures 5.14, 5.21, 5.22, 5.23, and 5.24 show the proximity of the nerve to the distal interphalangeal joint (DIPJ) capsule and explains why the palmar digital nerve block may abolish DIPJ pain.[1] The palmar digital nerve continues distally in the parietal groove of the distal phalanx beside the dorsal artery (Fig. 5.14) and thus innervates the coria of the medial and lateral hoof walls, toe, and sole. Solear foot pain induced by placement of set screws beneath the dorsal margin of the distal phalanx is abolished by the palmar digital nerve block.[2]

References

1. Bassage, L.H., Ross, M.W., 2011. Diagnostic analgesia. In: Ross, M.W., Dyson, S.J. (Eds.), Diagnosis and management of lameness in the horse. Elsevier, St Louis, pp. 100–135.

2. Schumacher, J., Steiger, R., Schumacher, J., de Graves, F., Schramme, M., Smith, R., Coker, M., 2000. Effects of Analgesia of the Distal Interphalangeal Joint or Palmar Digital Nerves on Lameness Caused by Solar Pain in Horses. Veterinary Surgery 29, 54–58.

SECTION 2

Conditions of the Foot

14 Laminitis

Laminitis is the most serious disease of the equine foot and causes pathologic changes in anatomy that lead to long-lasting, crippling changes in function (chronic laminitis or founder). It is the second-biggest killer of horses after colic.

In the normal horse or pony the distal phalanx (P3, coffin or pedal bone) is attached to the inside of the hoof by a tough, but flexible, suspensory apparatus. The surface of the inner hoof wall is folded into vertically oriented, leaflike lamellae (laminae) to increase the surface area of this suspensory apparatus of the distal phalanx. A horse has laminitis when these lamellae suddenly fail. Without the distal phalanx properly attached to the inside of the hoof, the weight of the horse drives the bone down into the hoof capsule (sinking) and the forces of locomotion lever the hoof capsule away (dorsally) from the distal phalanx (capsular rotation).

Important arteries and veins are sheared and crushed, and the dermis of the coronet and sole is damaged. There is unrelenting pain in the feet and a characteristic lameness.

Laminitis has a developmental phase during which lamellar separation is triggered. This precedes the appearance of the foot pain of laminitis. The developmental period lasts 40 to 48 hours in the case of laminitis caused by excessive, sudden ingestion of soluble, nonstructural carbohydrates, such as starch or fructan (the septic shock syndrome of laminitis). Sometimes no developmental phase can be recognized; the horse or pony is discovered with the clinical signs of laminitis with no apparent ill health or inciting problem occurring beforehand (the metabolic, hyperinsulinemic syndrome of laminitis).

Many people own and care for horses all their lives and never encounter a horse with laminitis. However, when it does strike, laminitis is heartbreaking. The pain and suffering are relentless, and sometimes euthanasia is the only responsible option for an owner, despite the stoic ability of many horses to live on as cripples. Formulating an effective management plan for a horse with laminitis is one of the most difficult tasks a horse owner can be confronted with. The owner, in consultation with a veterinary clinician and farrier, will have to decide if the investment of money, time, and energy is worthwhile while at the same time considering the welfare of the horse. After months of treatment and the expenditure of perhaps thousands of dollars, the horse in question may still be suffering severely. The clinical signs, the extent and severity of lamellar pathology, and the response to therapy vary unpredictably among individual horses, and this makes a rational treatment strategy, with an accurate prognosis, difficult to formulate. Severe damage to the internal anatomy of the hoof can occur within the space of a few hours, and the severity and extent of this initial damage is the single most important factor influencing the final outcome.[17]

LAMINITIS RADIOLOGY

As the histopathology of acute laminitis clearly shows, the major feature of acute laminitis is a progressive increase in the distance between the epidermal lamellae and their dermal connective tissue attachments. Initially, this distance is microscopic in scale but may rapidly progress to a separation measurable in millimeters. In radiologic terms, this translates to an increase in the distance between the dorsal hoof wall and the dorsal (parietal) cortex of the distal phalanx; for convenience, the hoof–distal phalangeal distance (HDPD). The HDPD never varies in normal horses (See Chapter 12 Radiography of the Horse's Foot). If the HDPD increases, laminitis is the likely cause and it is extremely important to know the rate and magnitude of the HDPD increase. Good-quality radiographs, documenting the shifting status of the distal phalanx within the hoof capsule, supply important diagnostic and prognostic information and should be part of the workup of every laminitis case.

Radiology of Acute/Early Chronic Laminitis

Radiographs of horses or ponies, in the acute/early chronic stage of laminitis, should be examined for an increase in the HDPD. An increase of just 2 to 3 mm is extremely significant in the context of early chronic laminitis. In the first few days of the chronic phase, the hoof wall and the distal phalanx will draw apart but remain parallel. Rotation of the distal phalanx, relative to the hoof wall, occurs later. A valid diagnosis of early chronic laminitis can be made on the basis of a small increase in the HDPD. With an early diagnosis, prevention of any further increase by the application of the correct medical and supportive shoeing strategies may be possible. It is a mistake to let rotation of the distal phalanx alone be the sole diagnostic criterion of chronic laminitis—the diagnosis can be made earlier than this with good-quality radiographs. Early diagnosis and early treatment can produce a better outcome. Additional diagnostic criteria are: 1. The appearance of a radiolucent line adjacent to the inner edge of the dorsal hoof wall; 2. Rotation of the hoof capsule away from the parietal surface of the distal phalanx (capsular rotation); 3. Palmar/plantar rotation of the distal phalanx off the phalangeal axis; 4. A decrease in the distance between the distal margin of the distal phalanx and the dorsal sole (or the ground surface). 5. An increase in the distance between the proximal edge of the hoof wall and the extensor process of the distal phalanx.

The rate at which the HDPD increases correlates with the severity of the acute lesion

When the entire lamellar attachment apparatus fails simultaneously and there is circumferential separation of hoof from the distal phalanx, the HDPD increases. The distal phalanx sinks vertically into the hoof capsule, without palmar rotation, and such cases are appropriately termed "sinkers." The distance from the proximal edge of the hoof wall to the extensor process also increases—the founder distance.[3] When sinkers are dissected, the hoof wall falls away free of its dermal connective tissue attachments to the distal phalanx. This most severe outcome of the laminitis process carries with it the gravest of prognoses, especially if it has occurred in all four feet. The animal suffers intense unrelenting pain, and there is virtually no hope of a satisfactory recovery; euthanasia is usually the only logical option. It is emphasized that severe, life-threatening laminitis can be diagnosed without palmar rotation of the distal phalanx being evident on lateromedial radiographs. Predicting when a horse will become a sinker is difficult. The radiolucent line that forms beneath the inner hoof wall is also an indicator of severity. Its presence means that considerable lamellar separation and stretching have occurred. Dissection and histopathology of lamellae, which display the linear radiolucency, show that the lucent zone corresponds to a zone of dorsal epidermal lamellae between which the dermal lamellae are absent. Air or gas is in the spaces once occupied by the dermal lamellae. The spaces between the lamellae are dry, and the lamellae readily peel apart. Usually, the tips of the epidermal lamellae are still connected to the lamellar dermis.

How the gas forms between the lamellae, when the hoof capsule and the surrounding tissues are still intact, is a mystery, but one explanation is that the gas is nitrogen, coming out of solution in the blood, as progressive lamellar separation creates a vacuum (a gradient of negative pressure). The linear, radiolucent zone is sometimes erroneously referred to as a seroma; however, serum is not radiolucent and not always present. In acute/chronic laminitis, lateromedial projections supply the most information. However, two other projections supply useful data and should be included in the radiographic examination. They supply reference information that could be useful later if the case deteriorates with the passage of time. The dorsal 65° proximal–palmarodistal ("upright pedal" or "high coronary") view, exposed to show the margin of the distal phalanx, records demineralization and progressive lysis of the tip of the distal phalanx. The dorsoproximal–palmarodistal ("standing") view, with the x-ray beam parallel to the ground, shows if the linear, radiolucent lines, usually beneath the dorsal hoof wall (as shown by the lateromedial projection), are also present beneath the lateral and medial hoof walls. If they are present, this means that separation is extensive (not just confined to the toe) and the gravity of the prognosis is increased. Dorsal hoof wall resection is contraindicated if radiolucent lines are visible at the quarters, under the lateral and medial hoof walls.

Radiology of Chronic Laminitis

With increasing chronicity, the dorsal hoof wall rotates further away from the distal phalanx and the solear surface of the distal phalanx begins to compress the dermis of the sole. The margin of the distal phalanx gets closer to the ground. As pressure between bone and sole increases, the sole undergoes necrosis and the distal margin of the bone is slowly lysed.[8] Lateromedial radiographs should be made to show the divergence between the angles of the dorsal hoof wall and distal phalanx. The amount of capsular rotation is correlated inversely with return to athletic performance. Horses with less than 5.5 degrees of rotation may return to athletic function. Those with more than 11.5 degrees lose their capacity to perform, remain crippled, and may have to be euthanized because of intractable pain. The degree of capsular rotation is calculated by subtracting the hoof angle from the angle of the parietal surface of the distal phalanx. The hoof angle is measured at the intersection of the line extended downward from the outer surface of the hoof wall (ideally, the radiopaque marker taped to the surface of the hoof) and the horizontal line at the bearing surface of the hoof (ideally, the radiopaque marker embedded in the edge of the wooden block). The angle of the distal phalanx is measured at the intersection of a line extended down from the parietal cortex of the distal phalanx and the horizontal line of the bearing surface of the hoof. The hoof angle and the angle of the distal phalanx are parallel in radiographs of normal feet. The finding that the severity of pain and lameness at the time of initial examination is in fact more reliable has challenged the concept that palmar rotation of the distal phalanx accurately predicts outcome for the horse. Most veterinarians agree that the Obel system for grading the lameness of laminitis takes precedence over the radiographic determination of capsular rotation as a means of predicting final outcome. Our good correlation between the extent and severity of histologic, lamellar damage and grade of lameness supports this view.[16] In addition to palmar rotation, the distal phalanx should be examined radiographically for bone modeling, osteolysis, distal margin fractures, and osteitis. These changes may take several weeks to develop after the onset of laminitis, and when present, indicate that the horse is well into the chronic stage and thus more difficult to rehabilitate. They are associated with the distal margin of the descended distal phalanx where downward pressure against the sole, or in severe cases the ground, is at its greatest. Ingrowing tubular and lamellar horn in the form of a lamellar wedge also triggers bone lysis and modeling proximal to the distal margin. In mild chronic laminitis, where capsular rotation is minimal (<5.5 degrees), the tip of the distal phalanx remodels and appears "ski-tipped" in lateromedial radiographs. In dorsal 65° proximal–palmarodistal oblique radiographs, the dorsal margin of the distal phalanx has a ragged appearance where bone has been lysed, making this projection more informative than the lateromedial. Rapid, extensive decalcification of bone accompanies severe capsular rotation of the distal phalanx (>11.5 degrees) and such horses are poor candidates for rehabilitation. Occasionally, the laminitis is triggered by trauma to the hooves (road founder) and the margin of the distal phalanx may be fractured. Severe palmar rotation and solar prolapse of the distal phalanx is usually accompanied by infection. The sole may be underrun, and gas lines delineating the solar corium may be visible on lateromedial radiographs. Osteitis of the distal phalanx and abscess formation may cause pus and gas to discharge from the coronet and can be monitored with dorsal 65° proximal–palmarodistal radiographs. In chronic laminitis of long standing, there can be spectacular demineralization of the distal phalanx.

VENOGRAPHY OF LAMINITIS

During the chronic phase of laminitis, the distal phalanx shifts from its normal position and descends in the hoof capsule. In severe cases pathologic changes continue to develop and worsen over time and venography enables early assessment of pathology that would otherwise remain undetected. In moderate to severe chronic laminitis, venography can detect structural changes to coronary, sublamellar, and solar tissues that have diagnostic and prognostic value. Venography has been used to investigate clinical case material and document vascular changes as horses progress from

normal into the acute and chronic phase of laminitis. Knowing when venographic compromise occurs in the acute or chronic phase of laminitis and linking this to the pathology of tissue obtained post-mortem provides a better understanding of the chronic laminitis process. Importantly, the information obtained from venography informs on remedial measures and whether they are successful or not.

Venography of Acute/Early Chronic Laminitis

Venography detected changes in hoof anatomy as early as five to seven days after laminitis development.[2] The severity and rate at which venographic changes developed correlated to the degree of lameness. Sequential venograms and measurements gave important information about the insidious pathology that chronic laminitis inflicts on foot structures within the hoof capsule.

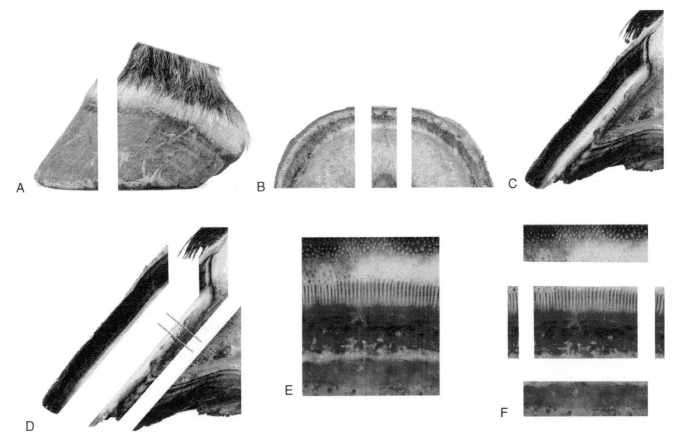

• **Figure 14.1** Feet destined for lamellar histopathology are disarticulated at the metacarpophalangeal joint (MCPJ) or proximal interphalangeal joint (PIPJ) and sectioned with a band saw. With the sole on the base plate of the band saw, the first saw cut is from lateral to medial, cutting just palmar to the proximal, dorsal hoof wall (**A**). Then, with the newly cut surface on the base plate and the sole facing the operator, the second and third saw cuts are made, 15 mm apart, on either side of the apex of the frog (**B**). The resultant wedge-shaped section of dorsal hoof wall, lamellae, sublamellar dermis, and distal phalanx is laid on its side (**C**) and further trimmed to remove the bulk of the outer hoof wall and all but the parietal cortex of the distal phalanx (**D**). Finally, two additional saw cuts are made (yellow lines in **D**), 20 mm apart, in the midwall region, to produce a tissue block consisting of inner hoof wall, lamellae, sublamellar dermis, and parietal cortex of the distal phalanx (**E**). Using a steel-backed razor blade or a disposable microtome blade and handle, all surfaces of the lamellar block are trimmed to remove tissue damaged by the teeth of the band saw blade (**F**). Extra care is taken to ensure only 1 mm of hoof wall adjoins the abaxial bases of the epidermal lamellae. Leaving more than 1 mm of hard hoof wall damages the microtome blade when sectioning. Finally, the trimmed block is reduced to one to two slices 5 mm thick that are placed in the tissue cassette. The hoof wall edge of the block is placed adjacent to the cassette hinge to ensure the dermal edge of the tissue block is sectioned first; this gives best results. Sections are fixed in 10% buffered formalin, dehydrated in alcohol, and embedded in paraffin wax. Sections 5 to 7 μm thick are cut and stained with haematoxylin and eosin (H&E) and periodic acid–Schiff (PAS) stains.

LAMINITIS HISTOPATHOLOGY

Most descriptions of laminitis histopathology derive from laminitis induced experimentally with either a single large dose of carbohydrate of either grain starch or oligofructose (OF)—the alimentary model[10,16,22,26]—or by infusing insulin into the blood for a prolonged period of time—the hyperinsulinemic model.[1,6] The sequence of microscopic events before the onset of clinical laminitis follows a consistent temporal pattern,[5] and the development of laminitis can be staged according to the degree of severity of these changes. Lamellar biopsies taken under local anesthesia from horses developing OF-induced laminitis at 12, 18, 24, 30, 36, and 48 hours after dosing were used to develop a laminitis histopathology timeline.[28] Taking multiple serial lamellar biopsies neither inflames adjacent tissues makes, nor it particularly painful for the horse.[11]

Making the lamellar basement membrane (BM) clearly visible is important and requires staining lamellar tissues with periodic acid–Schiff (PAS) stain[16] (see Figs. 8-6 and 8-7) or with immunohistochemical methods using a basement membrane–specific antibody such as collagen type IV, collagen type VII, or laminin 5[18] (see Figs. 8-12 and 8-13).

Grade 0: Normal Lamellar Histopathology

Normal lamellar anatomic characteristics, assessed before allocating a laminitis grade to a section of lamellar hoof tissue, are as follows (see Figs. 8-3, 8-4, 8-5, 8-6, and 8-7).

- The tips of the secondary epidermal lamellae (SELs) are always rounded (club-shaped) and never tapered or pointed.
- The basal cell nucleus is oval, with the long axis of the oval at a right angle to the long axis of the SEL. These parameters can be satisfactorily assessed using routine hematoxylin and eosin (H&E) staining of sections.
- The BM penetrates deeply into the crypts between the SELs and outlines the wafer-thin, but connective tissue–filled, secondary dermal lamellae.
- The BM tightly adheres to the basal cells of each SEL. The PAS or immunohistochemical stains show this best.

The length of a normal SEL is approximately 125 μm and its width 25 μm.[7]

Grade 1: Laminitis Histopathology

The earliest change attributable to laminitis is loss of shape and normal arrangement of the lamellar basal and parabasal cells. The basal cell nuclei become rounded instead of oval and take an abnormal position in the cytoplasm of the cell. The SELs become stretched, long, and thin, with tapering instead of club-shaped tips. SEL length increases to approximately 245 μm and decreases in width to 15 μm.[7] These changes were present at 12 hours in serial lamellar biopsies taken after oligofructose dosing.[28]

First noticeable at the tips of the SELs are teat-shaped bubbles of loose BM (see Fig. 14-36). Examination of laminitis tissues with the electron microscope confirms lysis and separation of the lamellar BM. The greater magnification shows widespread loss of basal cell adhesion plaques (hemidesmosomes) and contraction of the basal cell cytoskeleton away from the inner cell surface. Electron microscopy shows why the BM separates from the feet of the basal cells. The filaments that anchor hemidesmosomes to the lamina densa of the BM no longer bridge the dermal/epidermal interface.[9]

Grade 2: Laminitis Histopathology

Because the BM is no longer completely tethered to the basal cells, it slips farther away from SEL tips, with each cycle of weight bearing by the horse. Portions of the lamellar BM are lysed initially at the tips of secondary dermal lamellae (between the bases of SELs). Lamellar epidermal cells that lose their BM clump together to form amorphous, basement membrane–free masses on either side of the primary lamellar axis (see Fig. 14-37).

Electron microscopy of the attenuated lamellar tips of grade 2 histologic laminitis confirms BM separation from the plasmalemma of the lamellar epidermal basal cell. Usually the adjacent dermis seems unaffected by the laminitis process.[19]

Grade 3: Laminitis Histopathology

In laminitis the worst-case scenario is a rapid and near-total BM lysis and separation from all the epidermal lamellae of the hoof toe, quarters, heels, and bars. Sheets of BM are stripped away, forming aggregations of loose, isolated BM in the connective tissue adjacent to the lamellae (see Figures 14-38 ABC and 14-39). The stretched, thin BM-free lamellar epidermal cells are left as isolated columns on either side of the keratinized axis of the primary epidermal lamella, with little viable connection to the dermal connective tissue still attached to the distal phalanx. Similar lesions were described by Nils Obel in 1948.[15] The epidermal lamellar tips slip away from the BM connective tissue attachments, at first, microscopically. However, as the separation between hoof and distal phalanx increases, it becomes measurable in millimeters and can be detected radiographically (see Fig. 14-47). As the lamellae progressively lose their suspensory capacity, the distal phalanx sinks into the hoof capsule—a distance measurable on radiographs as the founder distance (see Fig. 14-47). Because the BM is the key structure bridging the epidermis of the hoof to the suspensory connective tissue of the distal phalanx, wholesale loss and disorganization of the lamellar basement membrane inexorably leads to the pathology of hoof and bone that characterizes the chronic stage of laminitis.

The laminitis process also affects the lamellar capillaries. As the BM and the connective tissue between the SELs disappear, so do the capillaries. They become obliterated, compressed against the edges of the primary dermal lamellae. Without a full complement of capillaries in the lamellar circulation, blood probably bypasses the capillary bed through dilated arteriovenous shunts changing the nature of the foot circulation. A bounding pulse becomes detectable by finger palpation of the digital arteries. Furthermore, epidermal cell necrosis, intravascular coagulation, and edema are not universally present in sections made from tissues in the early stages of laminitis. The vessels in the primary and secondary dermal lamellae, even the smallest, are predominantly open, without evidence of microvascular thrombi (see Fig.14-36).

In the days after the acute phase, the processes that caused lamellar BM dysadhesion and lysis, basal cell dislocation, and lamellar attenuation appear to abate. Epidermal compartments become enveloped in normal-appearing BM and the majority of epidermal basal cells (EBCs) are of normal shape and orientation. The major abnormality is the spectacular disarray of lamellar architecture. Epidermal islands form, and, no longer connected to their respective lamellar axis, lose their capacity to function as a suspensory apparatus between the dorsal hoof wall and the distal

phalanx. The resumption of athletic exercise and thus greater foot break-over strain, particularly in the forefeet, could conceivably rupture surviving lamellar attachments. This is likely the mechanism behind the notorious exacerbations that plague horses that appear to have recovered from a primary bout of laminitis. The small but significant increase in distance measurable on radiographs is a reflection of the stretching and attenuation of lamellae quantifiable histopathologically.[27] This emphasizes the importance of good-quality radiographs to assess the severity of the initial laminitis insult. Even a small increase in the dorsal hoof distal phalanx distance (HDPD) indicates to the practitioner that histopathological changes similar to those described here have occurred. Early radiographs can be used as a yardstick against which to measure any subsequent exacerbation (Fig. 14-36 to Fig. 14-43).

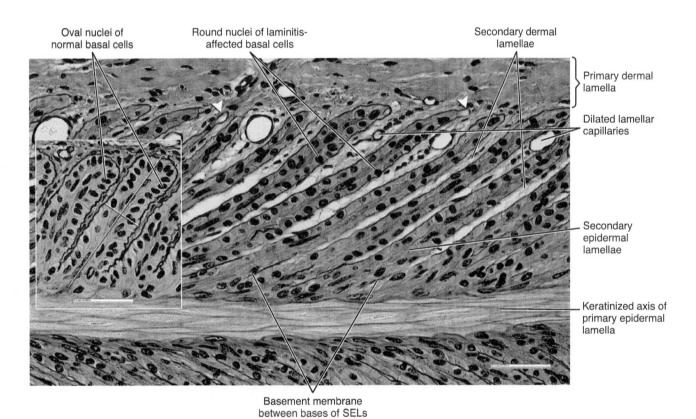

Oval nuclei of normal basal cells

Round nuclei of laminitis-affected basal cells

Secondary dermal lamellae

Primary dermal lamella

Dilated lamellar capillaries

Secondary epidermal lamellae

Keratinized axis of primary epidermal lamella

Basement membrane between bases of SELs

• **Figure 14.2** Grade 1 laminitis histopathology. Photomicrograph of transverse section of dorsal, midwall secondary epidermal lamellae (SELs) affected by oligofructose-induced laminitis (the sepsis-related laminitis model). The tissues are stained with periodic acid–Schiff's (PAS) reagent to highlight the carbohydrate-rich, magenta-colored, basement membrane (*arrows*). The inset shows normal SELs photographed to the same scale; the yellow line shows SEL length (approximately 125 μm), and the white line shows SEL width (approximately 25 μm). The histopathology is scored grade 1 because the SELs are stretched, long, and thin, with tapering instead of club-shaped tips. The laminitis-affected SELs are almost twice their normal length and half their width; approximately 245 μm and 15 μm, respectively. SEL stretching results in fewer basal cell nuclei per micrometer of SEL, and the basal cell nuclei are round instead of oval and positioned abnormally close to the lamellar basement membrane. Some cells retain an oval-shaped nucleus, but the long axis of the nucleus is parallel to the basement membrane (BM) instead of at right angles to it (compare with the normal nuclei in the inset). Teat-shaped bubbles of loose, detached BM are present at the tips of some SELs (*arrowheads*). Lamellar BM, although faded and blurred in places, is still present at the tips of secondary dermal lamellae, between the bases of SELs close to the keratinized axis of the primary epidermal lamella. The large diameter of the lamellar capillaries suggests the circulation was vasodilated at this stage of laminitis development. (Stain = periodic acid-Schiff (PAS). Bars = 50 μm.)

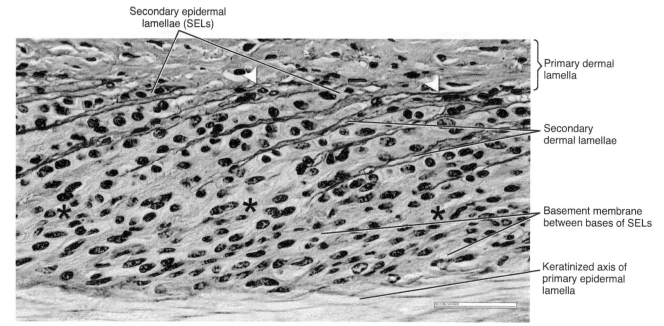

- **Figure 14.3** Grade 2 laminitis histopathology. Photomicrograph of transverse section of dorsal, midwall secondary epidermal lamellae (SELs) affected by oligofructose-induced laminitis (the sepsis-related laminitis model). The tissues are stained with periodic acid–Schiff's (PAS) reagent to highlight the carbohydrate-rich, magenta-colored, basement membrane. The histopathology is scored grade 2 because it is more advanced than the grade 1 histopathology shown in Figure 14-36. The teat-shaped bubbles of loose, detached BM that were present at the tips of some SELs in Figure 14-36 are now more extensive and have been drawn out into double-layered strands of BM (*arrowheads*). Lamellar BM is no longer present at the tips of secondary dermal lamellae, between the bases of SELs. Epidermal basal cells, without the controlling influence of an intact, functional basement membrane, are beginning to coalesce into an unstructured mass with compromised suspensory function (*asterisks*). (Stain = periodic acid Schiff (PAS).. Bar = 50 μm.)

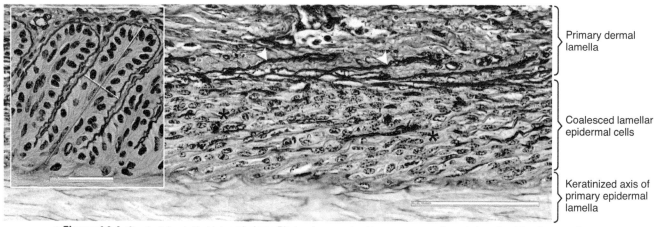

- **Figure 14.4** Grade 3 laminitis histopathology. Photomicrograph of transverse section of dorsal, midwall secondary epidermal lamellae (SELs) affected by oligofructose-induced laminitis (the sepsis-related laminitis model). The tissues are stained with periodic acid–Schiff's (PAS) reagent to highlight the carbohydrate-rich, magenta-colored, basement membrane. The histopathology is scored grade 3 because it is more advanced than the grade 2 histopathology shown in Figure 14-37. The drawn-out, double-layered strands of BM (*arrowheads*) are longer and now measure approximately 130 μm, which is equivalent to the length of a normal SEL (*inset*). Virtually all the BM has been stripped from each SEL and has been relocated to the edges of the primary dermal lamella. Secondary dermal lamellae are devoid of functional BM, and virtually all lamellar epidermal cells have coalesced into a multicellular, unstructured mass (*asterisks*). With the BM detached and epidermal lamellae reduced in surface area, the ability of the lamellae to suspend the distal phalanx is severely compromised. The distal phalanx sinks deeply into the hoof capsule in feet with grade 3 laminitis histopathology. Clinically, there is severe, crippling pain scoring Grade III or IV on the Obel laminitis pain scale. (Stain = periodic acid-Schiff [PAS]. Bar = 50 μm.)

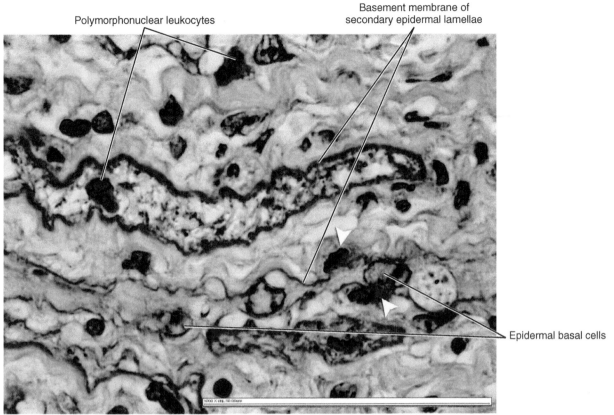

Polymorphonuclear leukocytes

Basement membrane of
secondary epidermal lamellae

Epidermal basal cells

● **Figure 14.5** Grade 3 laminitis histopathology. High-magnification photomicrograph of transverse section of dorsal, midwall secondary epidermal lamellae (SELs) affected by oligofructose-induced laminitis (the sepsis-related laminitis model). The tissues are stained with periodic acid–Schiff's (PAS) reagent to highlight the carbohydrate-rich, magenta-colored, basement membrane and the granules within polymorphonuclear leukocytes (PMNs). The high-magnification image shows the basement membrane (BM) that was stripped from the tips of SELs is the focus of an inflammatory response. Some PMNs have entered the empty BM compartment to lyse and phagocytise its contents, and others (*arrowheads*) are adjacent to the BM and appear to have lysed it. Not all the separated, double-stranded BM is devoid of lamellar epidermal basal cells (LEBCs). Some basal cells remain BM enclosed and survive, isolated in the lamellar dermis. In the days that follow the acute episode, these LEBCs proliferate and form BM-bound islands of epidermis (Figures 14-42 and 14-43) and, failing to connect to the lamellar axis, contribute little to the suspension of the distal phalanx within the hoof capsule. (Stain = periodic acid Schiff (PAS). Bar = 50 μm.)

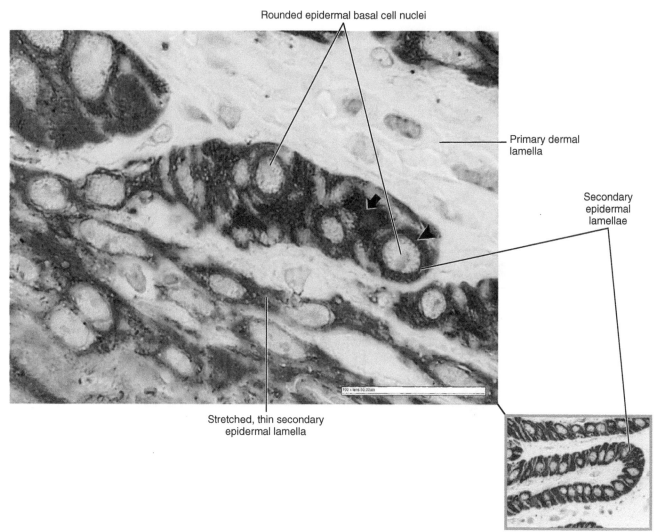

Rounded epidermal basal cell nuclei

Primary dermal lamella

Secondary epidermal lamellae

Stretched, thin secondary epidermal lamella

● **Figure 14.6** Grade 2 laminitis histopathology. Photomicrograph of transverse section of dorsal, midwall lamellae, immunostained for cytokeratin 14 (K14). Cytokeratin intermediate filaments form the majority of the lamellar epidermal basal cell (LEBC) cytoskeleton and localize to two attachment plaques: hemidesmosomes and desmosomes forming a multifilament suspensory cradle for the cell nucleus in the cytoplasm of the cell (Fig. 8-19). In laminitis-affected LEBCs, the dark brown immunostained K14 cytoskeleton (*arrowhead*) is no longer linked to attachment plaques and has condensed around the now rounded nucleus. In other LEBCs, the cytoskeleton has coalesced in the center of the LEBC (*arrow*) and is not connected to either the basal plasmalemma or the apical and lateral plasmalemma. Disintegration of both the LEBC cytoskeleton and the adhesion plaques between lamellar cells leads to thinning and stretching of secondary epidermal lamellae, ultimately compromising the suspension of the distal phalanx within the hoof capsule. The inset shows cytokeratin K14 staining of normal lamellae. (Bar = 50 µm.)

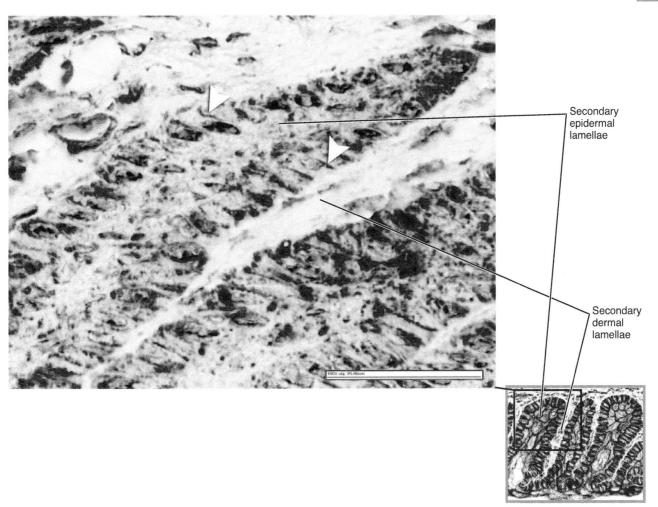

Secondary
epidermal
lamellae

Secondary
dermal
lamellae

●**Figure 14.7** Actin immunostaining of laminitis-affected lamellar epidermal basal cells (LEBCs) in transverse section. The laminitis was induced in Standardbred horses by the hyperinsulinaemic euglycaemic clamp technique. In transverse sections of normal lamellae, actin associates with adherens junctions, the attachment plaques bridging adjacent LEBCs and the dark-brown immunostaining due to actin characterizes the lateral boundaries of adjacent LEBCs (inset and Fig 8.20, 8.15 and 8.21). In lamellae affected by hyperinsulinaemia the normal pattern of actin immunostaining has been obliterated and the boundaries between adjacent LEBCs can no longer be distinguished by actin immunostaining. Disintegration of adherens junctions has dispersed actin and only remnants of organised actin remain (arrowheads). Lacking functional attachments between adjacent LEBCs the secondary epidermal lamellae are abnormally narrow and elongated. Bar = 25 μm (0.025 mm).

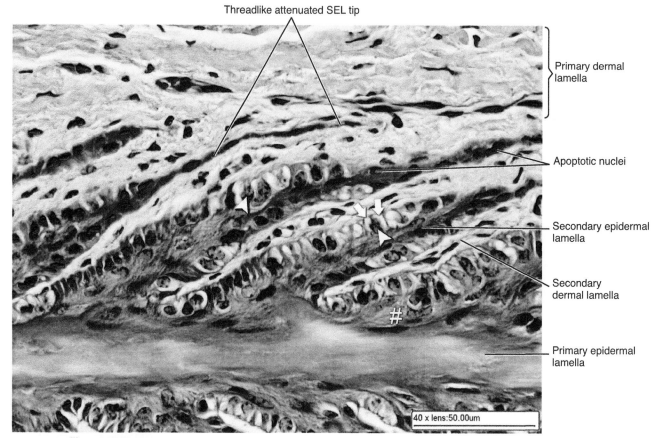

Threadlike attenuated SEL tip

Primary dermal lamella

Apoptotic nuclei

Secondary epidermal lamella

Secondary dermal lamella

Primary epidermal lamella

40 x lens:50.00um

● **Figure 14.8** Histopathology of laminitis induced by 48-hour hyperinsulinemia in an adult Standardbred (transverse section). The areas of clear cytoplasm (*arrows*) beside the nucleus (*arrowheads*) bordering the lateral walls of most of the lamellar epidermal basal cells suggest collapse of the actin cytoskeleton (see Fig. 14-34). However, the keratin intermediate filament cytoskeleton, an eosinophilic band between the nucleus and the basal plasma membrane, is still intact, suggesting that hemidesmosomes in some cells have survived. As a result of cytoskeleton and attachment plaque degradation, the tips of many secondary epidermal lamellae (SELs) are extremely attenuated and stretched into fine threads. The LEBC nuclei in the stretched tips are dark and condensed consistent with apoptosis. (Stain = haematoxylin and eosin. Bar = 50 µm.)

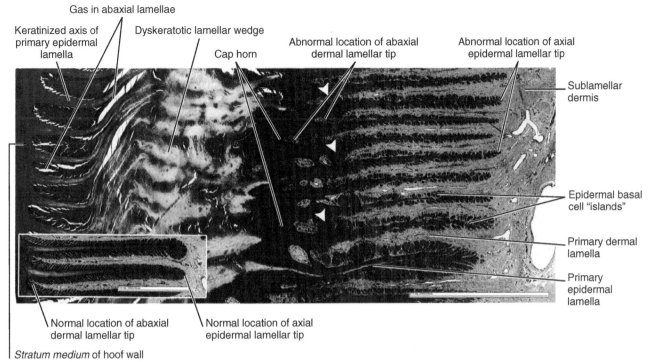

Gas in abaxial lamellae

Keratinized axis of primary epidermal lamella

Dyskeratotic lamellar wedge

Cap horn

Abnormal location of abaxial dermal lamellar tip

Abnormal location of axial epidermal lamellar tip

Sublamellar dermis

Epidermal basal cell "islands"

Primary dermal lamella

Primary epidermal lamella

Normal location of abaxial dermal lamellar tip

Normal location of axial epidermal lamellar tip

Stratum medium of hoof wall

• **Figure 14.9** Chronic laminitis histopathology in an adult Standardbred gelding seven weeks after oligofructose-induced laminitis (the sepsis-related laminitis model). At 48 hours after laminitis induction, a lamellar biopsy showed grade 3 laminitis histopathology (Figure 14-38 ABC). The inset shows normal lamellae, aligned with the inner hoof wall, at the same scale as the main image. The laminitis-affected epidermal lamellae are triple their normal length, approximately 4.3 mm longer than normal. Lamellar displacement of this magnitude is associated with dislocation of the distal phalanx and is reflected on lateromedial radiographs as an increase in the distance between the distal phalanx and the hoof wall and an increase in the "founder distance" (Figure 14-33). There is severe compromise to the suspensory apparatus of the distal phalanx (SADP) because most secondary epidermal lamellae (SELs) are no longer connected to the central keratinized axes of primary epidermal lamellae; the surface area of SADP attachment is thus significantly reduced. This disconnect between lamellae and hoof means that pain-free suspension of the distal phalanx within the hoof capsule is lost, evidenced clinically, in this case, by a score of Obel grade II on the laminitis pain scale. SELs are represented by irregularly shaped, ovoid, basement membrane–bound islands of epidermal basal cells lacking connection to the central lamellar axis. Cap horn has formed between more abaxial lamellae, as well as dyskeratotic tubules (*arrowheads*). During the acute phase, the abaxial dermal lamellae were stripped from their normal location, leaving the abaxial epidermal lamellae avascular. A large mass of radiopaque (Figure 11-4 and 14-9) dyskeratotic horn, the "lamellar wedge," now occupies this lamellar avascular zone. The lamellae adjacent to the *stratum medium* of the hoof wall are empty of tissue but contain gas (possibly air) that shows as a radiolucent line on lateromedial radiographs (Figure 14-2 AB). The isolated islands of epidermal basal cells form within seven days of laminitis induction.[1] Their presence here, seven weeks after induction, suggests that reconnection of basal cell islands to form normal SELs is not likely to happen. In the hours and days following the acute phase, LEBCs become enclosed by basement membrane and remain marooned in the lamellar dermis, unable to contribute effectively to the SADP. Stain = haematoxylin and eosin. Bar in main picture = 2000 μm (2.0 mm).

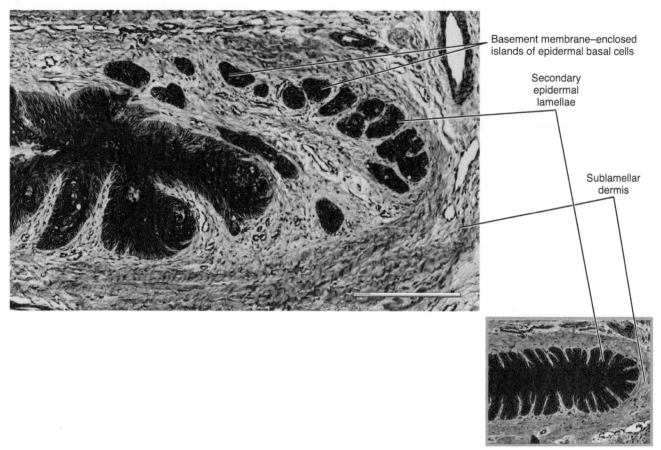

Basement membrane–enclosed
islands of epidermal basal cells

Secondary
epidermal
lamellae

Sublamellar
dermis

● **Figure 14.10** Chronic laminitis histopathology in an adult Standardbred gelding seven weeks after oligofructose-induced laminitis (same specimen as in Figure 14-42). The main photomicrograph shows the axial tip of a single, midwall epidermal lamella. The inset shows the tip of a normal axial lamella (not to scale). The epidermal lamellae are fragmented, and secondary epidermal lamellae are represented by irregularly shaped islands of basement membrane–bound epidermal basal cells no longer connected to the axis of its primary epidermal lamella. Thus the surface area available for suspension of the distal phalanx is significantly reduced. Stain = haematoxylin and eosin. (Bar in main picture = 200 μm (0.2 mm).

CASE HISTORY 1: PERACUTE, SEVERE LAMINITIS IN AN ARABIAN MARE

An adult Arabian mare developed severe colitis with pyrexia and systemic septicemia. Despite intensive care, clinical laminitis developed within 48 hours, and with the mare recumbent and serum oozing from the heels, she was euthanized. One front foot was CT scanned to create a Mimics® model of the foot. The other foot was radiographed, sectioned with a band saw, and photographed; tissues were prepared for histopathological examination and examined by light microscopy.

At first glance, the radiographic images were unremarkable. However, when measurements were made the distance between the outer hoof wall and the adjacent distal phalanx cortex was 22 mm instead of the expected 17 mm. The founder distance was 16 mm, more than double the upper limit of the normal—4.1 ± 2.17 mm.[4] Few horses with founder distances greater than 15.2 mm can be treated successfully and either die or are euthanized.[3] Remarkably,

considering the intensity of the clinical pain, there was no rotation of either the hoof or the distal phalanx.

When sectioned with a band saw, the lamellar dermis separated from the epidermal lamellae of the inner hoof wall. The distal phalanx was loose inside the hoof capsule and had sunk downward, crushing the dorsal solar dermis, which appeared blanched, as if blood had been compressed from it. There was a clear space between the lamellar dermis, which was still attached to the parietal cortex of the distal phalanx, and the epidermal lamellae of the inner hoof wall. The coronary papillae were distracted distally as if plucked from their epidermal sockets by the descent of the distal phalanx.

This indicated catastrophic failure of the suspensory apparatus of the distal phalanx and explained the severe and rapid development of the clinical signs and great pain suffered by the mare. Euthanasia was the only humane option.

The Mimics® model showed the distal phalanx, in separating from the inner hoof wall, had sunk onto the sole. The normal space between the margin of the distal phalanx and the horny sole was absent because the distal phalanx (DP) was no longer suspended by its suspensory apparatus. In this situation the margin of the DP crushes the nerves and blood vessels of the solear dermis and explains the intense pain and suffering.

Histopathology showed the dermal and epidermal lamellae as two separate entities, one degloved from the other. The axial tips of some epidermal lamellae had snapped off and were present, still in their original position, in the dermis. Many of the remnant epidermal lamellae were stripped of basal cells, while others were relatively unaffected. Isolated secondary epidermal lamellae, ruptured from their attachment to the keratinized axes of primary epidermal lamellae, lined the edges of primary dermal lamellae.

Most of the secondary epidermal lamellae had lost their detached basal and parabasal cell populations, leaving only the empty basement membrane "shell" embedded in the dermis. However, a few basal cells survived, and with many in mitosis, a healing response was already under way.

This case was instructive on several counts. It showed how rapidly colitis and the associated laminitis can destroy the suspensory apparatus of the distal phalanx. The cause of the colitis was not established, so we can only speculate which microbes and their toxins were involved. There were few outward signs that the hoof capsule was damaged—not enough time had elapsed for a "dropped" sole or a "laminitic" hoof ring to develop. However, the coronary cushion had sunk below the sharp proximal edge of the *stratum medium,* making the coronet concave instead of the normal convex. This tissue "deficit" in the entire coronary band, extending from heel to heel, is the hallmark of the "sinker," the worst-case scenario for laminitis. Even radiographs were unremarkable at first glance. The pain experienced by the mare was intense, demonstrating the consequences of pressure between bone and sole. The importance of an intact functional suspensory apparatus of the distal phalanx cannot be overestimated. When it fails, as this case shows, the consequences are catastrophic. Interestingly, laminitis associated with colitis has been successfully prevented using distal limb cooling in an equine hospital. The odds of developing laminitis from colitis were reduced 10 times if effective distal limb cooling was part of the treatment regimen (Fig. 14-44 to Fig. 14-45).

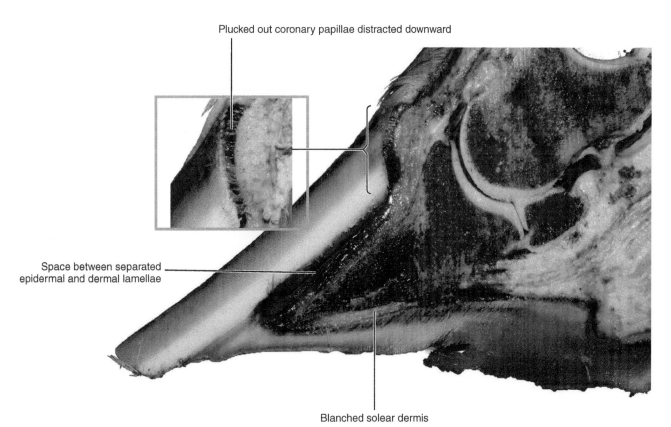

Plucked out coronary papillae distracted downward

Space between separated epidermal and dermal lamellae

Blanched solear dermis

• **Figure 14.11** Front foot sagittal section from colitis-affected mare with severe, rapid-onset laminitis. The lamellar dermis has separated from the epidermal lamellae of the inner hoof wall, leaving a clear space. The distal phalanx has sunk downward onto the dorsal solar dermis, which appears blanched, as if blood has been compressed from it. The inset shows the coronary papillae distracted distally and plucked from their epidermal sockets by the descent of the distal phalanx.

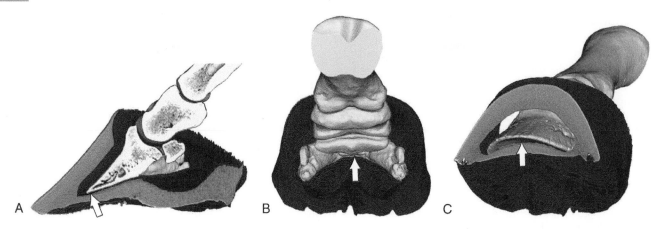

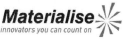

• Figure 14.12 Mimics model of the front foot from the colitis-affected mare with severe, rapid-onset laminitis, showing the anatomic relationship between the distal phalanx (DP) and the hoof capsule. The DP margin is in abnormally close contact with the sole. The arrows, in **A, B,** and **C,** show the absence of the "space," in life, the dermis, normally between the distal phalanx and the horny sole (compare with normal Mimics models in Figure 6.12). The DP distal margin, in contact with the sole, crushes the solear dermis, causing severe pain. With each step the horse attempts, breakover levers the bone down onto the contused dermis. Hence, the laminitis gait: shuffling, with the feet kept forward to avoid the posterior, breakover phase of the stride.

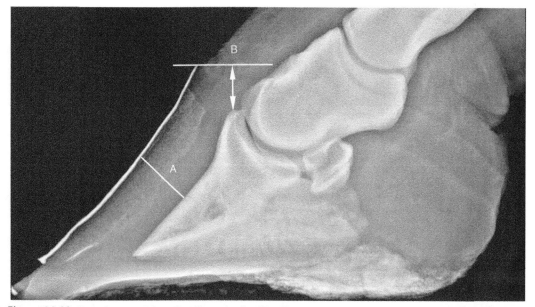

• Figure 14.13 Front foot mediolateral radiograph of colitis-affected mare with severe, rapid-onset laminitis. The distance **A** is 22 mm instead of the expected 17 mm. There is no rotation of either the hoof or the distal phalanx. The sublamellar and solear dermis, normally a radiolucent zone adjacent to the dorsal distal phalanx, is absent, especially beneath the solear distal margin. The distance between line **B**, the proximal border of the *stratum medium*, and the proximal extensor process (the "founder distance") is 16 mm, more than double the normal 4 to 6 mm. The distal phalanx has sunk and is dislocated within the hoof capsule (Compare with normal radiographs in Figs 12.1 and 12.4). (Radiograph by Tori McGuire, WestVETS Equine Hospital.)

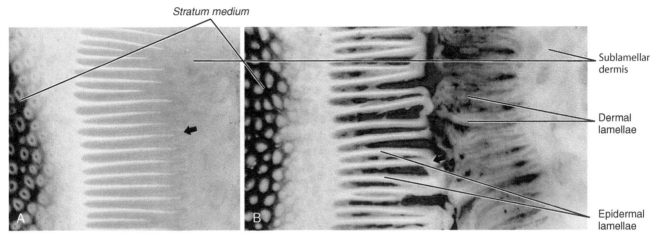

Stratum medium

Sublamellar dermis

Dermal lamellae

Epidermal lamellae

• Figure 14.14 Photographs of unstained sections cut from the midwall lamellae of a normal horse (**A**) and from the colitis-affected mare with severe, rapid-onset laminitis (**B**). The axial tips of normal lamellae are transparent (*arrow*). In the laminitis-affected tissue (**B**), the axial tips are blood-stained and displaced (*arrow*); there is a clear space between the lamellar dermis and the epidermal lamellae of the inner hoof wall.

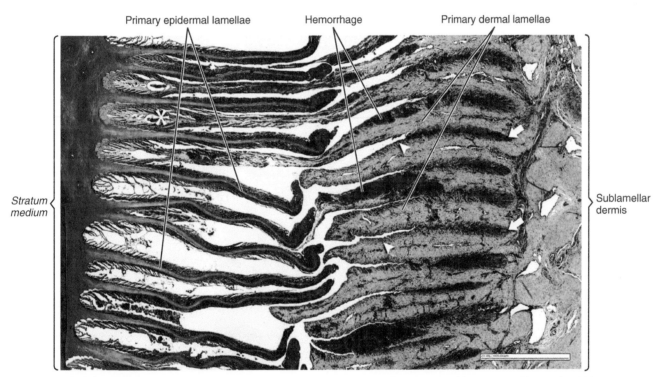

Primary epidermal lamellae   Hemorrhage   Primary dermal lamellae

Stratum medium

Sublamellar dermis

• Figure 14.15 Photomicrograph of midwall lamellae from the colitis-affected mare with severe, rapid-onset laminitis. The detachment between epidermal and dermal lamellae is near complete. The axial tips of some epidermal lamellae appear to have snapped off and are still present in their original position in the dermis (*arrows*). Many of the remnant epidermal lamellae are stripped of basal cells while others are relatively unaffected (*asterisk*). Secondary epidermal lamellae, ruptured from their attachment to the keratinized axes of primary epidermal lamellae, line the edges of primary dermal lamellae (*arrowheads*). (Stain = haematoxylin and eosin. Bar = 1000 μm [1 mm].)

Hemorrhage replacing absent
primary epidermal lamellae

Primary dermal lamella

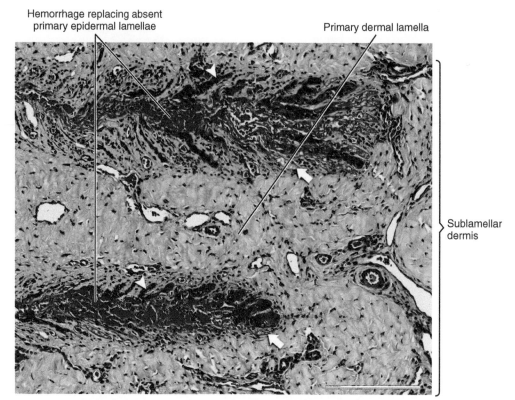

Sublamellar
dermis

● **Figure 14.16** Photomicrograph of midwall lamellae from the colitis-affected mare with severe, rapid-onset laminitis. Secondary epidermal lamellae (*arrowheads*), without attachment to the keratinized axes of primary epidermal lamellae (PELs), line the edges of primary dermal lamellae. Hemorrhage has filled the spaces created by the traumatic exit of the PELs. Many secondary epidermal lamellae are devoid of basal cells but are represented by the remnants of their basement membranes. Many newly arrived inflammatory cells are already within damaged lamellae. (Stain = haematoxylin and eosin. Bar = 200 μm [0.2 mm].)

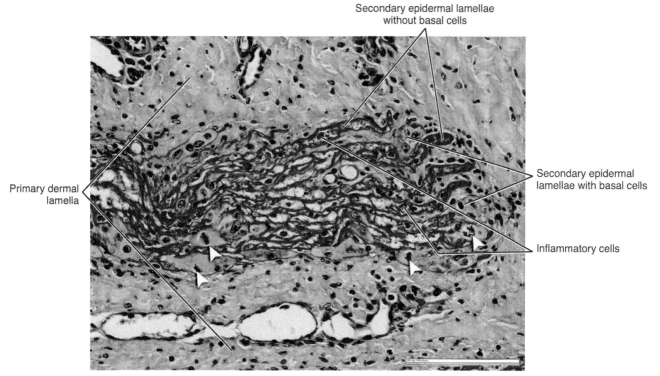

Secondary epidermal lamellae
without basal cells

Secondary epidermal
lamellae with basal cells

Primary dermal
lamella

Inflammatory cells

● **Figure 14.17** Photomicrograph of the axial tip of a midwall lamella from the colitis-affected mare with severe, rapid-onset laminitis. The lamellar basement membrane is colored magenta by periodic acid Schiff staining. Most of the secondary epidermal lamellae have lost their detached basal and parabasal cell populations, leaving only the empty basement membrane embedded in the dermis. However, a few basal cells survived and the numerous mitotic figures (*arrowheads*) among their nuclei suggest epidermal proliferation is under way. Many inflammatory cells have infiltrated the damaged lamellae. (Stain = periodic acid–Schiff. Bar = 150 μm [0.15 mm].)

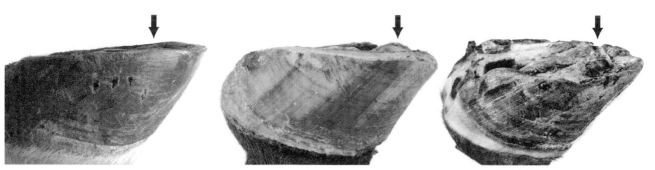

● **Figure 14.18** The convex "dropped" sole (*arrows*) of chronic laminitis is generally a grave clinical finding. It indicates that the distal phalanx has descended into the hoof capsule and crushed the solear dermis, causing varying degrees of necrosis of the horny sole. In severe cases (far right) there is prolapse of the distal phalanx and its associated dermis through the crescent-shaped zone of horny sole necrosis. Although the foot on the far left seems a relatively mild example, there was nevertheless extensive lysis of the distal phalanx and distortion of tubular horn growth (Fig. 14-51).

CASE HISTORY 2: SEVERE CHROINIC LAMINITIS IN A THOROUGHBRED COLT

A young Thoroughbred colt, in preparation for race training, developed a relatively mild colitis that responded to therapy. Intermittent lameness followed, but foot radiographs showed only "mild" changes. Five months later the colt was again ill and inappetant with moderate 3/5 lameness; hoof testing over the sole provoked a brisk, positive pain response. Radiographs were still considered unremarkable. Six months after the initial episode of colitis new radiographs showed capsular rotation, modeling and lysis of the distal phalanx with "ski-tip" formation. Support shoes with silicone packing to the palmar sole had little clinical impact.

Nine months after the initial colitis, radiographs and venograms showed severe distal phalanx modeling and lysis and significant deficits in the contrast medium filling of sublamellar vessels. With permanent damage to the suspensory apparatus of the distal phalanx and to the distal phalanx itself, as well as unremitting pain, the colt was euthanized on humane grounds. The feet were submitted for gross pathology, histopathology, and CT examinations. The results illustrate the difficulty of diagnosing the insidious progression of a destructive lamellar wedge. Understanding the destructive consequences of lamellar wedge development in this case emphasizes the importance of early detection and effective corrective strategies. (Fig. 14-52 to Fig. 14-7).

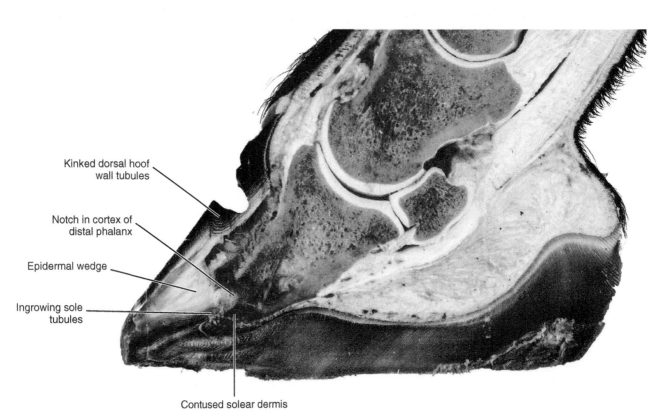

Kinked dorsal hoof wall tubules

Notch in cortex of distal phalanx

Epidermal wedge

Ingrowing sole tubules

Contused solear dermis

● **Figure 14.19** Sagittal section of the front foot of the Thoroughbred colt with severe chronic laminitis. The dorsal hoof wall has been trimmed away distally but still shows tubule kinking in the midwall region, suggesting the major laminitis episode, in terms of SADP failure and sinking of the distal phalanx (DP), occurred four to five months earlier. The coronary dermis and coronary horn production appear normal. The dorsal hoof wall is not parallel to the parietal DP surface, indicating some rotation of the hoof capsule. The DP margin is abnormally close to the dorsal sole; the solear dermis in this region is contused. There is a lytic notch in the distal parietal cortex of the DP, just proximad to the distal margin, that is occupied by in-growing epidermal tissue. The source of the epidermal tissue is a large toe wedge consisting of dysplastic lamellae, terminal (white line), and dorsal sole tubules.

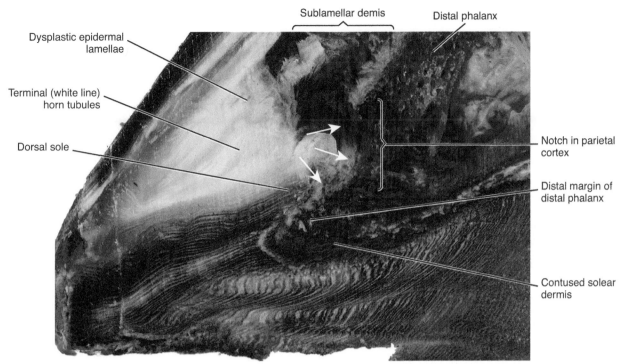

Sublamellar demis

Distal phalanx

Dysplastic epidermal lamellae

Terminal (white line) horn tubules

Dorsal sole

Notch in parietal cortex

Distal margin of distal phalanx

Contused solear dermis

• **Figure 14.20** Closeup photograph of the toe in Figure 14.9. Higher magnification shows the notch in the parietal cortex of the distal phalanx (proximad to the distal margin) and the tubular epidermal tissue occupying the notch. Pigmented dorsal sole and nonpigmented terminal (white line) tubule horn are displaced proximally and have grown into the DP notch (arrows show the direction of growth). The sole tubules beneath the DP margin and the contused solear dermis are kinked and dysplastic.

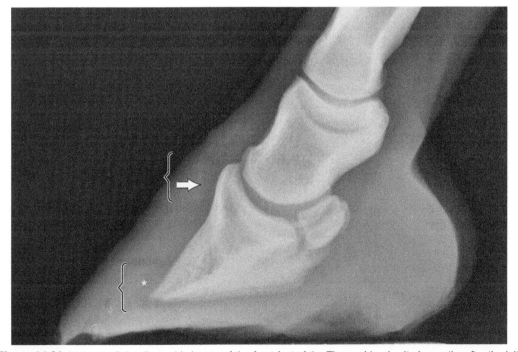

• **Figure 14.21** Lateromedial radiographic image of the front foot of the Thoroughbred colt six months after the initial colitis. The hoof distal phalanx distance (HDPD) is markedly increased and the radiolucent zone, normally present around the DP, is largely absent (see normal radiographs in figures 12.1 and 12.4). In particular, radiodense material is closely associated with the distal 25% of the DP dorsal cortex and lytic notch (*asterisk*) formation has commenced. There is remodeling of the DP distal margin. The DP is aligned with the phalangeal axis (not rotated). The orientation of the proximal hoof wall is abnormal and directed toward the DP extensor process, in the direction of the arrow. Venography may have detected the encroaching tubular hoof material, and strategic hoof resection (in the zones bracketed) may have prevented what happened next.

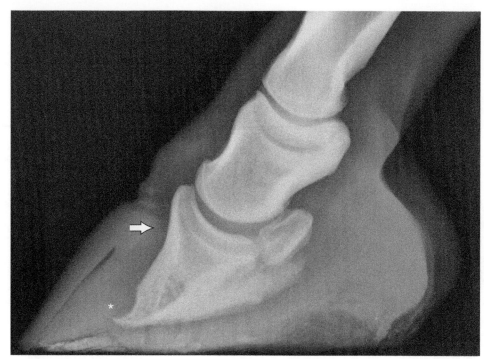

• **Figure 14.22** Lateromedial radiographic image of the front foot of the Thoroughbred colt foot nine months after the initial colitis. The appearance of a lucent line beneath the hoof wall, absent three months earlier, suggests a second episode superimposed on an earlier episode(s). The hoof distal phalanx distance (HDPD) has continued to increase, and radiodense material occupies a notch that has formed in the distal 25% of the distal phalanx (DP) dorsal cortex (*asterisk*). Note the lytic notch is proximal to the DP distal margin. The DP is not aligned with the phalangeal axis (an example of phalangeal rotation). The radiopaque proximal hoof wall is abnormally close to the proximal distal phalanx (*arrow*).

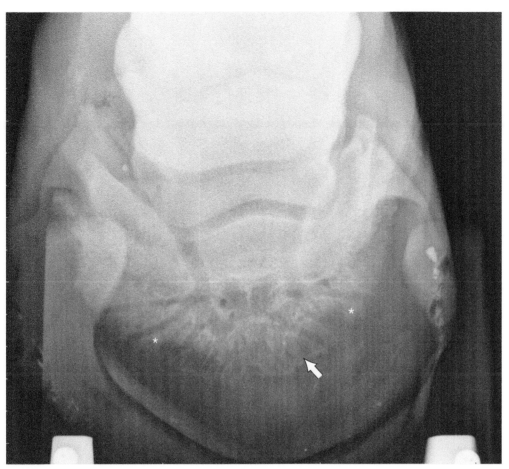

● **Figure 14.23** Dorsal 65° proximal–palmarodistal oblique radiographic image of the Thoroughbred colt foot nine months after the initial colitis. The lysis of the distal phalanx, manifest as a notch in the dorsal cortex in the lateromedial projection, extends medially and laterally as a lucent shadow (*between asterisks*). The extent of this bone lysis is greater medially. Interestingly, the DP distal margin (*arrow*) is still present (compare with normal radiograph in figure 12.2).

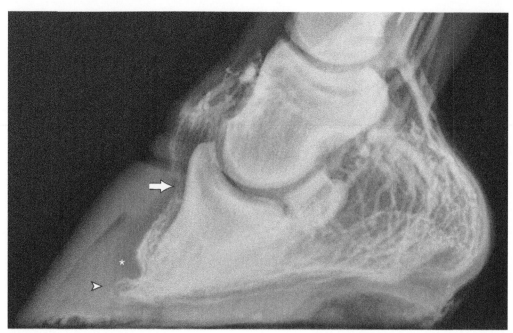

• **Figure 14.24** Lateromedial contrast-enhanced radiographic image (venogram) of the Thoroughbred colt front foot nine months after the initial colitis. The radiodense material occupying the notch in the distal phalanx is outlined by contrast medium (*asterisk*). The absence of contrast in the space-occupying mass suggests an epidermal origin. The abnormal location and orientation of contrast-filled terminal and solar papillae (*arrowhead*) indicates the presence of dislocated tubular horn. The proximal hoof wall, abnormally close to the DP extensor process (*arrow*), is not associated with bone lysis but has compressed the veins in this region and prevented their filling with contrast medium (compare with normal radiographs in figures 12.5 and 12.6).

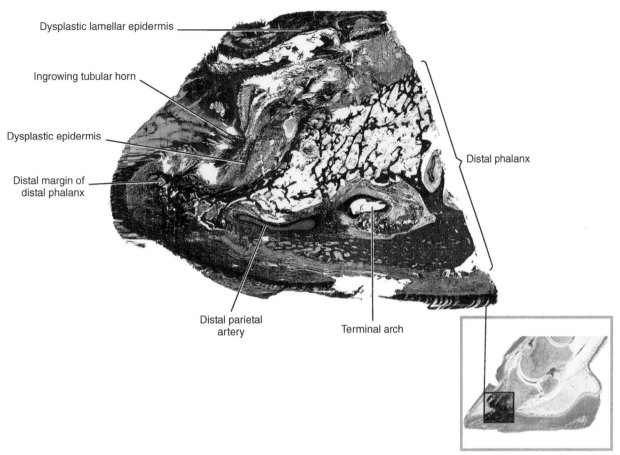

Dysplastic lamellar epidermis

Ingrowing tubular horn

Dysplastic epidermis

Distal margin of
distal phalanx

Distal phalanx

Distal parietal
artery

Terminal arch

• **Figure 14.25** Decalcified histologic section of the Thoroughbred colt dorsal, distal phalanx (DP) stained with Masson's trichrome. Bone and epidermis are stained red and connective tissue is stained blue. The parietal DP cortex lacks an organized cortex and is extremely porotic, evidence of active lysis. Bone lysis has created a deep notch in the distal parietal cortex proximad to the distal margin. Connective tissue and dysplastic epidermis occupies the notch, and dorsal to the notch there is displaced, tubular dorsal sole and terminal (white line) horn; the lamellar wedge. The palmar solear cortex of the distal phalanx is normal, but dorsally, it is encircled by tubular epidermis and is extensively remodeled. The box in the inset shows the provenance of the section.

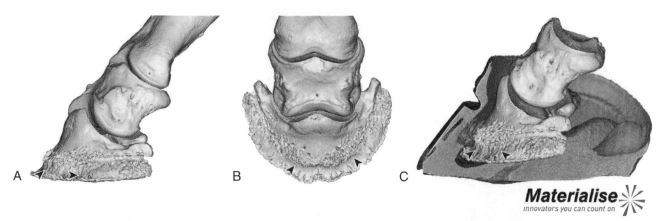

● Figure 14.26 Mimics models of CT data from the foot of the Thoroughbred colt with severe chronic laminitis. There is extensive modeling of the distal phalanx and what appeared to be a "ski-tip" notch on lateromedial radiographs is actually a broad zone of bone lysis that has created a deep groove (*arrowheads*) in the distal bone, extending over the dorsal half of the bone (**A** and **B**). Proximad to the notch the parietal cortex is characterized by spicules of new bone formation. The relationship between the hoof capsule and the remodeled distal phalanx is shown in **C.** Ridges of hard tubular horn project toward the groove in the distal parietal cortex of the distal phalanx.

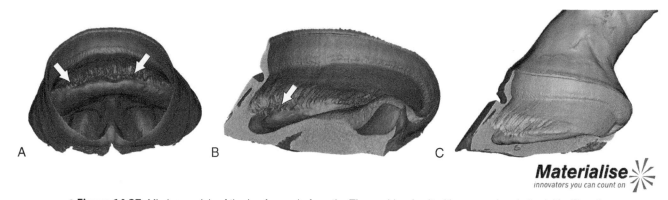

● Figure 14.27 Mimics models of the hoof capsule from the Thoroughbred colt with severe chronic laminitis. The dislocation of the distal phalanx that accompanied the initial episode of laminitis has caused significant changes to hoof architecture. The palmar view of the empty hoof capsule (**A**) shows a ridge of hard horn (*arrows*) projecting inwards from the distal third of the dorsal hoof wall. The sagittal view of the hoof capsule (**B**) shows the ridge (*arrow*) extending over the dorsal half of the inside hoof wall. The relationship between the lamellar dermis is shown in **C.** The horny ridge impinges and compresses the dermis distally but not proximally.

INSULIN AND LAMINITIS

All tissues need glucose (blood sugar) for energy, but most tissues, including the lamellae of the horse's hoof, can only take up glucose from the bloodstream with the help of glucose transport proteins (GLUTs). There are a number of different GLUT proteins. The glucose transport for the equine hoof epidermal lamellae is GLUT1, which is not affected by insulin. The GLUT4 proteins of muscle and other tissues are switched on by insulin, and when they become unresponsive, the body makes more insulin to compensate. Insulin concentrations in the blood are a good diagnostic marker (or risk factor) for laminitis.

Equine Metabolic Syndrome

The term *equine metabolic syndrome* refers to horses with a history of laminitis, insulin resistance, cresty necks, and increased adipose tissue deposits in the withers and dorsal area of the back.[12] Elevated serum insulin concentrations distinguish ponies that are susceptible to dietary pasture-associated laminitis.[24,25] Furthermore, insulin concentrations are markedly elevated in ponies that develop laminitis after consuming high-energy diets, while their glucose, free fatty acid, and cortisol concentrations remain normal. In contrast to humans, insulin-resistant horses rarely develop pancreatic exhaustion and are capable of producing exceptionally high serum insulin concentrations.[14] Hyperinsulinemia is a key factor in triggering equine laminitis (endocrinopathic laminitis). The onset of laminitis is associated with plasma insulin concentrations exceeding 100 μIU/ml (normal range = 8 to 30 μIU/ml).[29]

Hyperinsulinemic Laminitis

To test the hypothesis that hyperinsulinemia triggers laminitis, normal, lean ponies and Standardbred horses, with no prior history of insulin resistance or laminitis were subjected to prolonged hyperinsulinemia and euglycemia. All of the ponies developed laminitis within 72 hours of hyperinsulinemia.[1,6] This highlights the importance of insulin in the pathogenesis of endocrinopathic laminitis. Horses and ponies at risk of laminitis should be blood tested for the early detection of hyperinsulinemia. Before sampling, access to grain or other soluble carbohydrate must be prevented for three hours. A single blood sample showing elevated insulin predicts that laminitis will occur or may become worse.[29] Techniques should be employed to lower insulin concentrations and restore insulin sensitivity. A weight-reducing diet with a low glycemic index and physical exercise reduce insulin resistance in horses.[20] The search is on to find insulin-sensitizing drugs, of the type given to human patients with type 2 diabetes, that will reduce hyperinsulinemia in ponies and horses and thus the likelihood of developing endocrinopathic laminitis.

CASE HISTORY 3: HYPERINSULINEMIC LAMINITIS IN AGED PONY

A sedentary 17-year-old Australian Pony at pasture suddenly developed clinical laminitis. The pony was insulin resistant with a fasting blood insulin concentration of 300 μIU/ml at the time of onset. Normal blood insulin concentration for ponies is less than 30 μIU/ml. The foot pain experienced by the pony was difficult to control with nonsteroidal antiinflammatory drugs and progressively worsened over time. A variety of support shoes and pads were tried, but none made any lasting difference. On humane grounds the pony was euthanized and the feet collected for gross and histologic examination (Fig. 14-8 to Fig. 14-16 ABC).

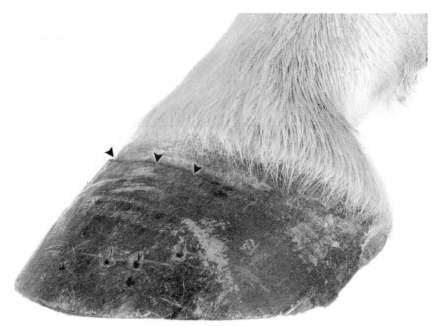

• **Figure 14.28** Photograph of the foot of the 17-year-old Australian Pony with hyperinsulinaemic laminitis 10 weeks after the first clinical signs. The deep groove (*arrowhead*) in the dorsal hoof wall developed shortly after laminitis onset. The hoof wall between the groove and the coronary band hairline has grown in the 10 weeks since the original incident. Note that the normally parallel hoof growth rings converge dorsally in this case. Compared with the quarters and heels, hoof growth in the dorsal half of the hoof appears retarded. However, this appearance is misleading, and, as the following gross sagittal sections show, the dorsal hoof wall is in fact kinked and deformed and producing normal amounts of tubular horn.

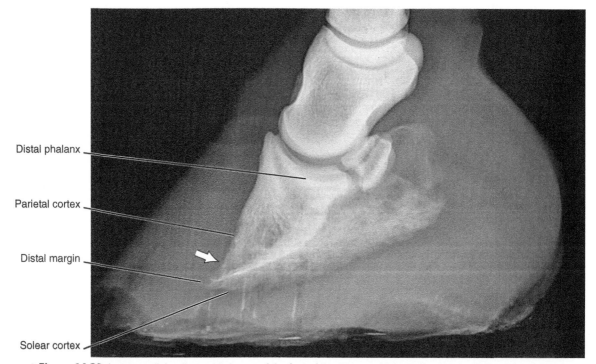

Distal phalanx

Parietal cortex

Distal margin

Solear cortex

• **Figure 14.29** Lateromedial radiographic image of the foot of the 17-year-old Australian Pony with hyperinsulinaemic laminitis of 10 weeks' duration. The hoof distal phalanx distance is double normal, and the hoof wall has rotated away from the distal phalanx (capsular rotation). The arrow locates an abnormal radiopaque mass dorsal to the distal margin of the distal phalanx that has obliterated the normally radiolucent zone around the distal margin (Compare with normal radiographs in Figure 12.1 and 12.4). There is considerable modeling and lysis of the dorsal parietal and solear cortices of the distal phalanx. The distal margin of the distal phalanx is fragmented. The solear cortex of the distal phalanx is abnormally close to the horny sole. (Radiograph Emily Mabbott, WestVETS Equine Hospital.)

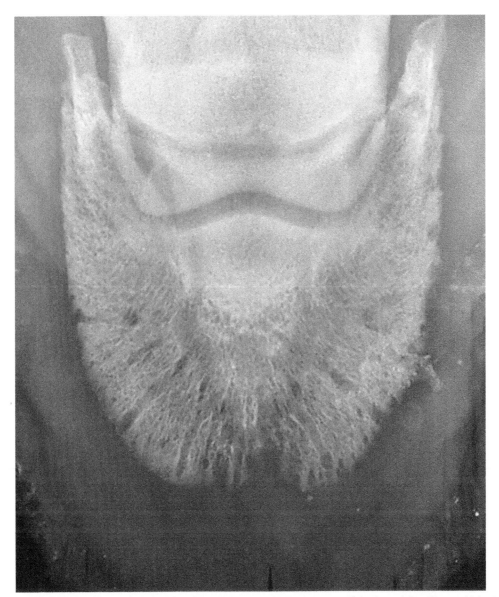

• **Figure 14.30** Dorso 65° proximal-palmarodistal oblique radiographic image of the foot of the 17-year-old Australian Pony with hyperinsulinaemic laminitis of 10 weeks' duration. The modeling and lysis of the distal margin of the distal phalanx are shown to be more extensive in this projection than in the lateromedial projection and indicate a poor likelihood of recovery to soundness. Assessing the extent of distal phalanx modeling and lysis is important in laminitis case management, and this projection should be routinely included in the laminitis radiographic protocol (Compare with normal radiograph in Figure 12.2).

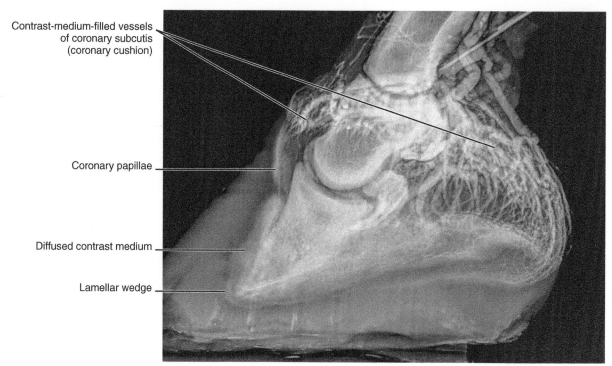

Contrast-medium-filled vessels
of coronary subcutis
(coronary cushion)

Coronary papillae

Diffused contrast medium

Lamellar wedge

● **Figure 14.31** Lateromedial contrast-enhanced radiographic image (venogram) of the 17-year-old Australian pony with hyperinsulinaemic laminitis. The palmar digital vein of the left forelimb was infused with 20 ml iodinated contrast medium. The only vessels clearly defined by contrast medium are the venous plexi of the coronary subcutis, the ungular cartilages, and the bulbs of the heels. The dorsal half of the foot lacks clear filling of veins in the coronary, sublamellar, and solear dermis (Compare with normal radiographs in Figures 12.5 and 12.6). Clear filling of veins is prevented by compression of the dermis by displaced proximal and distal tubular horn and lamellar wedge enlargement. Axial to the radiopaque epidermal lamellar wedge, contrast medium has diffused from vessels in the lamellar dermis, creating a cloudy, opaque pattern corresponding to the lamellar dermis shown in the gross sagittal section (Fig. 14-12). The vascular pattern of the contrast medium in the coronary papillae also corresponds to the direction of the proximal dorsal hoof wall tubular horn in the gross sagittal section. (Radiography Emily Mabbott, WestVETS Equine Hospital.)

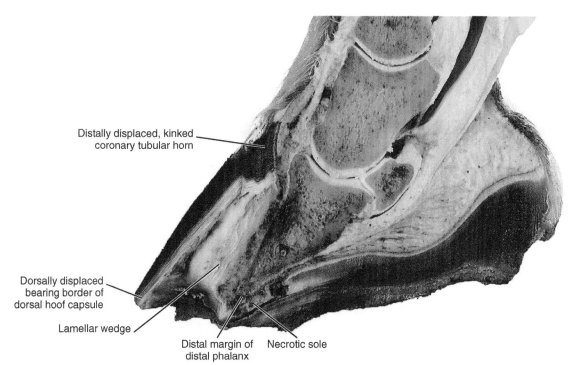

Distally displaced, kinked
coronary tubular horn

Dorsally displaced
bearing border of
dorsal hoof capsule

Lamellar wedge

Distal margin of
distal phalanx

Necrotic sole

• **Figure 14.32** Sagittal section of the foot of the 17-year-old Australian Pony with hyperinsulinaemic laminitis of 10 weeks' duration. The distal phalanx has sunk deep into the hoof capsule, and its dorsal solear margin is in contact with the now necrotic horny sole. The founder distance is twice normal, and the coronary horn tubules are kinked and displaced distally, explaining the apparent retardation of dorsal hoof growth shown in Figure 14-8. There is a large lamellar wedge between the dorsal hoof wall and the parietal surface of the distal phalanx. The distal part of the wedge is made up of tubular terminal horn and dorsal sole that is likely proliferating, expanding, and growing palmarly in the direction of the distal margin of the distal phalanx. The bearing border of the dorsal hoof wall is distracted so far dorsally from the distal phalanx that it is unable to bear weight. This forces the foot to be loaded on the dorsal sole directly beneath the dislocated distal phalanx. This explains the bone lysis and modeling, the contused solear dermis, the pressure necrosis and infection of the sole, and the intractable pain suffered by the pony.

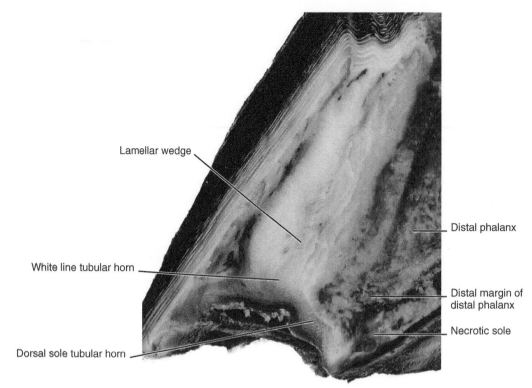

Lamellar wedge

White line tubular horn

Dorsal sole tubular horn

Distal phalanx

Distal margin of distal phalanx

Necrotic sole

• **Figure 14.33** Sagittal section of the foot of the 17-year-old Australian Pony with hyperinsulinaemic laminitis of 10 weeks' duration. The macrophotograph shows the detail of the lamellar wedge and necrotic sole. The growth of the tubular terminal horn and dorsal sole has been redirected by the dislocated distal phalanx. It is now expanding and "growing" toward the distal margin of the distal phalanx, accelerating bone lysis and modeling and contributing to palmar rotation of the distal phalanx. The density of the epidermal wedge explains the radiopaque mass, dorsal to the distal margin of the distal phalanx, noted in the lateromedial radiograph (Fig. 14-9).

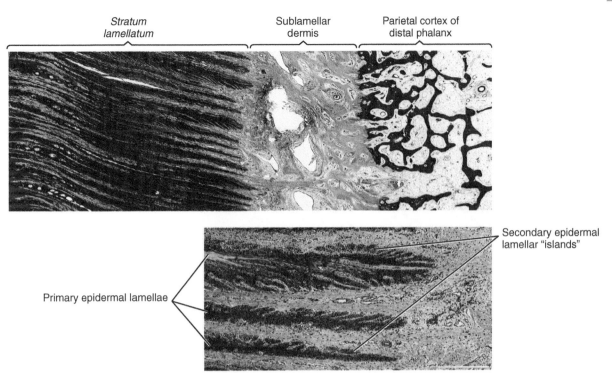

• Figure 14.34 Photomicrograph of transverse sections of lamellae and distal phalanx of the 17-year-old Australian Pony with hyperinsulinaemic laminitis of 10 weeks' duration. The epidermal lamellae are typical of chronic laminitis. The lamellar axial tips have abnormal shapes and are reduced in surface area, thus compromising the suspensory function for the connective tissue attachment of the distal phalanx. The abaxial lamellae are fused together, forming extensive cap horn between heavily keratinized primary epidermal lamellae. Stain = Masson's trichrome. The inset shows the axial tips of three lamellae. Many of the secondary epidermal lamellae are isolated islands no longer connected to the malformed primary epidermal lamellae. The islands were formed from basal cells proliferating within remnants of basement membrane that survived the inciting episode of laminitis. Stain = haematoxylin and eosin. Scale = 100 μm (0.1 mm).

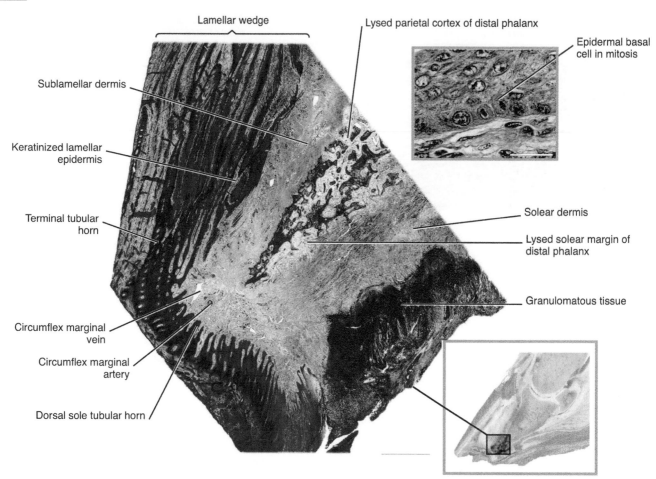

Lamellar wedge

Sublamellar dermis

Keratinized lamellar epidermis

Terminal tubular horn

Circumflex marginal vein

Circumflex marginal artery

Dorsal sole tubular horn

Lysed parietal cortex of distal phalanx

Epidermal basal cell in mitosis

Solear dermis

Lysed solear margin of distal phalanx

Granulomatous tissue

● **Figure 14.35** Photomicrograph of a decalcified sagittal section of the foot of the 17-year-old Australian Pony with hyperinsulinaemic laminitis of 10 weeks' duration. Stained with Masson's trichrome, epidermis and bone are red, connective tissue is blue. The section shows the distal margin of the distal phalanx surrounded by dystrophic lamellae and displaced tubular horn of the white line and dorsal sole; the lamellar wedge. There is also a granulomatous mass in the zone of necrotic sole noted on the gross sagittal section (Fig. 14-12 and Fig. 14-13). Extensive osteolysis has destroyed the solear margin of the distal phalanx and much of the parietal cortex. The dorsoproximally displaced tubules of terminal (white line) and dorsal sole epidermis are approximately 2 mm from the distal margin instead of the usual 20 mm. There is dyskeratosis among the distorted epidermal lamellae adjacent to the distal parietal cortex with regions of hard keratinized material abnormally close (1.8 mm) to the bone. The lamellar wedge epidermis is proliferating, as evidenced by mitosis among the epidermal basal cells (*upper inset*). The box in the lower inset shows the provenance of the specimen. (Stain = Masson's trichrome. Bar = 2 mm.)

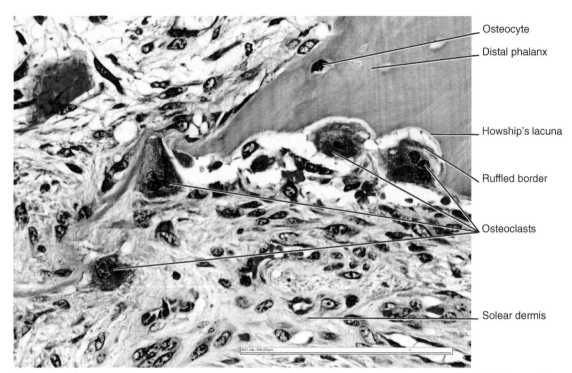

Osteocyte

Distal phalanx

Howship's lacuna

Ruffled border

Osteoclasts

Solear dermis

• **Figure 14.36** Photomicrograph of a decalcified sagittal section of the distal margin of the distal phalanx of the **17-year-old Australian Pony with hyperinsulinaemic laminitis of 10 weeks' duration.** Large multinucleate osteoclasts are resorbing bone from the solear cortex of the distal phalanx. The depressions in the bone created by osteoclastic bone resorption are called *Howship's lacunae.* Adjacent to the bone, the osteoclast has a ruffled border that secretes organic acids to dissolve the mineral contents of the bone and lysosomal collagenases to degrade the osteoid, organic matrix. (Stain = haematoxylin and eosin. Bar = 100 μm [0.1 mm].)

CASE HISTORY 4: TRAUMATIC LAMINITIS (ROAD FOUNDER) IN A SEVEN-YEAR-OLD THOROUGHBRED GELDING

A Thoroughbred gelding was purchased fresh from the race-track with the owner planning a sporting career for the horse. At the time of purchase the feet of the gelding were "filed" back short; the frogs had been removed, and the shoes were too small. The horse was released into a round yard with a hard rocky substrate and observed exercising freely with "incredible energy." Two days later the horse was walking tentatively and despite treatment with nonsteroidal antiinflammatories, the gait and stance became progressively worse. Eight days after purchase the gait was typical of laminitis with the front legs outstretched. Hoof testers applied to the front toes produced sharp withdrawal. Eighteen days after purchase, after being transported indoors onto deep sawdust bedding, the distressed horse became recumbent, unable to stand, and was euthanized on humane grounds.

After euthanasia one forefoot was immediately examined, dissected, and photographed; the other was frozen for computed tomography (CT) scanning at a later date. A superficial examination of the foot showed two abnormalities. First, the proximal edge of the hoof wall was sharp on palpation, with a pronounced deficit in the coronary subcutis extending circumferentially from toe to both heels. This is the hallmark abnormality of a severe "sinker," the worst manifestation of acute laminitis. The second abnormality was a convex, instead of the normally concave, sole. The distal phalanx had sunk into the hoof capsule, pushing the sole downward, creating a bulge. There was a palpably soft, crescent-shaped zone in the sole corresponding to the distal margin of the distal phalanx.

When the forefoot was cut with a band saw in the sagittal plane, bloodstained fluid was released from a large cavity between the distal phalanx and the inner hoof wall. The fluid did not resemble pus, and there was no abcessation or evident infection of the foot contents. The distal phalanx is normally firmly attached to the inner lamellar layer of the hoof wall by the connective tissue of the suspensory apparatus of the distal phalanx (SADP). In this case only remnants of the SADP remained; the majority of the connective tissue remained attached to the distal phalanx and had completely separated from the lamellae of the inner hoof wall. The distal phalanx had sunk deeply into the hoof capsule and had crushed the solear dermis. The toe of the hoof capsule was an abnormally large distance from the tip of the distal phalanx. The separation between hoof lamellae and bone was present from toe to heel.

The tubules of the proximal hoof wall were severely kinked. The abrupt and severe descent of the distal phalanx had distorted the hoof wall growth zone, redirecting it upward instead of the normal downward. The length of the kinked tubules (3 to 4 mm) suggested that the initial laminitis episode occurred about 14 days before euthanasia.

A similar distortion of tubular hoof growth had occurred distally. The tubules of the white line and dorsal sole were kinked and directed inward toward the distal phalanx instead of downward toward the ground. The solear dermis beneath the margin of the distal phalanx was crushed and separated from the adjacent solear horn.

Examination of the inner hoof wall of the specimen gave a clear view of epidermal lamellae free of virtually all dermal attachments. The lamellae were near normal in appearance but had totally separated from their dermal counterparts. Laminitis of such severity is rare and indicates that a catastrophic inflammatory event had occurred in the 18 days before euthanasia. The attachment between epidermis and dermis had been destroyed with remarkable completeness. Current research thinking is that enzymatic activation, triggered by inflammation, is responsible for the cleaving of epidermal from dermal lamellae. Without lamellar attachments, the distal phalanx was free to rapidly sink into the capsule, crushing the solear dermis and causing the horny sole to bulge downward, giving the dropped sole appearance.

CT scans of the second foot showed similar pathology. Three-dimensional models constructed from the CT data using Mimics® Materialise software showed the extent of the dislocation of the distal phalanx within the hoof capsule. Further analysis showed numerous margin fractures of the distal phalanx (Fig. 14-17 ABC to Fig. 14-25).

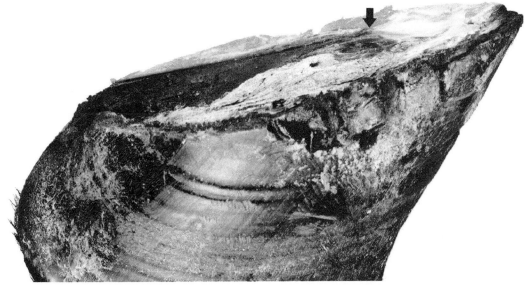

• Figure 14.37 The foot of the road founder case at the time of euthanasia showing a convex, "dropped" sole (*arrow*) instead of the normal concave sole. The distal phalanx had sunk into the hoof capsule, forcing the sole to bulge downward. The margin of the distal phalanx was on the verge of prolapsing through a crescent-shaped zone of necrotic sole.

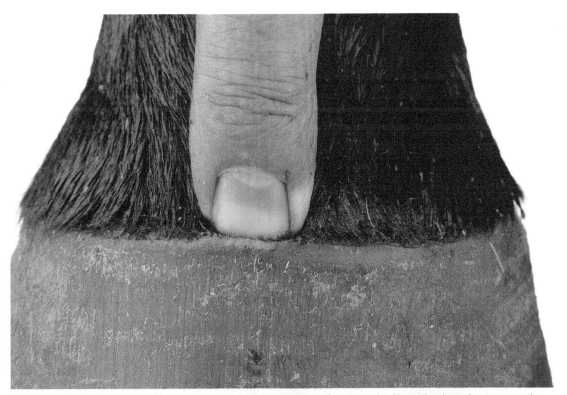

• Figure 14.38 The foot of the road founder case at the time of euthanasia. Normally, the subcutaneous tissue adjoining the proximal edge of the hoof wall is solid and full and cannot be compressed with the finger. With the rapid development of severe laminitis, the skeletal structures inside the hoof capsule sink deeply, creating a palpable coronary band deficit and a sharp edge to the proximal hoof wall.

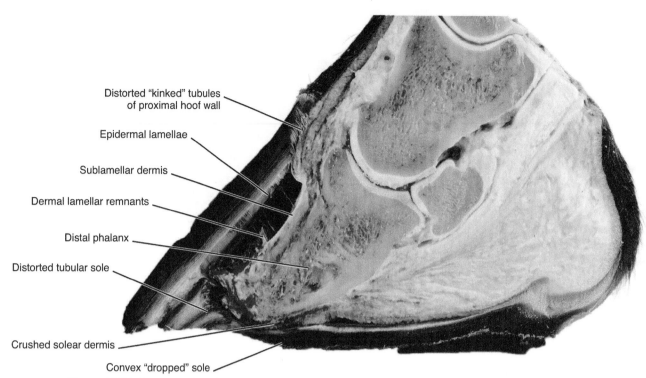

Distorted "kinked" tubules
of proximal hoof wall

Epidermal lamellae

Sublamellar dermis

Dermal lamellar remnants

Distal phalanx

Distorted tubular sole

Crushed solear dermis

Convex "dropped" sole

● **Figure 14.39** Sagittal section of the foot of the road founder case, showing severe downward dislocation of the distal phalanx. The cavity between bone and hoof contained blood-stained fluid. The solear dermis beneath the margin of the distal phalanx is crushed and separated from the adjacent solear horn.

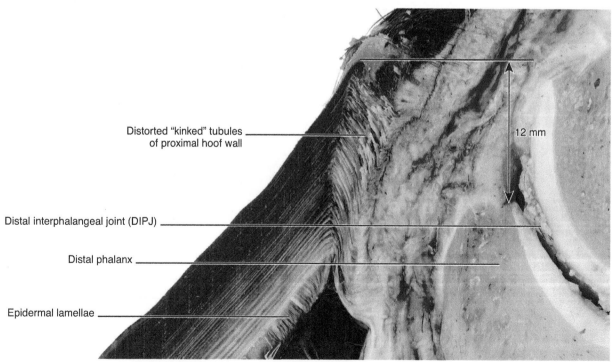

Distorted "kinked" tubules
of proximal hoof wall

12 mm

Distal interphalangeal joint (DIPJ)

Distal phalanx

Epidermal lamellae

● **Figure 14.40** Close-up photograph of the sagittal section of the foot of the road founder case showing the kinked proximal hoof wall tubules. There is a sharp boundary between normal and kinked hoof wall tubules (*asterisk*). The double-ended arrow, between the hard edge of the proximal hoof wall and the extensor process of the distal phalanx, shows a "founder distance" of 12 mm, which is approximately twice the normal.

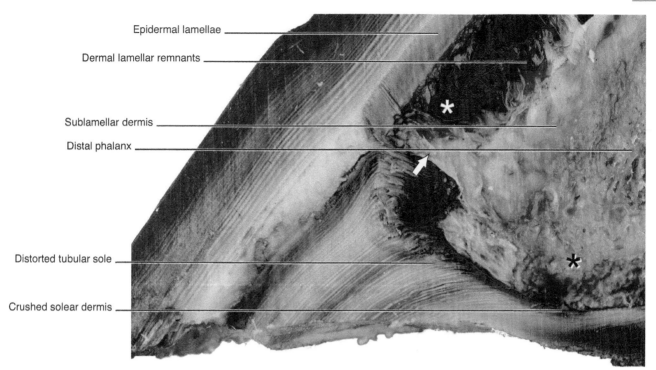

Epidermal lamellae

Dermal lamellar remnants

Sublamellar dermis

Distal phalanx

Distorted tubular sole

Crushed solear dermis

• **Figure 14.41** Close-up photograph of the sagittal section of the foot of the road founder case showing the white line, dorsal sole region. The asterisks show the before laminitis (*white asterisk*) and after laminitis (*black asterisk*) of the distal phalanx. The tubules of the dorsal sole are kinked and directed inward toward the distal phalanx instead of downward toward the ground. The band of tissue between the margin of the distal phalanx and the hoof wall (*arrow*) contains terminal papillae and remnants of terminal horn. The solear dermis beneath the margin of the distal phalanx is crushed and separated from the adjacent solear horn.

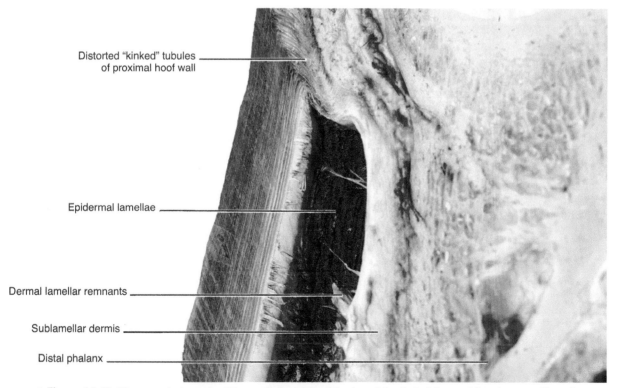

Distorted "kinked" tubules of proximal hoof wall

Epidermal lamellae

Dermal lamellar remnants

Sublamellar dermis

Distal phalanx

• **Figure 14.42** Close-up photograph of the sagittal section of the toe of the foot of the road founder case. There is near-complete separation between epidermal lamellae and the sublamellar dermis still attached to the parietal surface of the distal phalanx. It is rare to observe such complete lamellar separation in a clinical case; the epidermal lamellae are near normal in shape and size, resembling lamellae from an exungulated hoof.

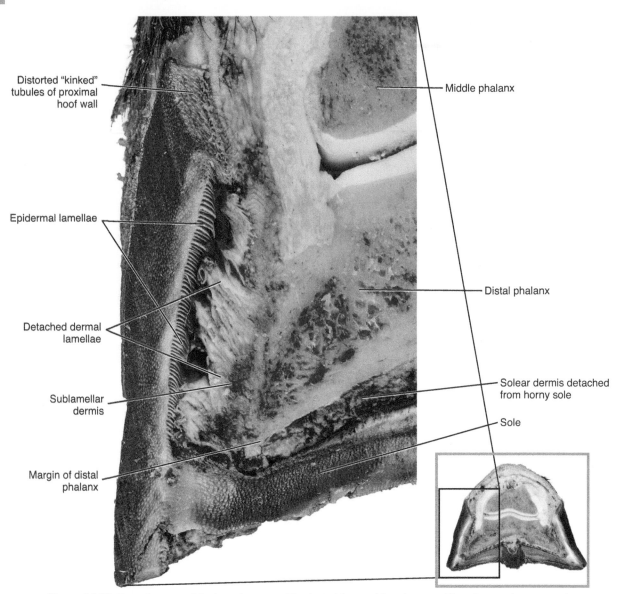

Distorted "kinked" tubules of proximal hoof wall

Middle phalanx

Epidermal lamellae

Distal phalanx

Detached dermal lamellae

Solear dermis detached from horny sole

Sublamellar dermis

Sole

Margin of distal phalanx

● **Figure 14.43** Frontal section of the lateral quarter of the foot of the road founder case. There is complete separation between the hoof lamellae and the suspensory connective tissue attached to the parietal cortex of the distal phalanx. Note the solear dermis is also detached from the horny sole. Without functional lamellar attachments at the toe, quarters, and heels the distal phalanx is "free" inside the hoof capsule, crushing the solear dermis whenever the foot is loaded.

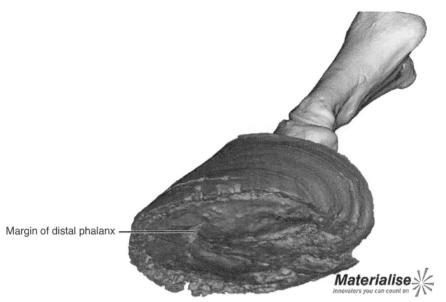

Margin of distal phalanx

● **Figure 14.44** Three-dimensional Mimics model from CT data of the foot of the road founder case. The distal phalanx has perforated the horny sole and the sole is convex, or "dropped."

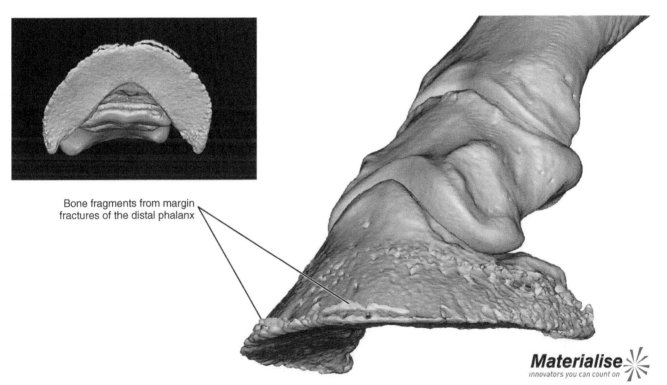

Bone fragments from margin fractures of the distal phalanx

● **Figure 14.45** Three-dimensional Mimics model from CT data of the foot of the road founder case. There are several fractures of the distal margin of the distal phalanx. The fragments appear to have occurred simultaneously and have been distracted upward by the pull of the still attached suspensory apparatus of the distal phalanx. Inset: solear view of distal phalanx, highlighting the margin fractures.

CONCLUDING REMARKS

At the time of euthanasia, the gelding had severe, extensive laminitis with no chance of recovering to a pain-free existence and a normal life. Euthanasia was the only humane option, and the decision was correctly taken. The sharp demarcation between normal and kinked proximal hoof wall tubules marks the onset of the distal phalanx sinking into the hoof capsule. Severe and rapidly developing laminitis had caused near total failure of the SADP. Without a functional SADP, the distal phalanx was free of its suspensory connections and sank deeply into the hoof capsule, crushing the sole and distorting both the proximal and distal tubular growth zones of the hoof. The extent and completeness of the lamellar failure and SADP were remarkable. Laminitis does not occur spontaneously, and the history provides some clues to the causation. The fractures to the distal margin of the distal phalanx are significant. Bone fractures trigger a marked inflammatory response, recruiting many of the cells and enzyme systems known to be associated with laminitis. It is possible that the trauma that crushed the solar corium and caused multiple fractures of the margin of the distal phalanx triggered a massive inflammatory response that "overflowed" to adjacent lamellae, effecting massive enzymatic destruction of lamellar architecture. Thus a "tsunami" of laminitis spread up the lamellae from the epicenter of sole trauma and fractured, inflamed bone. The history of "filing back short" the hoof wall and "pony-sized" shoes too small for the feet of a Thoroughbred could have contributed to sole trauma and margin fractures of the distal phalanx. Exercising with "incredible energy" when released from confinement could have coincided with the traumatic fracturing of the margin of the distal phalanx, especially if the ground was hard enough to directly impact the soles of the feet. Short hoof walls and small shoes applying sole pressure could have been contributing factors.

It is also possible that the sudden onset of laminitis and sinking of the distal phalanx had nothing to do with sole trauma and the distal margin fractures. Fracturing of the distal margin could have occurred *after* the laminitis and sinking of the distal phalanx had occurred when the bone came close to ground contact. This seems unlikely, as the majority of severe laminitis cases in the author's records, examined using CT, do not exhibit margin fractures. There are cases of global severe laminitis, also with the catastrophic sinking into the hoof capsule, that had no margin fractures when euthanized. In chronic laminitis, bone remodeling of the distal margin certainly develops, but not with the abrupt fracture line and fragment dislocation that characterized the feet of this gelding. In hindsight, it will be difficult to establish the true timeline of events. This case is as severe as laminitis gets, and the horse appears to have suffered the bad luck of a confluence of events that aligned to trigger an unusual inflammatory explosion that destroyed his lamellar attachments and so crippled him.

CASE HISTORY 5: CHRONIC LAMINITIS IN AN ARABIAN ENDURANCE HORSE

A mature Arabian mare developed clinical laminitis 3 days after being ridden in a 100-km endurance competition. Four months later the mare still displayed a typical forelimb laminitic gait with exaggerated digital pulses and deformed proximal hoof wall growth dorsally. Lateromedial radiographic images of the front feet showed capsular rotation of the hoof and a significant lamellar wedge dorsal to the parietal surface of the distal phalanx. There was early modeling of the distal phalanx dorsal to the distal margin. The deep groove, present in the dorsal proximal hoof wall, indicated that considerable sinking of the distal phalanx had occurred at the time of the inciting incident. A venographic image showed reasonably good filling of the veins in the dermis of the coronary band, sublamellar and solear dermis, suggesting the absence of major filling defects due to lamellar wedge formation and/or deformed tubular hoof wall growth. Thus, with a prognosis favorable for life as a broodmare, the agreed treatment plan included deep digital flexor tendon tenotomy (to normalize the elevated palmar angle of the distal phalanx), resection of the proximal dorsal hoof wall (to redirect coronary tubular horn growth), and resection of the dorsal toe (to remove the lamellar wedge and displaced terminal horn and dorsal sole). At all times the feet were supported with shoeing devices that prevented the dorsal sole, beneath the distal margin of the distal phalanx, from making ground or shoe contact. Initially, the shoeing device was the Steward Clog[23] and later bespoke aluminium heart bar shoes. The shoes were reset every four weeks, and each time, the resections in the dorsal hoof wall were deepened to their starting levels. The front feet recovered to a near-normal shape and appearance. Radiographs and venograms, eight months after onset, show near-normal parameters. At the time of writing the mare is "paddock sound," beginning light trail rides, without the clinical lameness due to laminitis (Fig. 14-26 to Fig. 14-35).

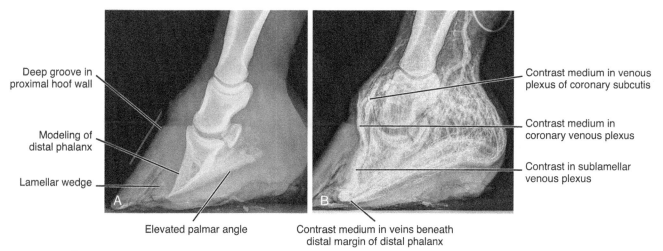

Deep groove in proximal hoof wall

Modeling of distal phalanx

Lamellar wedge

Elevated palmar angle

Contrast medium in venous plexus of coronary subcutis

Contrast medium in coronary venous plexus

Contrast in sublamellar venous plexus

Contrast medium in veins beneath distal margin of distal phalanx

• **Figure 14.46** Radiographic images of the foot of the Arabian endurance horse with chronic laminitis. Four months after the initial episode of laminitis, the lateromedial radiographic image of the right front foot (**A**) shows capsular rotation of the hoof and a significant lamellar wedge dorsal to the parietal surface of the distal phalanx. There is early modeling of the distal phalanx dorsal to the distal margin. The deep groove in the dorsal proximal hoof wall indicates that considerable sinking of the distal phalanx occurred at the time of the inciting incident. The venographic image (**B**) shows reasonably good filling of the veins in the dermis of the coronary band, sublamellar, and solear dermis, suggesting the absence of major filling defects due to distal phalanx dislocation, lamellar wedge formation and/or deformed tubular hoof wall growth. (Radiograph and venogram by Kylie Schaaf, WestVETS Equine Hospital.)

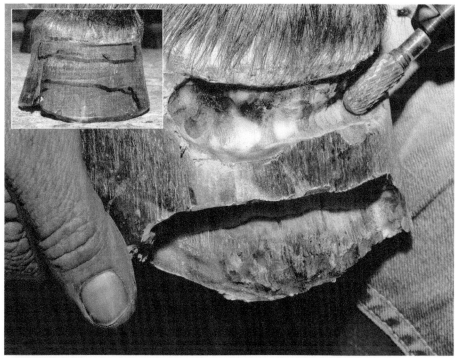

• **Figure 14.47** The foot of the Arabian endurance horse photographed during strategic resection of the dorsal hoof. An abrasive rotating burr was used to resect a window in the proximal dorsal hoof wall from the medial quarter to the lateral. The inset shows the foot before resection, with the resection plan marked in red. The depth of the resection was judged by thumb pressure; when the resected area could be compressed, the resection was stopped, usually with zero or minor hemorrhage. The coronary resection followed the contours of the internal coronary groove just distad to the periople. The same principle was applied to the distal half of the dorsal hoof wall, removing discolored lamellar wedge and distorted dorsal sole. The band of hoof between the proximal and distal resections was left as a bridge to prevent possible medial and lateral collapse of the foot.

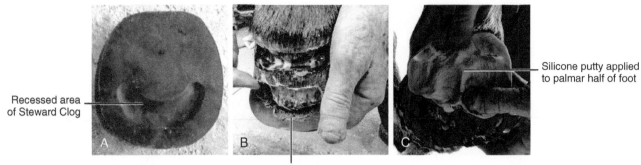

Recessed area of Steward Clog

Silicone putty applied to palmar half of foot

Recessed area enlarged to avoid dorsal sole contact

• **Figure 14.48** A plastic Steward Clog* was applied to the foot of the Arabian endurance horse with chronic laminitis and attached with resin casting tape.[†] To minimize contact between the clog and the dorsal sole, the recessed area of the Clog was enlarged with a rotating bur tool. The heels and quarters were trimmed with nippers and rasp thereby becoming the principal bearing border of the foot. The palmar half of the sole was packed with silicone putty and allowed to set under load. The dorsal half of the foot was trimmed to relieve it of load bearing. Thus the palmar half of the foot was recruited for load bearing while the dorsal half was rehabilitated.
* http://www.hopeforsoundness.com/cms/steward-clog-instruction-guide.html
[†] 3M™ Scotchcast™ Plus Casting Tape 82002 or Equicast support tape, http://www.equicast.com/

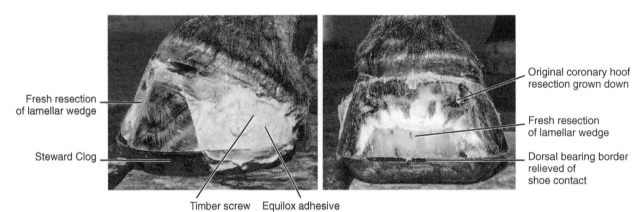

Fresh resection of lamellar wedge

Steward Clog

Original coronary hoof resection grown down

Fresh resection of lamellar wedge

Dorsal bearing border relieved of shoe contact

Timber screw   Equilox adhesive

• **Figure 14.49** The foot of the Arabian endurance horse photographed at the third shoeing. The Steward Clog* was reapplied to the foot at monthly intervals by fixing timber screws to the clog beside the heels and quarters and applying polymethylmethacrylate (Equilox)[†] to bond screws, clog, and the hoof together. The initial coronary hoof wall resection has grown distally by 30 to 35 mm, and the distal dorsal hoof wall has been rasped to the point of giving to thumb pressure as before. This minimizes the influence of the lamellar wedge on the dorsal distal phalanx and dermal tissue surrounding it. Note that heel preparation has relieved the dorsal bearing border of loading pressure.
* http://www.hopeforsoundness.com/cms/steward-clog-instruction-guide.html
[†] http://www.equilox.com/

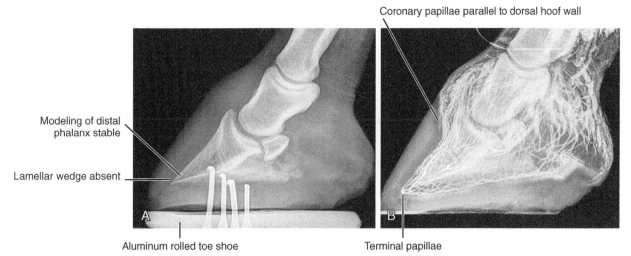

Coronary papillae parallel to dorsal hoof wall

Modeling of distal phalanx stable

Lamellar wedge absent

Aluminum rolled toe shoe

Terminal papillae

● **Figure 14.50** Radiograph and venogram of the front foot of the Arabian endurance horse eight months after the initial episode. Eight months after the initial episode, the front feet were radiographed again and a venogram performed. The lateromedial radiographic image (**A**) shows restoration of a normal palmar angle to the distal phalanx. The modeling of the distal parietal cortex is now virtually undetectable. Notably, the lamellar wedge, so evident eight months earlier, is absent and the radiolucent zone representing the sublamellar dermis now has normal proportions. The distance between the outer hoof wall and the parietal surface of the distal phalanx is still greater than normal by 15%. However, capsular rotation is now absent, and the dorsal hoof wall and parietal surface of the distal phalanx are approximately parallel. The dorsal solear dermis is still radiopaque and has not completely recovered. The venogram of the same foot is close to normal (**B**). Note the angle of the coronary papillae is parallel to the dorsal hoof wall and parietal surface of the distal phalanx. The dorsal terminal papillae are obscured, perhaps because the terminal horn in this area is still deformed. The vessels of the remaining terminal papillae are well filled and correctly oriented. Radiograph and venogram by Kylie Schaaf, WestVETS Equine Hospital.

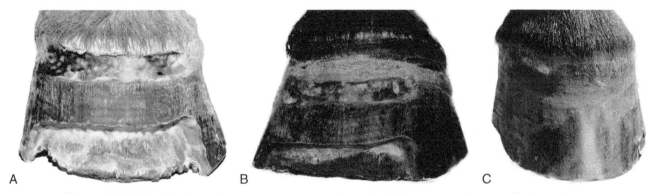

A   B   C

● **Figure 14.51** The foot of the Arabian endurance horse photographed at three stages of recovery. On the anniversary of the original resection, the mare's foot was trimmed and photographed (**C**). The mare was walking normally, free of the clinical signs of laminitis, and being introduced to light trail riding. The resected zones of hoof wall had progressed distally as new coronary hoof was produced from the now normalized proximal growth zone (as corroborated by the radiographs and venograms in Figure 14-30). Notably, new hoof growth was parallel to the hairline. For comparison, the original resection (**A**) and the foot three months later (**B**) are shown. Radical as the original hoof resections may appear, they seem to correct the deformed proximal hoof growth and lamellar wedge formation problems of chronic laminitis, and, along with careful "shoeing," contribute to foot rehabilitation. It is likely irrelevant which "type" shoe is used as long as it protects the dorsal sole, uses the palmar half of the foot for weight bearing, and mechanically aids easy break-over.

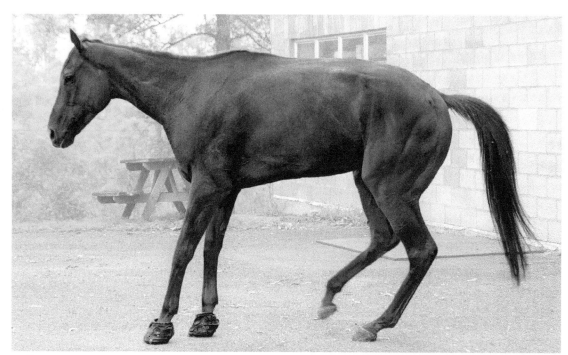

● **Figure 14.52** **The gait of a horse with severe laminitis.** When a horse develops laminitis, the front feet are invariably the most severely affected. With the distal phalanx dislocated downward and compressing the dorsal sole, it becomes extremely painful for the horse to load and break over at the toe. If forced to walk, it will bring its hind legs forward, under its abdomen, and half rear (as if attempting a "levade") before stepping forward in front. The posterior phase of the front stride is thus very much shortened. Although the relief of pain is ethically important, it may be detrimental to abolish it completely with peripheral nerve blocks and large doses of analgesics, because walking without the warning signal of pain is believed to worsen the mechanical destruction of the already compromised suspensory apparatus of the distal phalanx.

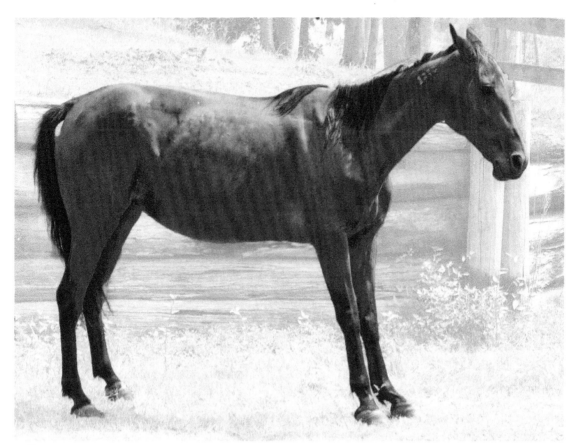

• **Figure 14.53** The stance of a horse with severe laminitis. To ease the pain of loading the dorsal solear dermis after downward dislocation of the distal phalanx, horses will stand with their feet forward of the normal vertical stance phase, shifting weight from one foot to the other. Laminitis usually affects the forefeet more severely than the hind, presumably because the forequarters carry a greater proportion of the horse's weight (about 65%). Often, the hind feet appear to be spared completely. In the chronic laminitis case pictured, the mare is shifting weight from one forefoot to the other. The shifting weight behavior of horses with laminitis is assumedly performed to relieve pain. The common explanation is that when the pain in one foot becomes unbearable, that foot is lifted off the ground. Pain then mounts in the weight-bearing foot until the horse feels compelled to relieve it by shifting weight to the other foot. Horses with chronic laminitis shift weight like this for months, sometimes years.

References

1. Asplin, K. E., Sillence, M. N., Pollitt, C. C., & McGowan, C. M. (2007). Induction of laminitis by prolonged hyperinsulinaemia in clinically normal ponies. *Veterinary Journal, 174,* 530–535.

2. Baldwin, G. I., & Pollitt, C. C. (2010). Progression of venographic changes after experimentally induced laminitis. *Veterinary Clinics of North America. Equine Practice, 26,* 135–140.

3. Cripps, P. J., & Eustace, R. A. (1999). Factors involved in the prognosis of equine laminitis in the UK. *Equine Veterinary Journal, 31,* 433–442.

4. Cripps, P. J., & Eustace, R. A. (1999). Radiological measurements from the feet of normal horses with relevance to laminitis. *Equine Veterinary Journal, 31,* 427–432.

5. Croser, E. L., & Pollitt, C. C. (2006). Acute laminitis: Descriptive evaluation of serial hoof biopsies. In *52nd Annual Convention of the American Association of Equine Practitioners.* San Antonio, Texas, U.S.A. (pp. 542–546).

6. de Laat, M. A., McGowan, C. M., Sillence, M. N., & Pollitt, C. C. (2010). Equine laminitis: Induced by 48 h hyperinsulinaemia in Standardbred horses. *Equine Veterinary Journal, 42,* 129–135.

7. de Laat, M. A., van Eps, A. W., McGowan, C. M., Sillence, M. N., & Pollitt, C. C. (2011). Equine laminitis: Comparative histopathology 48 hours after experimental induction with insulin or alimentary oligofructose in Standardbred horses. *Journal of Comparative Pathology,* 145, 399–409.

8. Engiles, J. B. (2010). Pathology of the distal phalanx in equine laminitis: More than just skin deep. *Veterinary Clinics of North America. Equine Practice, 26,* 155–165.

9. French, K. R., & Pollitt, C.C. (2004). Equine laminitis: Loss of hemidesmosomes in hoof secondary epidermal lamellae correlates to dose in an oligofructose induction model: An ultrastructural study. *Equine Veterinary Journal, 36,* 230–235.

10. Garner, H. E., Coffman, J. R., Hahn, A. W., Hutcheson, D. P., & Tumbleson, M. E. (1975). Equine laminitis of alimentary origin: An experimental model. *American Journal of Veterinary Research, 36,* 441–444.

11. Hanly, B. K., Stokes, A. M., Bell, A. M., Johnson, J. R., Keowen, M. L., Paulsen, D. B., Sod, G. A., & Moore, R. M. (2009). Use of serial laminar tissue collection via biopsy in conscious healthy horses. *American Journal of Veterinary Research, 70,* 697–702.

12. Johnson, P. J. (2002). The equine metabolic syndrome peripheral Cushing's syndrome. *Veterinary Clinics of North America. Equine Practice, 18,* 271–293.

13. Kullmann, A., Holcombe, S. J., Hurcombe, S. D., Roessner, H. A., Hauptman, J. G., Geor, R. J., & Belknap, J. (2013). Prophylactic

digital cryotherapy is associated with decreased incidence of laminitis in horses diagnosed with colitis. *Equine Veterinary Journal. 46*, 554–559.

14. McGowan, C., Frost, R., Pfeiffer, D., & Neiger, R. (2004). Serum insulin concentrations in horses with equine Cushing's syndrome: Response to a cortisol inhibitor and prognostic value. *Equine Veterinary Journal, 36*, 194–198.

15. Obel, N. (1948). *Studies of the Histopathology of Acute Laminitis.* PhD thesis. Almgvist and Wilcsells Bottrykeri Ab Uppsala, Uppsala.

16. Pollitt, C. C. (1996). Basement membrane pathology: A feature of acute equine laminitis. *Equine Veterinary Journal, 28*, 38–46.

17. Pollitt, C. C. (2008). *Equine laminitis*: Current concepts, RIRDC Publication No.08/062, Canberra, Australia.

18. Pollitt, C. C., & Daradka, M. (1998). Equine laminitis basement membrane pathology: Loss of type IV collagen, type VII collagen and laminin immunostaining. *Equine Veterinary Journal, 26* (Suppl.), 139-144.

19. Pollitt, C. C., & Visser, M. B. (2010). Carbohydrate alimentary overload laminitis. *Veterinary Clinics of North America. Equine Practice, 26*, 65–78.

20. Pratt, S. E., Geor, R. J., & McCutcheon, L. J. (2006). Effects of dietary energy source and physical conditioning on insulin sensitivity and glucose tolerance in Standardbred horses. *Equine Exercise Physiology, 36*, 579–584.

21. Redden, R. F. (2001). A technique for performing digital venography in the standing horse. *Equine Veterinary Education, 13*, 128–134.

22. Sprouse, R. F., Garner, H. E., & Green, E. M. (1987). Plasma endotoxin levels in horses subjected to carbohydrate induced laminitis. *Equine Veterinary Journal*, 19, 25–28.

23. Steward, M. L. (2003). How to construct and apply atraumatic therapeutic shoes to treat acute or chronic laminitis in the horse. In *American Association of Equine Practitioners 49th Annual Convention.* New Orleans, Louisiana, U.S.A. (pp. 337–346).

24. Treiber, K. H., Kronfeld, D. S., & Geor, R. J. (2006). Insulin resistance in equids: Possible role in laminitis. *Journal of Nutrition, 136*, 2094S–2098S.

25. Treiber, K. H., Kronfeld, D. S., Hess, T. M., Byrd, B. M., Splan, R. K., & Staniar, W. B. (2006). Evaluation of genetic and metabolic predispositions and nutritional risk factors for pasture-associated laminitis in ponies. *Journal of the American Veterinary Medicine Association, 228*, 1538–1545.

26. van Eps, A. W., & Pollitt, C. C. (2006). Equine laminitis induced with oligofructose. *Equine Veterinary Journal, 38*, 203–208.

27. van Eps, A. W., & Pollitt, C. C. (2009). Equine laminitis model: Lamellar histopathology 7 days after induction with oligofructose. *Equine Veterinary Journal, 41*, 735–740.

28. Visser, M. B., & Pollitt, C. C. (2011). The timeline of lamellar basement membrane changes during equine laminitis development. *Equine Veterinary Journal, 43*, 471–477.

29. Walsh, D. M., McGowan, C. M., McGowan, T., Lamb, S. V., Schanbacher, B. J., & Place, N. J. (2009). Correlation of plasma insulin concentration with laminitis score in a field study of equine Cushing's disease and equine metabolic syndrome. Journal of Equine Veterinary Science, 29, 87–94.

15 Navicular Disease

Chronic forelimb lameness due to pain arising from degenerative changes in the distal sesamoid (navicular) bone, suspensory ligaments of the navicular bone, the distal sesamoidean impar ligament, the navicular bursa, and the deep flexor tendon was described in the eighteenth century when Bridges wrote his treatise "No Foot No Horse" in 1752. The German equerry von Sind vaguely referred to "the little shuttle-like bone which could be injured in the horses foot" in 1775. It wasn't until the early nineteenth century that skepticism was overcome and veterinary surgeons and farriers in England and in the rest of Europe began to use experience and precise observations to diagnose navicular disease as a cause of equine lameness. Today, with the aid of radiography, nuclear scintigraphy, magnetic resonance imaging (MRI), and regional anesthesia, navicular disease is estimated to account for one third of all chronic forelimb lameness in horses.

Before the arrival of MRI, many veterinarians accepted that pain in the distal sesamoid region was a syndrome rather than a specific disease entity.[3] It was considered that navicular "syndrome" more accurately described a chronic, progressive degeneration of the navicular bone, the navicular bursa, the deep digital flexor, and the associated ligaments.

The term *syndrome* implied a spectrum of changes— some of these changes having the potential of being diagnosed early enough to respond to management procedures that permitted horses to return to normal levels of performance or alternative work.

The development of MRI enabled diagnosis of disease in the components of the podotrochlear apparatus a reality, making use of the term *syndrome* redundant.[1] The podotrochlear apparatus consists of the collateral sesamoidean ligaments (CSLs), the distal sesamoidean impar ligament (DSlL), and the navicular bursa, along with the navicular bone, and clinicians using MRI can now locate lesions in each of them. When MRI is beyond a client's budget or is unavailable, navicular bursography supplies more diagnostic information than radiography alone.[4]

Navicular disease can appear suddenly as an acute, severe condition in relatively young horses (especially Quarter Horses). It can also develop insidiously, as a chronically progressive disease in older mature horses. It is usually a bilateral forelimb problem but can be unilateral.

It is a common condition in Quarter Horses, which tend to have narrow, upright, boxy feet, small relative to their body size, and also in European Warmblood horses, many of which have relatively tall, narrow feet. It is also common in Thoroughbred horses, which frequently have rather flat feet, with low collapsed heels, often associated with a broken back hoof pastern axis.[1] Interestingly, a one-degree decrease in the angle of the solar cortex of the distal phalanx increased compressive forces on the navicular bone by 4%,[2] perhaps explaining the link between low heels and palmar foot pain.

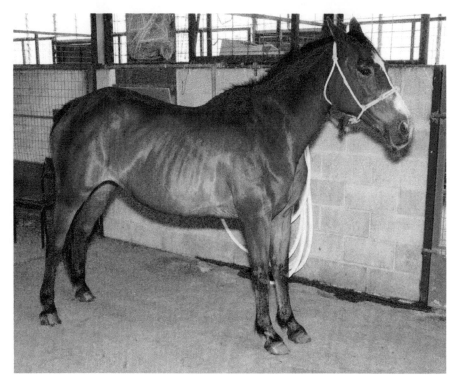

● **Figure 15.1** Stance of an Australian Stock Horse mare with advanced navicular disease. Horses with advanced navicular disease often stand with their forefeet "in front", more forward than normal. This posture is believed to ease the pain and fits the hypothesis that the disease is associated with the pressure the deep flexor tendon exerts on the flexor surface of the distal sesamoid (navicular) bone.

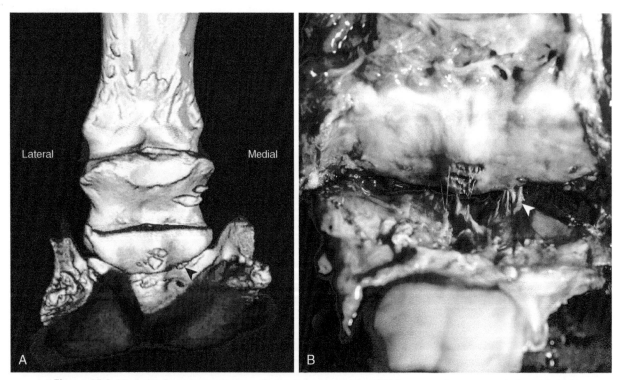

● **Figure 15.2** Navicular flexor cortex lesions. Computed tomography (CT) image and necropsy photograph of the navicular bone and deep digital flexor tendon of the Australian Stock Horse mare with advanced navicular disease. The CT image (**A**) is from the left front foot and shows multiple pathologies of the podotrochlear apparatus. There is a large enthesophyte of the lateral collateral sesamoidean ligament, a bone fragment in the distal border (arrowhead) and deep erosions of the distal flexor cortex. The necropsy photograph (**B**) shows the central flexor cortex lesions, detected in the CT image, adhered to the deep digital flexor tendon (DDFT). The surface of the DDFT, adjacent to the flexor cortex, was discolored and fibrillated. There was also an adhesion from the DDFT to the distal border fragment (arrowhead), suggesting pathology more significant than expected from a simple border fracture. In fact, a frontal plane CT image (Fig. 15.3) showed radiolucent areas in the cortex and medulla of the navicular bone surrounding the fragment.

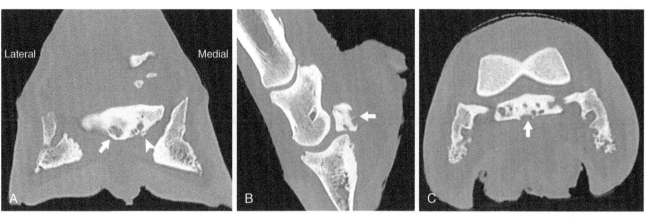

• **Figure 15.3** Three computed tomography (CT) images of the foot of the Australian Stock Horse mare with advanced navicular disease. The frontal image (**A**) shows a distal border fracture of the navicular bone associated with adjacent radiolucent areas. At necropsy there were adhesions between the deep digital flexor tendon (DDFT) and the large radiolucent area (*arrow*). The radiolucent areas penetrate deeply into the flexor cortex (arrows in **B** and **C**). The transverse image (**C**) is roughly equivalent to a palmar 45° proximal-palmarodistal oblique (skyline) radiograph and shows the value of this projection in detecting the presence of full-thickness flexor cortex lesions. Flexor cortex lesions carry a grave prognosis. Note the fragment in the medial distal border is associated with cortical and medullary radiolucencies, a finding often associated with lameness.

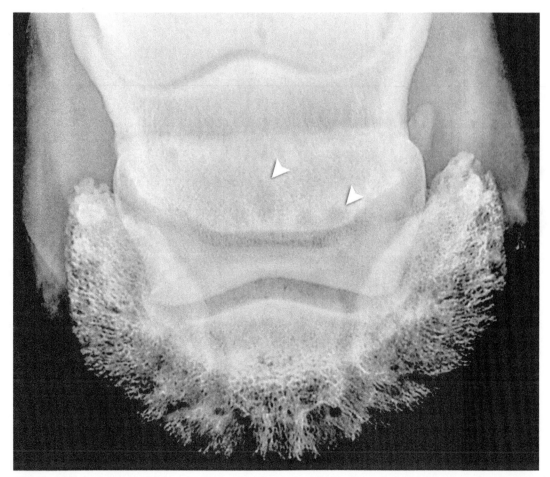

• **Figure 15.4** Radiographic image of a foot with advanced navicular disease; dorsal 65° proximal-palmarodistal oblique projection. The large, radiolucent, cystlike lesions within the spongiosa of the bone (*arrowheads*) penetrated the flexor cortex; the horse had a bilateral forelimb lameness. At necropsy there were adhesions between the flexor cortex lesions and the deep digital flexor tendon (DDFT). (Radiograph: Kylie Schaaf, WestVETS Equine Hospital.)

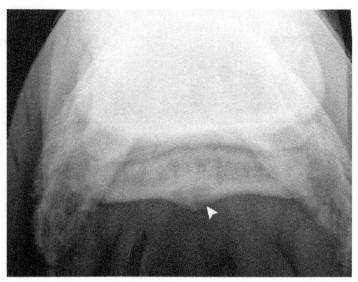

• **Figure 15.5** Radiographic image of a foot with advanced navicular disease; palmar 45° proximal-palmarodistal oblique (skyline) projection. There is a large lucent area (arrowhead) penetrating the flexor cortex of the bone. There were multiple adhesions between the bone lesion and the deep flexor tendon. (Radiograph: Kylie Schaaf, WestVETS Equine Hospital.)

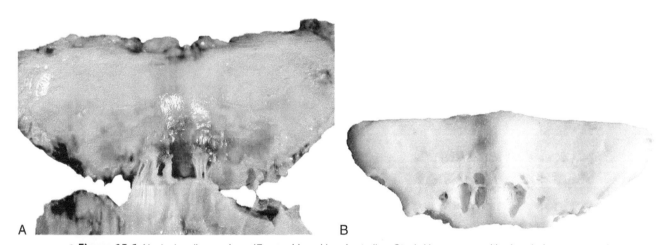

A   B

• **Figure 15.6** Navicular disease in a 17-year-old working Australian Stock Horse mare with chronic lameness and intractable pain, euthanized on humane grounds. At necropsy the flexor surface of the distal sesamoid (navicular) bone was exposed and the deep digital flexor tendon (DDFT) reflected down (**A**). The fibrocartilage of the distal sesamoid flexor surface is thinned, eroded, and discolored. There are adhesions from the deep flexor tendon attached to large lesions on the flexor surface of the distal sesamoid bone. The cleaned navicular bone (**B**) shows the lesions to be cavities in the flexor cortex that penetrate deeply into the spongiosa of the bone; they correspond precisely with the adhesions sites in **A**. Note that the lesions are clustered around the central ridge and the distal half of the bone: the predilection sites for the development of navicular disease pathology.

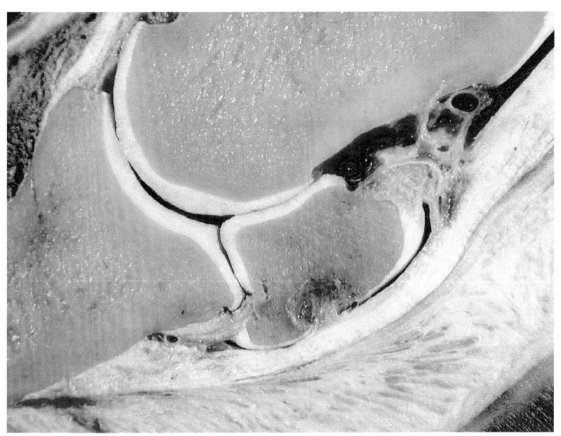

• **Figure 15.7** Sagittal section photograph of the navicular bone of the 17-year-old working Australian Stock Horse mare with advanced navicular disease in figure 15.6. The large lesion in the flexor cortex penetrates into the medulla of the distal sesamoid bone and is adhered to the deep digital flexor tendon (DDFT). The flexor surface fibrocartilage surrounding the lesion is thin and discolored yellow. Similar discoloration is mirrored on the apposing surface of the DDFT.

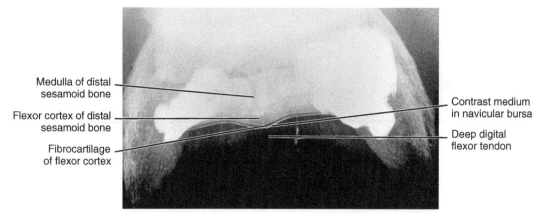

Medulla of distal sesamoid bone

Flexor cortex of distal sesamoid bone

Fibrocartilage of flexor cortex

Contrast medium in navicular bursa

Deep digital flexor tendon

• **Figure 15.8** Palmar 45° proximal-palmarodistal oblique radiographic image of a navicular bone with contrast medium (3 ml) injected into the navicular bursa. The contrast medium is juxtaposed between the distal sesamoid flexor cortex and the deep digital flexor tendon (DDFT). The fibrocartilage on the surface of the flexor cortex shows as an even, radiolucent line, highlighted by the contrast medium, without filling gaps due to adhesions or corrugations due to fibrillation of the DDFT.

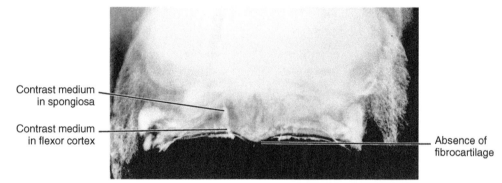

Contrast medium in spongiosa

Contrast medium in flexor cortex

Absence of fibrocartilage

• **Figure 15.9** Navicular bursography of the 17-year-old working Australian Stock Horse mare shown in Figure 15-6 and Figure 15-7. The palmar 45° proximal-palmarodistal oblique radiographic image with contrast medium (3 ml) injected into the navicular bursa. The absence of contrast medium over the central ridge of the flexor surface indicates erosion of the fibrocartilage in this area. The irregular outline and gaps in the contrast medium are consistent with adhesions between the flexor cortex and the deep digital flexor tendon (DDFT) (confirmed at necropsy Figure 15-6). Focal areas of contrast medium in the flexor cortex and spongiosa show there is communication between the bursa and medulla of the bone. The cystlike lesions on the flexor surface, noted at necropsy, align with the focal areas of contrast medium, an indication of the depth and severity of the pathology.

References

1. Dyson, S. J. (2011). Navicular disease. In M. W. Ross & S. J. Dyson (Eds.), *Diagnosis and management of lameness in the horse* (2nd ed., pp. 324–342). St. Louis, MO: Elsevier.
2. Eliashar, E., McGuigan, M. P., & Wilson, A. M. (2004). Relationship of foot conformation and force applied to the navicular bone of sound horses at the trot. *Equine Veterinary Journal, 36,* 431–435.
3. Turner, T. A. (1989). Diagnosis and treatment of the navicular syndrome in horses. *Veterinary Clinics of North America. Equine Practice, 5,* 131–144.
4. Turner, T. A. (2013). How to perform and interpret navicular bursography. *Proceedings of the 59th Annual Convention of the American Association of Equine Practitioners, Nashville, Tennessee, U.S.A., 7–11 December 2013,* 197–202.

16 Midline Toe Cracks

CASE HISTORY 1: FULL-LENGTH TOE CRACKS IN THE FOREFEET OF A MATURE THOROUGHBRED MARE

A mature Thoroughbred mare presented with large toe cracks centered close to the midline of the hoof capsule on both front feet, more severe on the right fore. The cracks extended from the coronary band to the bearing border of both hooves. Close examination of the right fore showed the hoof defect penetrated deeply into the dorsum of the foot with granulation tissue present in the coronary band above the crack. Finger pressure of the coronary band above the crack evoked a prompt pain response.

This hoof capsule showed signs of other pathology. Hoof growth rings were not parallel with the coronary band; they diverged from the dorsum and were wider apart at the heels. In addition, the sole of the right fore was convex instead of the normal concave and was markedly flattened. The sole was protruding below the bearing border of the hoof wall, suggesting that the margin of the distal phalanx (DP) was compressed against the sole horn, and close to physically penetrating the sole. The dorsal aspect of the hoof wall was distorted and dished.

With the exception of the toe crack, these features are often seen in the feet of chronic laminitis cases and reflect failure of the suspensory apparatus of the distal phalanx (SADP), the hallmark of laminitis. This could be the case here, and the presence of the toe crack may be an incidental finding. However, the toe crack itself could have caused the failure of the SADP, resulting in pathology and clinical signs indistinguishable from chronic laminitis.

This raises clinical questions regarding the way in which we manage horses with similar toe cracks. They can be catastrophic, especially in broodmare feet already compromised by endocrinopathic laminitis. This case highlights the need to not only stabilize the hoof but also to mechanically support the foot to prevent mechanical failure of the SADP.

The radiographs of the right forefoot showed significant pathology to both the distal phalanx and the normal anatomic relationship between the DP and the hoof capsule.

The mare was euthanized on humane grounds, and the foot was further evaluated by computed tomography (CT) scanning. The resultant images were used to generate 3-D reconstruction (Mimics models) of the foot using Mimics Materialise software. The generation of Mimics models allowed better assessment of the internal structures of the foot, identification of the full nature and extent of the foot pathologies, and exploration of their interrelationships. The findings were also linked to the clinical signs and the radiographic images.

The Mimics model revealed the presence of extensive divergence between the dorsal aspect of the distal phalanx as well as the dorsal aspect of the hoof wall (so-called capsular rotation). This change to the normal anatomic relationship between bone and hoof wall (anatomic dislocation) was marked by the presence of extensive bone modeling, and bone loss to the distal margin of the DP, seen as the ski-tip at the DP margin.

Mimics models of the distal phalanx revealed the full extent of both the bone modeling and the fracture that had occurred medially around the margin of the bone.

The solear cortex of the DP also displayed marked modeling and bone loss, with a corresponding reduction in the distance between the solear cortex of the bone and the sole horn. There was also a pronounced bulging of the sole horn in the region of the DP distal margin (dropped sole), suggesting imminent penetration of the bone through the sole.

The DP was anatomically dislocated; it had dropped downward into the hoof capsule following failure of the SADP. Either chronic laminitis or the severe toe crack could have caused this, and it is impossible to be certain which at this late stage.

The Mimics model also confirmed that the toe crack extended to the full thickness of the hoof wall in the region of the coronary band. It was also associated with an abnormal, hoof horn, keratoma-like mass, on the inner surface of the hoof capsule. The horn mass may have resulted from the altered pattern of hoof growth due to the toe crack.

There was pronounced new bone formation on either side of the toe crack, which extended into the soft tissues overlying the parietal surface of the DP. Presumably, this occurred in response to increased mechanical loading of the suspensory apparatus on either side of the crack, in an attempt to strengthen these structures in compensation for the absence or reduction of mechanical support in the immediate vicinity of the crack.

In conclusion, although the case displayed a wide range of pathologies consistent with chronic laminitis, it was probably the severe toe crack that compromised the normal mechanical support between the DP and hoof wall, dislocated the bone, and triggered the painful pathologic consequences demonstrated here.

The take-home message is that toe cracks are not minor problems that can be ignored. They should be treated promptly and thoughtfully, correcting the causal dorsopalmar hoof imbalance and stabilizing the crack to prevent its further development.

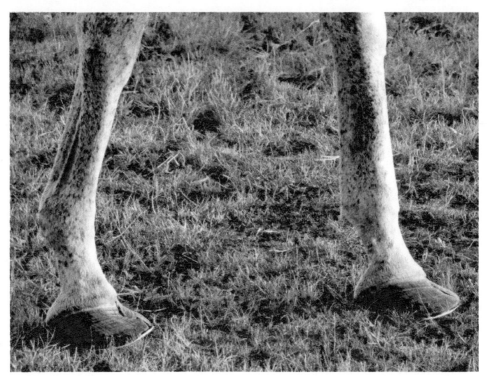

• **Figure 16.1** Case history 1: Toe cracks in the forefeet of a mature Thoroughbred mare. Large midline cracks of the hoof capsule were present in both front feet, more severe on the right. The cracks extended from the coronary band to the bearing border on each hoof.

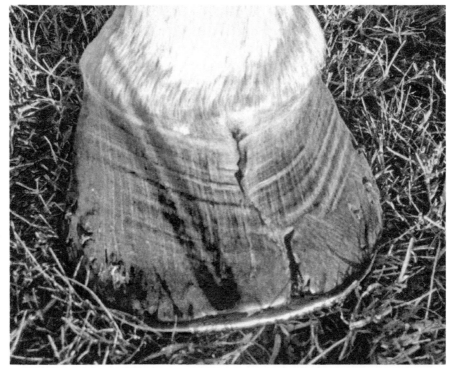

• **Figure 16.2** Case history 1: Toe cracks in the forefeet of a mature Thoroughbred mare. Closer examination of the right forefoot showed that the hoof defect penetrated deep into the hoof wall with granulation tissue present at the coronary band. Pressure on the coronary band above the toe crack evoked a prompt pain response.

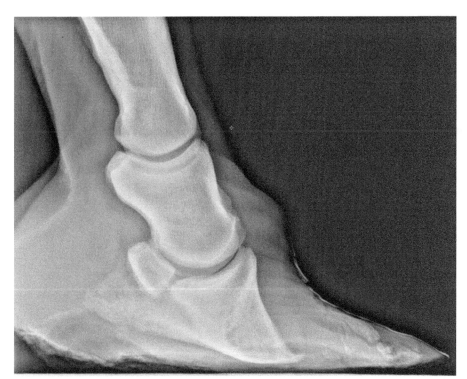

• **Figure 16.3** Case history 1: Toe cracks in the forefeet of a mature Thoroughbred mare. The radiographic image of the right forefoot shows significant pathology to both the distal phalanx and the normal anatomic relationship between the distal phalanx (DP) and the hoof capsule. There is wide separation between the DP and dorsal hoof wall, compression and flattening of the sole by the DP, and remodeling of the margin and solear aspect of the DP. The DP has developed a "ski-tip" at its distal margin. In addition, there is significant angular deviation between the dorsal aspect of the DP and the dorsal aspect of the hoof wall (so-called capsular rotation). In the normal foot the dorsal hoof wall and the parietal dorsal DP are parallel. Capsular rotation is commonly seen in chronic laminitis cases. The radiograph also highlights the dished appearance of the dorsal hoof wall. Note the abnormally close proximity of the solear aspect of the DP and the sole of the hoof capsule, which is in contact with the ground surface. In other words, there is almost zero "sole depth." The solear surface of the bone is abnormally curved and indicates that the compression of bone against the sole has resulted in severe bone modeling and bone loss as a consequence of increased mechanical pressure in this region.

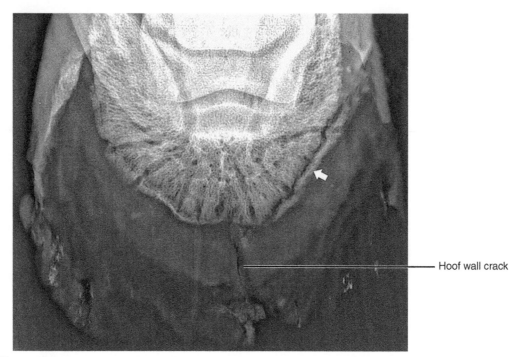

Hoof wall crack

• **Figure 16.4** Case history 1: Toe cracks in the forefeet of a mature Thoroughbred mare. The dorsal 65° proximal-palmarodistal oblique radiographic image further highlights the pathologic changes to the distal margin of the distal phalanx (DP). The bone pathology is due to the increased mechanical pressure among bone, the sole, and the ground surface. The radiograph shows severe bone modeling and bone loss along the distal margin of the DP. The DP is also fractured severely on the medial side (*arrow*) and partially on the lateral side. The fractures are due to the abnormal ground contact pressure. The radiograph also showed the extensive nature of the toe crack; it extends as a black line from the bearing border of the hoof wall, close to the midline of the foot, in the direction of the bone.

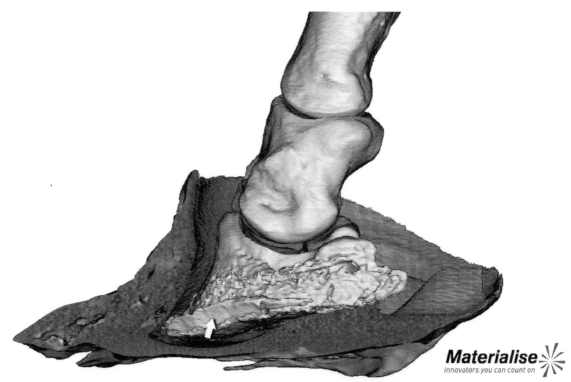

Materialise
innovators you can count on

• **Figure 16.5** Case history 1: Toe cracks in the forefeet of a mature Thoroughbred mare. Mimics reconstruction of the hoof capsule and distal phalanx, shows the rotation of the dorsal hoof wall away from the distal phalanx (capsular rotation). Note flattening of the horny sole and bone modeling and bone loss at the distal margin of the distal phalanx. This image equates to that seen in the lateromedial radiograph. The distal margin of the distal phalanx appears "ski-tipped." However, the Mimics model reveals the size and extent of the medial solear margin fracture (*arrow*), noted in Figure 16-4.

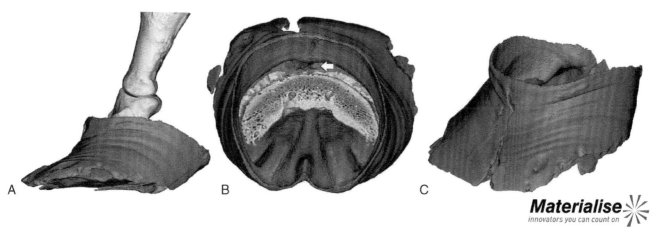

● **Figure 16.6** Case history 1: Toe cracks in the forefeet of a mature Thoroughbred mare. Mimics models of the hoof capsule show its anatomic interrelationships with the osseous structures of the distal limb. Note the partial solear prolapse beneath the dislocated distal margin of the distal phalanx (**A**), the presence of a midline, keratoma-like horn mass on the inner surface of the hoof capsule (*arrow* in **B**) and the full extent of the toe crack proximally (**C**).

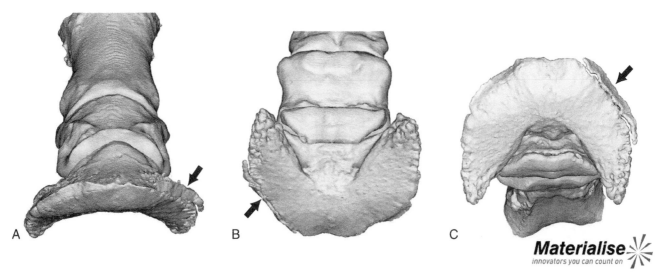

● **Figure 16.7** Case history 1: Toe cracks in the forefeet of a mature Thoroughbred mare. Mimics models of the bones of the distal limb show pronounced new bone formation, apparent as a roughened parietal surface of the distal phalanx (**A**), distal margin bone modeling, bone loss and fracture of the medial (*arrows*) and lateral border of the distal phalanx, and new bone formation (**B** and **C**). The models also revealed other pathologies within the foot, including a small distal border fracture of the navicular bone (**B**).

CASE HISTORY 2: DISTAL TOE CRACKS IN THE FOREFEET OF A THOROUGHBRED BROODMARE

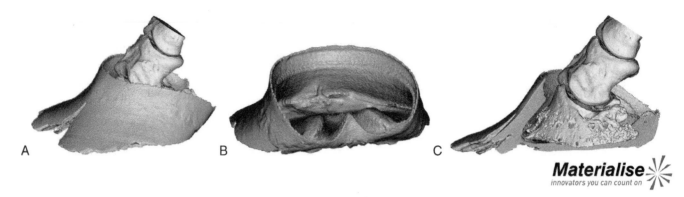

• **Figure 16.8** Case history 2: distal toe crack in the foot of a Thoroughbred broodmare. Mimics models of the hoof capsule with a midline distal toe crack shows the obvious cause of the toe crack; overgrowth of the toe has allowed a midline split to develop (**A**). Viewed from the inside, the crack is more than superficial. Along the crack line internally, a keratoma-like mass is present, involving the distal wall and dorsal sole (**B**). The influence of the epidermal mass has created a "kissing lesion" of bone lysis on the adjacent distal phalanx (**C**).

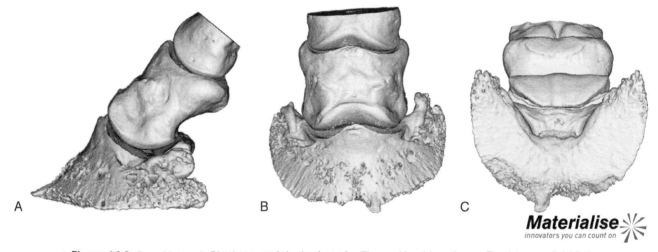

• **Figure 16.9** Case history 2: Distal toe crack in the foot of a Thoroughbred broodmare. The lateromedial Mimics model (**A**) shows a "ski-tip" appearance to the distal phalanx (DP) distal margin: a view replicated by a lateromedial radiograph. However, the dorsal (**B**) and palmar (**C**) views of the model show the true extent of the bone lysis and modeling. A large proportion of the distal margin is missing due to its lysis. In particular, the dorsal solear cortex is destroyed where ground/sole pressure has been applied to the bone.

CASE HISTORY 3: FULL LENGTH TOE CRACKS IN THE FOREFEET OF A QUARTERHORSE STALLION

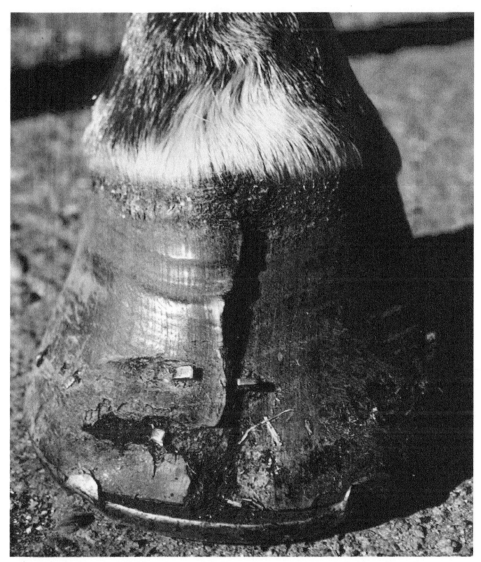

● **Figure 16.10** Case history 3: Full length toe crack in the forefeet of a Quarterhorse stallion. This heavily muscled, bilaterally lame, Quarter Horse stallion had deep cracks in the dorsal hoof walls extending from the hairline to the ground surface of both front feet. In the foot illustrated, the medial and lateral sides of the hoof are moving independently of one another, causing chronic, painful inflammation to the dermal tissues beneath the crack and preventing any hope of healing. The coronet, above the crack, is chronically inflamed and in danger of losing its ability to generate normal hoof wall. A futile attempt has been made to stabilize the crack with a side-clipped shoe and sutures made of horseshoe nails. However, the fault causing this toe crack lies with the style of horseshoeing, which is shown in Figure 16-11.

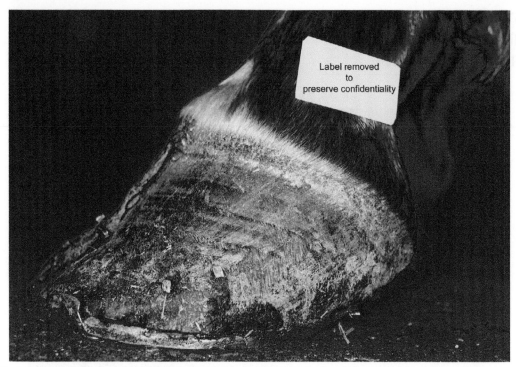

Label removed
to
preserve confidentiality

● **Figure 16.11** Case history 3: Full length toe crack in the forefeet of a Quarterhorse stallion. The toe is too long and has become flared close to the ground surface. The long flared toe has caused the proximal hoof wall to fold inward and develop a central fault line, manifesting as the toe crack. The heels are underrun and growing forward at an acute angle. The shoe is at least one size too small for the foot.

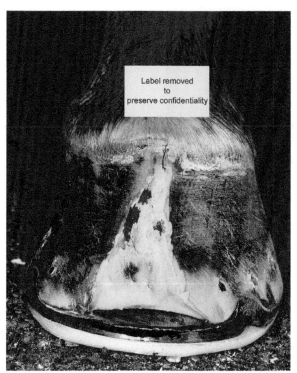

• **Figure 16.12** Case history 3: Full length toe crack in the forefeet of a Quarterhorse stallion. The crack in the dorsal hoof wall was entirely resected using half-round nippers, a motorized rotating bur, and a loop knife. A wide zone of necrotic and degenerate epidermal material was removed as close to the dermis as possible. Side clips were drawn on a shoe to support the medial and lateral halves of the foot. A polyurethane hospital plate has been fitted to the shoe.

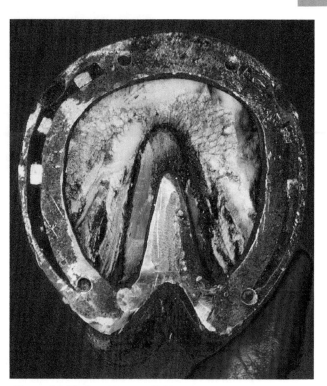

• **Figure 16.13** Case history 3: Full length toe crack in the forefeet of a Quarterhorse stallion. Because a large portion of the toe had been removed, thus weakening the suspensory function of the dorsal hoof wall, a heart bar shoe was fitted to the foot to provide additional foot support. Note the four drilled and tapped holes in the shoe: two at the toe and two at the heels.

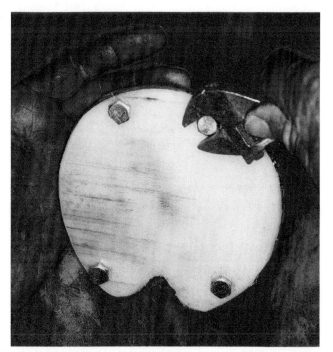

• **Figure 16.14** Case history 3: Full length toe crack in the forefeet of a Quarterhorse stallion. The space between the resected toe and the shoe was in danger of becoming filled with dirt, stones, and other contaminating material. If this occurred, pressure could have developed and damaged the solear dermis and the distal margin of the distal phalanx. In addition, the distal phalanx was close to the surface because of the resection and was in need of protection. To protect the sole of the foot, a dense, polyurethane hospital plate was bolted to the shoe via the holes previously drilled and tapped (Figure 16-13).

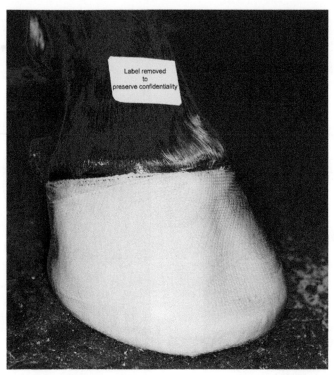

• **Figure 16.15** Case history 3: Full length toe crack in the forefeet of a Quarterhorse stallion. For the coronary epidermis to successfully generate new tubular hoof to replace resected hoof it is essential to stabilize the medial and lateral halves of the foot. This is usually achieved by making a metal rim shoe, a time-consuming process requiring considerable skill. A useful, alternative method is to simply encase the foot and the shoe in a cast made with resin casting tape (Equicast support tape, http://www.equicast.com/). The resin-impregnated tape is activated by immersion in water and wrapped around the foot. Within a few minutes the tape sets hard and effectively immobilizes the entire hoof. Note the felt padding at the heels. This is essential to prevent the tape from causing pressure necrosis at the bulbs of the heels.

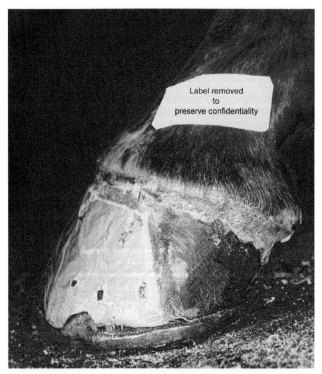

• **Figure 16.16** Case history 3: Full length toe crack in the forefeet of a Quarterhorse stallion· Six weeks later the resin cast was removed and the hoof was healing well. The coronet appeared normal and was generating a band of new hoof wall growing distally, replacing the resected deficit. The resected area of toe was no longer inflamed and cracked and was covered with a thin layer of keratinized epidermis. The owner of the Quarter Horse was eager to commence competition, so the toe was reconstructed with Equilox http://www.equilox.com/. A lateral view of the Equilox-reconstructed toe shows the new, more functional shape of the foot. Compare this view with Fig 16.11.The dorsal hoof wall is now the correct length and shape (not flared), and the heels are growing at an angle parallel to the toe. The shoe is the correct size and is set full at the heels to provide good heel support. A year later, with regular trimming, the hooves of the stallion had recovered to near normal.

CASE HISTORY 4: FULL LENGTH TOE CRACKS IN THE FOREFEET OF A THOROUGHBRED FILLY

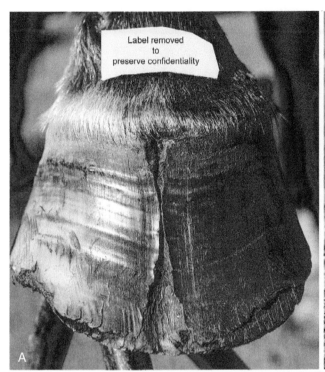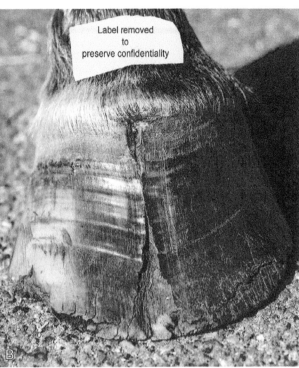

• **Figure 16.17** Case history 4: Full length toe crack in the foot of a Thoroughbred filly. This large, rapidly growing Thoroughbred filly developed dorsal hoof wall cracks in both front feet. The bloodline of this horse contained many horses with similar foot problems, suggesting that poor hoof quality and conformation are heritable. The heels were run-under, and the toe was long and flared. The toe crack was deepest and most severe, 3–4 cm below the coronet; the distal one third of the toe was virtually unaffected. The central fault line, which developed into a crack, appears due to a folding inward of the proximal and middle hoof wall. This principle is illustrated in the photographs **A** and **B**. In **A**, the foot is non–weight bearing and a space separates the medial and lateral halves of the foot. When the foot is weight bearing (**B**), one half of the foot overlaps the other and causes pain and chronic inflammation at the site of the crack. The overlap is greatest in the proximal half of the foot. While this independent movement of each half of the foot is allowed to occur, there is little chance that the toe crack will heal. Equilox (http://www.equilox.com) was used to reconstruct and stabilize the medial and lateral halves of the foot (as shown in Fig 16.6).

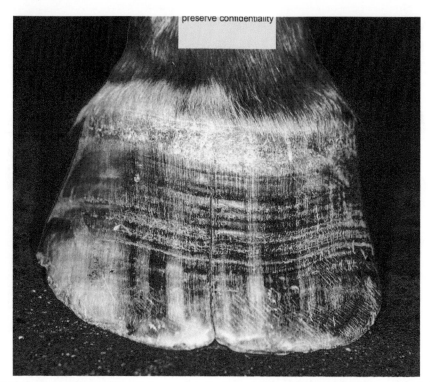

• **Figure 16.18** Case history 4: Full length toe crack in the foot of a Thoroughbred filly. Eight months later the crack and the Equilox (http://www.equilox.com) have grown out, and the mare is sound without shoes. A residual defect remains in the dorsal hoof wall because the original lesion damaged the coronary hoof growth zone of the coronary groove.

17 Seedy Toe ("White Line Disease")

Seedy toe, or "white line disease," is a term describing a separation progressing proximally up the nonpigmented inner hoof wall. The true white line (tubular terminal horn) is not actually involved; however, the misnomer "white line disease" (WLD) has become the accepted term. Pathology is confined to the nonpigmented inner hoof wall epidermis, sparing the epidermal lamellae (the *stratum internum*) and the dermis. Unlike penetrating foreign body infections (e.g., nail pricks), the microorganisms of WLD do not cause abscessation at the coronary band. The hollow cavitation that characterizes WLD can be localized to a small area (a seedy toe) or involve the entire toe from quarter to quarter. Generally, there is no lameness, but severe infections, progressively undermining much of the dorsal hoof wall, may trigger capsular rotation and a dropped sole and

resemble feet with chronic laminitis. Many types of microorganisms (bacteria and fungi) have been cultured from the leading edges of the infection with no clearly defined causative agent. The organisms are keratinophilic and have a predilection for the keratin-rich, soft, moist tubules of the nonpigmented inner hoof wall, a semianaerobic environment. The guiding principles of therapy are to debride and remove the affected hoof wall and clean the diseased epidermis, removing every last contaminated fissure. Support shoeing that recruits the palmar half of the foot for loading and relieves or spares the toe will be required in severe cases. Because the epidermal lamellae are not affected (the opposite of laminitis) and the proximal coronary hoof remains intact, the prognosis associated with prompt and judicious therapy is reasonably good.

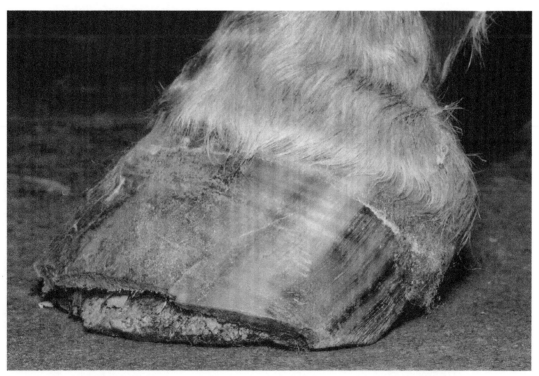

• **Figure 17.1** Australian Stock Horse colt with unilateral white line disease (WLD). There was cavitation beneath the entire dorsal hoof wall of the left forefoot, extending from the bearing border to 2 cm below the coronary band. The distorted, separated hoof capsule was non–weight bearing, and the horse was walking painfully on the exposed sole. The heels and frog of the foot were relatively normal.

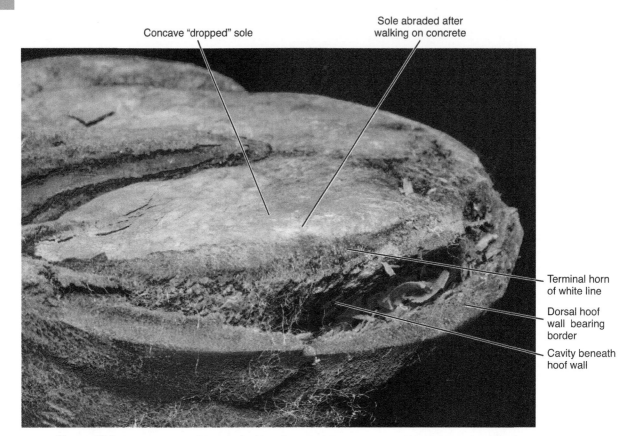

Concave "dropped" sole

Sole abraded after walking on concrete

Terminal horn of white line

Dorsal hoof wall bearing border

Cavity beneath hoof wall

• **Figure 17.2** Australian Stock Horse colt with unilateral white line disease (WLD). The sole of the foot was convex and completely detached from the hoof wall except at the heels. The horn at the circumference of the exposed sole was the dark-yellow color of terminal horn, suggesting that the separation process had affected the nonpigmented inner hoof wall and not the terminal horn of the true white line (i.e., abaxial to the white line). The sole was abraded where it had made contact with the concrete of the examination area.

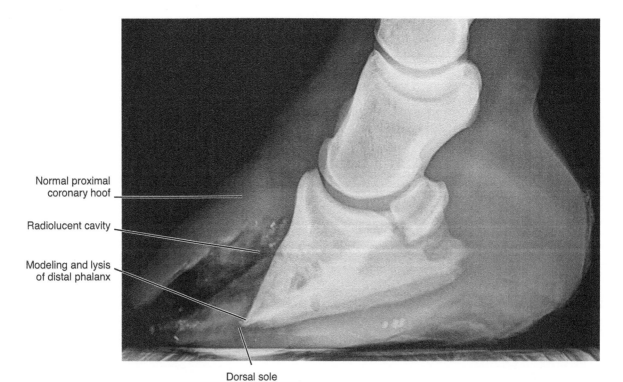

Normal proximal coronary hoof

Radiolucent cavity

Modeling and lysis of distal phalanx

Dorsal sole

• **Figure 17.3** Australian Stock Horse colt with unilateral white line disease (WLD). Latero-medial radiographic image of the foot affected by severe, extensive white line disease. There is capsular rotation of the dorsal hoof wall, and the distal phalanx is abnormally close to the dorsal sole, which is in contact with the ground. There is modeling and lysis of the dorsal margin of the distal phalanx. A large radiolucent cavity is present between the dorsal cortex of the distal phalanx and the inner hoof wall. The proximal extent of the cavity is 2 to 3 cm below the coronary band. (Radiograph by Kylie Schaaf, WestVETS Equine Hospital.)

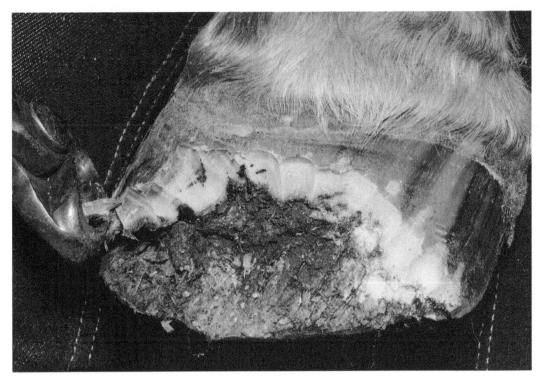

• **Figure 17.4** Australian Stock Horse colt with unilateral white line disease (WLD). Half-round nippers were used to resect the separated dorsal hoof wall. The proximal leading edge of the infection exuded black moist material. Mud and organic debris occupied the cavity.

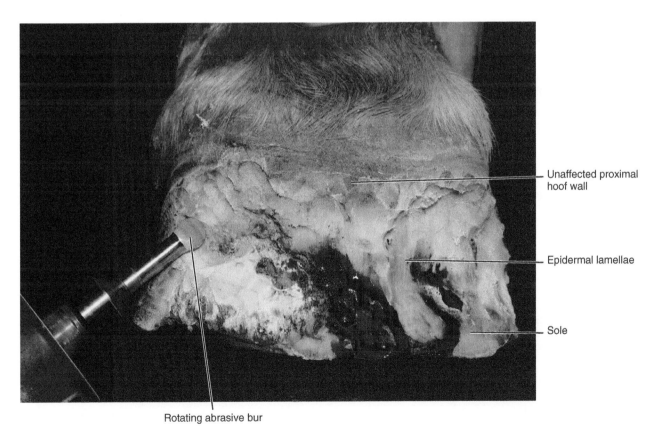

Unaffected proximal hoof wall

Epidermal lamellae

Sole

Rotating abrasive bur

• **Figure 17.5** Australian Stock Horse colt with unilateral white line disease (WLD). A rotating abrasive bur was used to complete the resection, removing all traces of the black infected material noted in Figure 17-3. The depth that the infection penetrated into the lamellar horn varied, and occasional hemorrhage was inevitable. Even minor dermal trauma invoked a sharp pain response, necessitating deep sedation or regional anesthesia to complete the resection procedure safely. The vertical linear pattern of normal epidermal lamellae was visible in some resected zones, corroborating that the lamellar hoof segment is not involved in white line disease. Note the proximal 2 to 3 cm of the coronary hoof is unaffected and available for use in the supportive shoeing strategy.

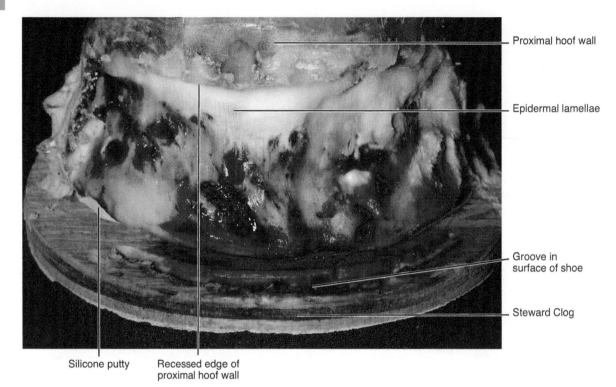

Proximal hoof wall

Epidermal lamellae

Groove in
surface of shoe

Steward Clog

Silicone putty   Recessed edge of
                 proximal hoof wall

• **Figure 17.6** Australian Stock Horse colt with unilateral white line disease (WLD). A wooden Steward Clog* was the initial support shoe chosen to rehabilitate the foot. The heels of the foot were trimmed for weight bearing and attached to the clog using the screw and Equilox technique shown in Figure 14-39. Silicone putty was set beneath the palmar half of the foot. To prevent the dorsal sole from weight bearing, a prosthetic dorsal hoof wall was designed to bridge the proximal hoof wall to the shoe. In preparation for fitting the prosthesis, a semicircular groove was cut into the bearing surface of the shoe and the leading edge of the coronary hoof wall was recessed. (http://www.hopeforsoundness.com/cms/steward-clog-instruction-guide.html)

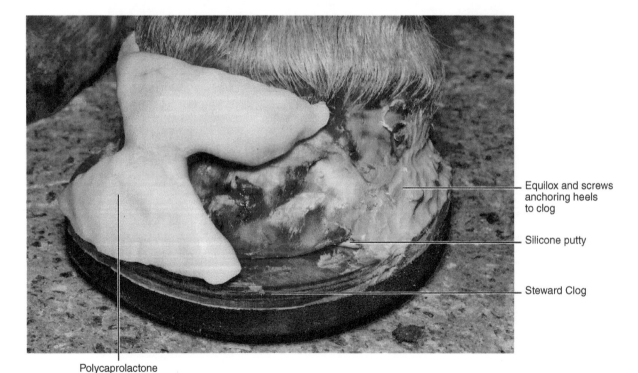

Equilox and screws
anchoring heels
to clog

Silicone putty

Steward Clog

Polycaprolactone
prosthesis

• **Figure 17.7** Australian Stock Horse colt with unilateral white line disease (WLD). A prosthetic dorsal hoof wall was prepared from cold-curing polycaprolactone plastic beads.*† The white beads were placed in hot water and, when transparent, were removed and shaped into a prosthesis that fit between the recess in the proximal hoof wall and the groove in the Steward Clog. When the shape was satisfactory, ice water was applied, curing the plastic into a white, durable, exactly fitting prosthesis. A space was left between the prosthesis and the remaining hoof wall so that medication could be applied in the interval between revisits for reshoeing. (*https://www.instamorph.com/; †http://www.imprintshoes.co.uk/imprint_hoof_repair.htm)

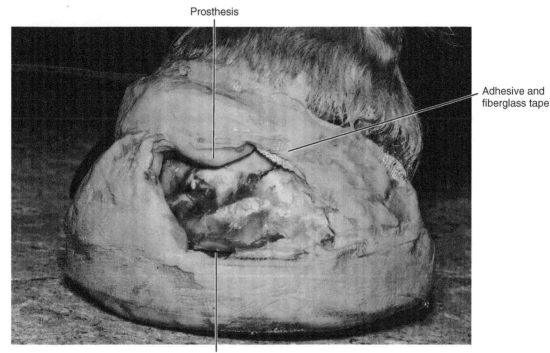

Prosthesis

Adhesive and
fiberglass tape

Space relieving sole pressure
on distal phalanx

● **Figure 17.8** Australian Stock Horse colt with unilateral white line disease (WLD). With the prosthesis in place methylmethacrylate adhesive (Equilox*) and fiberglass tape were applied to secure the prosthesis to both the shoe and the proximal hoof wall. Extra resin and tape anchored the heels to the prosthesis and dorsal hoof wall. Note the space between the dorsal sole and the shoe to relieve sole pressure on the dorsal margin of the distal phalanx. (*http://www. equilox.com/)

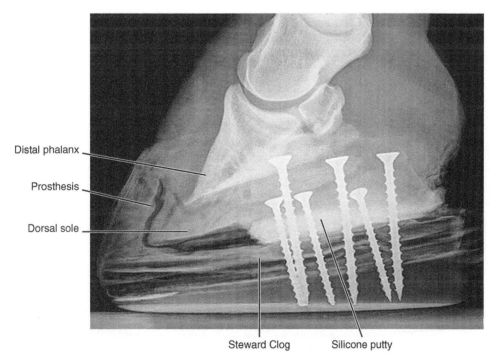

Distal phalanx

Prosthesis

Dorsal sole

Steward Clog   Silicone putty

● **Figure 17.9** Australian Stock Horse colt with unilateral white line disease (WLD). Progress radiographic image of the foot with the prosthesis and therapeutic shoe in place. The shoe has been compressed and worn away dorsally, leaving the heels unintentionally raised. The silicone putty is supporting the palmar half of the foot, relieving the load beneath the dorsal distal phalanx. The original cavity beneath the dorsal hoof wall has been eliminated, and the new dorsal hoof wall growth appears near normal. (Radiograph by Kylie Schaaf, WestVETS Equine Hospital.)

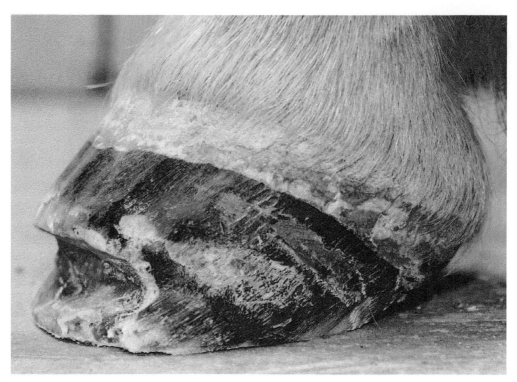

● **Figure 17.10** Australian Stock Horse colt with unilateral white line disease (WLD). Progress photograph taken four months after the initial presentation. Dorsal wall hoof growth is satisfactory with no sign of the cavity caused by the original infection. With sufficient hoof wall now available, the hoof has been prepared for attachment of an aluminium support plate and heart bar shoe.

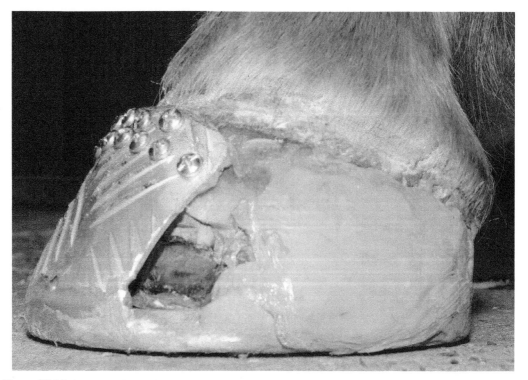

● **Figure 17.11** Australian Stock Horse colt with unilateral white line disease (WLD). An aluminium support plate designed to conform to the proximal dorsal hoof wall has been screwed into place. The base of the plate was welded to the toe of a custom-made aluminium heart bar shoe that has been glued in place at the heels and quarters. Fitted with this support shoe, lameness was abolished at the walk. The stallion was confined to a small yard throughout the eight-month treatment period. Aluminium heart bar shoe and support plate manufactured and fitted by Bruce Donaldson, Australian Certified Farrier.

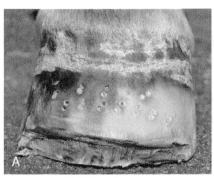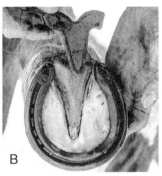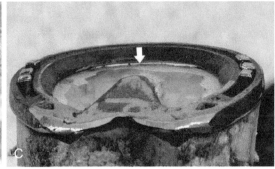

● **Figure 17.12** Australian Stock Horse colt with unilateral white line disease (WLD). Eight months after the initial presentation the dorsal hoof wall was distal to the margin of the distal phalanx (**A**). There was sufficient healthy hoof at the heels and quarters for the nailing on of a steel heart bar shoe. A factory-made steel shoe and frog plate insert were fitted to the bearing border of the hoof (**B**). When welded together the frog plate and shoe formed a heart bar shoe that was nailed in place (**C**). Note the space between the shoe and the hoof toe (*arrow*). This relieved the toe of weight bearing, thus protecting the margin of the distal phalanx. Toe relief was maintained throughout the treatment period. Heart bar shoe manufactured and fitted by Bruce Donaldson, Australian Certified Farrier.

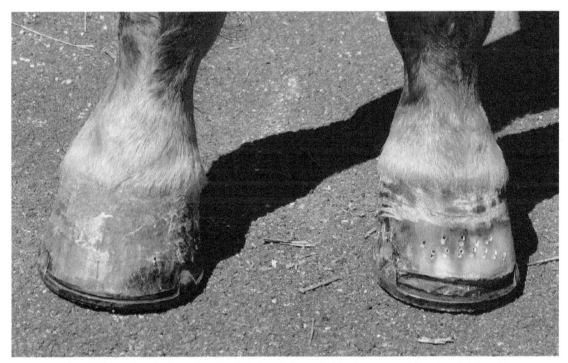

● **Figure 17.13** Australian Stock Horse colt with unilateral white line disease (WLD). Eight months after the initial presentation, with the dorsal hoof wall distal to the margin of the distal phalanx, the horse was shod with a side-clipped heart bar shoe nailed in place. There was no lameness at the walk or trot. The stallion is now a barefoot, working stock horse with a fully recovered left front foot. Farriery by Bruce Donaldson, Australian Certified Farrier.

Ossification of the ungular cartilages is called *sidebone*. Normal cartilages are palpable proximal to the palmar coronary band and, composed of hyaline cartilage, can be flexed with the fingertips. When ossified, the cartilages are palpably hard and rigid. The degree of ossification varies between individual horses. Sidebone is considered rare in light breeds, but common amongst the draft breeds. The cause is speculative, but likely associated with the chronic trauma resulting from unbalanced feet, faulty shoeing, and poor conformation. Ossified ungular cartilages are generally asymptomatic, but may cause lameness if fractured.

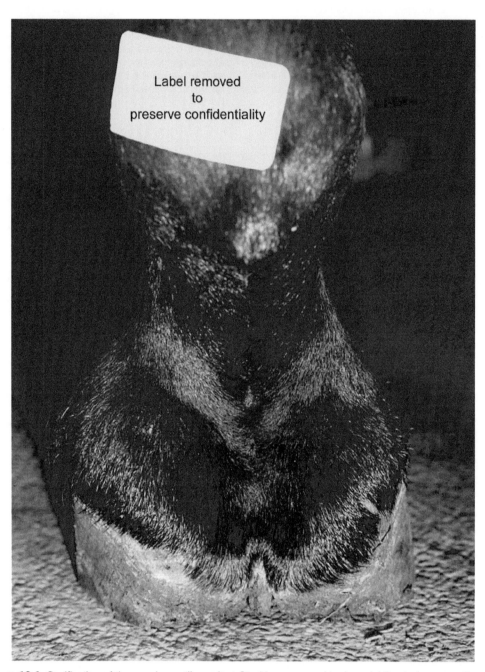

Label removed
to
preserve confidentiality

• **Figure 18.1** Ossification of the ungular cartilages in a Stockhorse mare. Hard, unyielding bulges over the medial and lateral coronets characterize ossification of the ungular cartialges (sidebone). The horse is lame because the medial sidebone has been fractured recently. The mare was put in foal and was able to return to work, free of lameness, when the fracture in the sidebone had re-ossified.

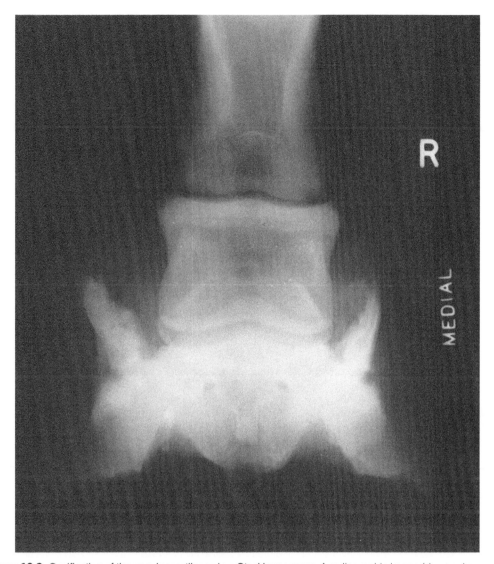

Figure 18.2 Ossification of the ungular cartilages in a Stockhorse mare. A radiographic image (dorsopalmar projection) of the foot in figure 18.1 shows the extensive ossification of both ungular cartilages. The medial sidebone was fractured. Compare this with the radiograph of a foot without ossification of the ungular cartilages in Fig 12.3.

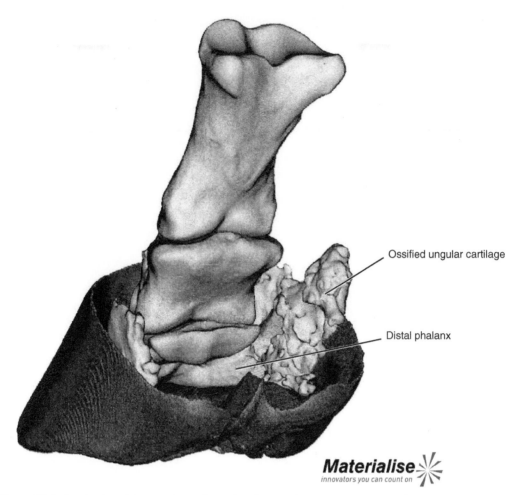

Ossified ungular cartilage

Distal phalanx

Materialise
innovators you can count on

● **Figure 18.3** Ossification of the ungular cartilages in a feral stallion. The replacement of the ungular cartilage with bone (ossification) usually starts along the proximal border of the distal phalanx and is not palpable in its early stages. However, when the ossification becomes extensive the sidebones can be palpated above the coronary border. Generally, sidebones are not a cause of lameness unless trauma causes them to become fractured. Even feral horses develop cartilage ossification, an incidental finding in a brumby stallion in our survey of the feet of 100 feral horse feet.[1,2]

References

1. Hampson, B. A., de Laat, M. A., Mills, P. C., & Pollitt, C. C. (2013). The feral horse foot. Part A: Observational study of the effect of environment on the morphometrics of the feet of 100 Australian feral horses. *Australian Veterinary Journal, 91,* 14–22.

2. Hampson, B. A., de Laat, M. A., Mills, P. C., Walsh, D. M., & Pollitt, C. C. (2013). The feral horse foot. Part B: Radiographic, gross visual and histopathological parameters of foot health in 100 Australian feral horses. *Australian Veterinary Journal, 91,* 23–30.

19 Coronary Band Injury

CORONARY BAND STAKE WOUNDS

Horses competing or working in timbered country are at risk of coronary band stake wounds. When the distal limb is flexed and moving forward, hardwood splinters or small branches enter the coronary band and are deflected beneath the hard proximal edge of the hoof wall. Breaking off short, the stake is sometimes barely visible at the entry site and initially may cause only mild lameness. If left *in situ*, the foreign body soon becomes a painful focus of inflammation and sepsis, and may permanently damage normal hoof wall production. A coronary band stake wound should be regarded as a veterinary emergency, with prompt removal of the foreign body a priority.

Case History 1: Coronary Band Stake Wound to the Foot of an Endurance Horse

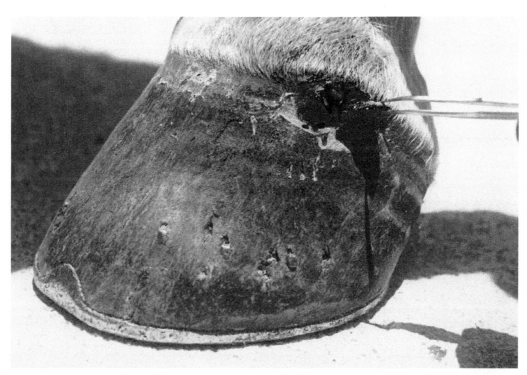

● **Figure 19.1** Coronary band stake wound to the foot of an endurance horse. During training through wooded country, this endurance horse brushed a tree stump and a splinter of wood was driven deep into the coronet of the quarter. The horse did not become lame until after the training ride was completed when the rider broke off a piece of wood projecting from the now obvious wound. Unfortunately, the remainder of the wood (a large piece as it turned out) remained lodged deep in the coronary groove, and the horse remained lame despite antibiotic therapy and rest. Two weeks after the initial injury the palmar nerve on the side of the injury was infiltrated with local anesthetic. The corrupt hoof, around the now discharging sinus, was pared away to expose the wooden stake. The photograph shows it being removed from the wound in the coronet with forceps.

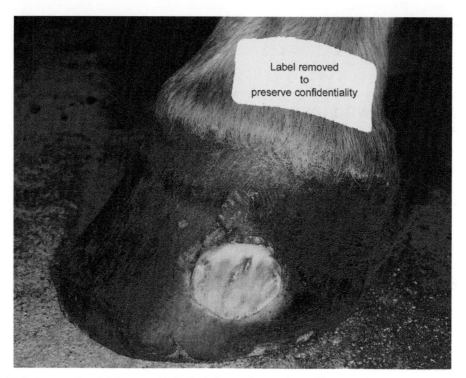

● **Figure 19.2** Coronary band stake wound to the foot of an endurance horse. The same foot as in Fig 19.1 four months later; the trauma and infection of the chronic stake wound to the coronet have left a large defect in the hoof wall. The defect is large because of the sepsis and necrosis that developed while the foreign body remained undetected, deep in the tissues of the coronet. Prompt removal of penetrating foreign bodies and effective treatment of the wound is vital if damage to the sensitive papillae of the coronet is to be avoided.

Case History 2: Coronary Band Stake Wound to the Foot of a Trail Riding Pony

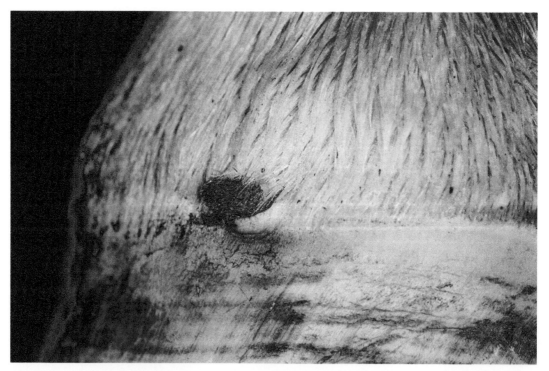

● **Figure 19.3** Coronary band stake wound to the foot of a trail riding pony. A coronary band stake wound occurred to this Pony Club horse during a trail ride in the forest. A piece of wood is visible at the hairline of the coronet; the length of the stake cannot be ascertained at this stage. The horse was quite lame, and veterinary attention was sought later the same day.

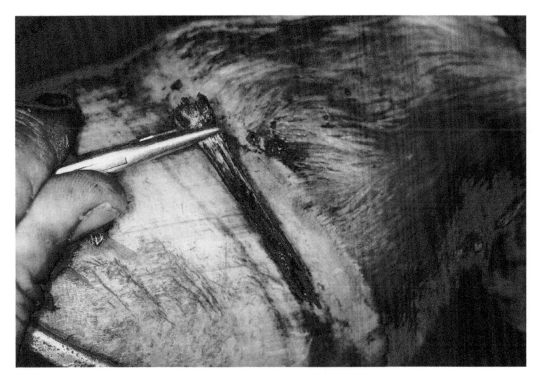

• **Figure 19.4** Coronary band stake wound to the foot of a trail riding pony. The palmar nerve (abaxial sesamoid site) on the side of the wound was infiltrated with local anesthetic, and the stump of the stake was grasped with needle holders. Considerable force was required to extricate the stake, which was notable for its length. After, treatment consisted of a topical dressing, tetanus prophylaxis, and a 3-day course of procaine penicillin, injected intramuscularly twice a day for 3 days. The lameness disappeared within two days. (Photo: Sandra Pollitt.)

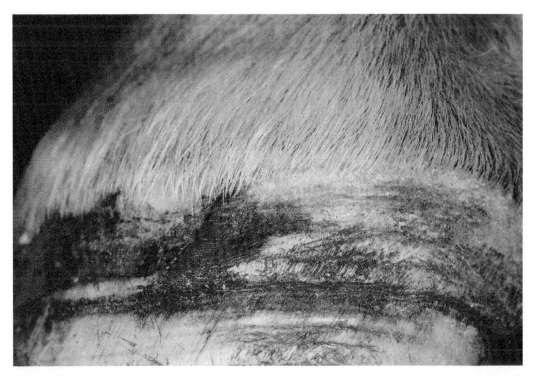

• **Figure 19.5** Coronary band stake wound to the foot of a trail riding pony. Several months later only a small defect is present in the hoof. Prompt, complete removal of the stake and prevention of infection has produced a far better outcome than the neglected case shown in Fig. 19.1.

Horse shoe nails are hammered up into the bearing border of the hoof wall to attach metal horse shoes to the feet of horses. The nails are precisely designed and manufactured, and, when correctly placed and driven, enter and exit the bearing border of the hoof wall without material harm. The sharp tip of the nail is bevelled and, when placed just abaxial to the yellow-colored "white line" (terminal horn) with the bevel facing axially (inwards), each hammer strike drives the shank of the nail obliquely through the hoof wall to exit approximately 20 mm above the bearing border. With the hoof correctly prepared and the nail holes in the fuller of the shoe located according to hoof wall thickness, horseshoes are "nailed on" daily to the feet of thousands of horses around the world with no adverse consequences. However, the horseshoe nail passes close to the terminal and solear papillae in the dermis (corium) of the "white line" and sole respectively, and inadvertent foreign body punctures of these structures leads to infection and abscess formation. Sometimes, the lameness is out of proportion to the size of the lesion and "pricked" horses may hold the infected foot off the ground and be "three-legged" lame.

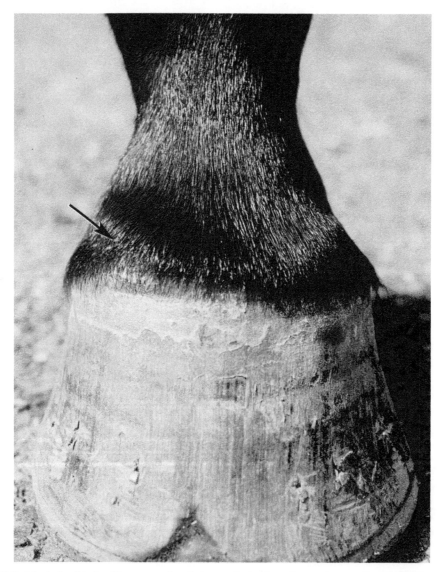

● **Figure 20.1** Infected nail hole with coronary band abscess in the foot of an endurance horse. Five days after shoeing, an acute, severe lameness developed in the right forefoot. The horse was treated for a further three days with intramuscular injections of procaine penicillin and prophylactic tetanus antitoxin, but the degree of lameness worsened. Examined from a distance, the horse was toe pointing and there was a suspicious swelling in the coronet above the lateral toe (*arrow*). In the region of the swelling, the hair of the coronet was erect, exposing the proximal border of the periople. Palpation of the swelling evoked a sharp pain response from the horse.

CASE HISTORY 1: INFECTED NAIL HOLE WITH CORONET ABSCESS

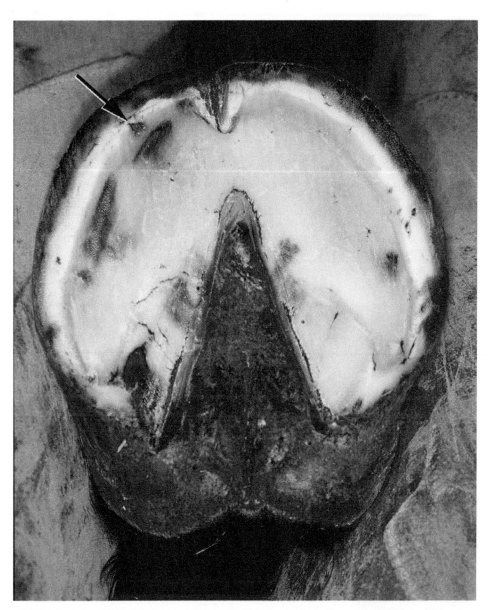

• **Figure 20.2** Infected nail hole with coronary band abscess in the foot of an endurance horse. The shoe was removed, and the sole was carefully pared with a sharp hoof knife. Paying particular attention to the nail holes, any suspicious foci of black necrotic sole were explored and removed with a loop knife. Paring of these suspicious spots was discontinued when removal of the necrotic material revealed normal sole. When paring of the sole was complete, two areas that had obvious deep necrosis remained. One was the central toe crack, and the other was the first nail hole (*arrow*) on the lateral side (directly aligned with the swelling in the coronary band).

Yellow pus flowing from nail hole

Nail incorrectly centered on
the "white line" instead of
the white inner
hoof wall.

Hoof tester

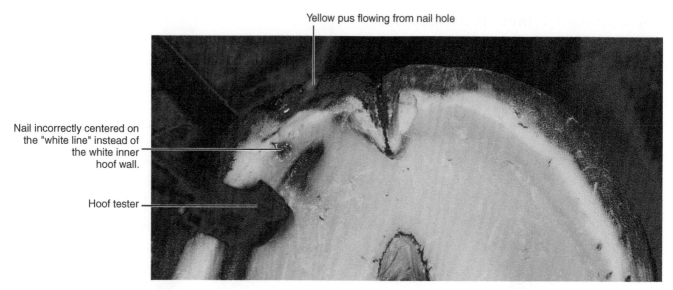

• **Figure 20.3** Infected nail hole with coronary band abscess in the foot of an endurance horse. Using hoof testers to compress the sole, one region at a time, the entire sole was tested. Only the region of the suspect first nail hole caused a pain response from the horse. In fact, sole compression beside the nail hole caused a flow of bubbling, yellow pus from the nail hole. The nail had been incorrectly centered on the yellow terminal horn "white line" and, when driven, had penetrated terminal and solear papillae, thus introducing infection. The nail should have been placed abaxial to the "white line" in the white inner hoof wall.

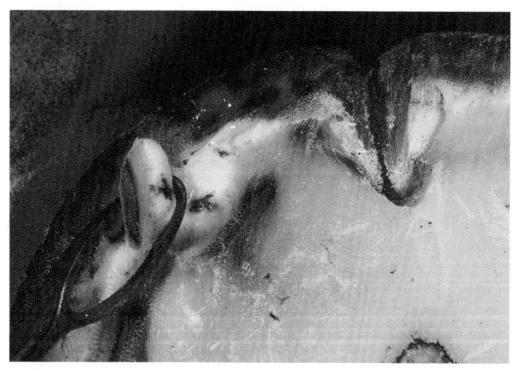

• **Figure 20.4** Infected nail hole with coronary band abscess in the foot of an endurance horse. Drainage of the abscess was established by paring away the hoof adjacent to the nail hole with a sharp loop knife. However, leaving a small drainage hole and calling a halt to proceedings at this stage could have led to an unsatisfactory outcome. The keratinolytic bacteria that establish themselves in hoof abscesses have strict growth requirements, and exposure to air is not one of them. Bearing in mind the likely commitment to protecting the sole with a hospital plate or at least a pad, it is best to continue resection around the abscess until all necrotic, underrun wall and sole are removed.

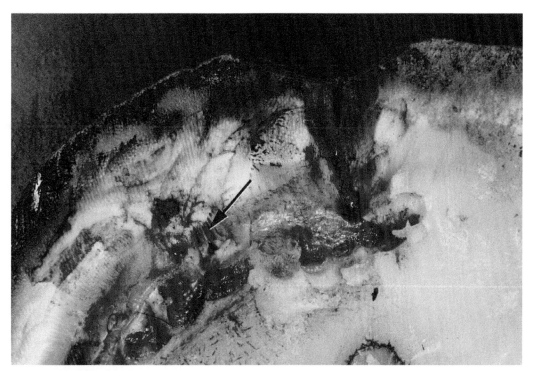

• **Figure 20.5** Infected nail hole with coronary band abscess in the foot of an endurance horse. As is often the case, a surprisingly large area of the sole was underrun by the infection. From one infected nail prick a zone of sole 10 mm × 70 mm was destroyed (almost the entire lateral perimeter of the sole). This is why it is important to fully resect underrun sole infections. It is difficult to predict their full extent, and any pockets left behind have a tendency to seal off and reestablish themselves. The sole resection in this case was done without sedation or local anesthesia. As long as the exposed solar corium is not treated roughly, most horses will tolerate the procedure well. The arrow points to a zone of hoof wall epidermal lamellae, which have been stripped of their dermal attachments by enzymes produced by the infection. These infected lamellae explain the painful swelling at the hairline of the coronet. The bacteria introduced by the nail prick are able to lyse keratin, and they have not only underrun the sole but also used the lamellae as an elevator and gained access to the coronet. It was a safe prediction that the coronary swelling would discharge pus from the hairline within the next few days. The exposed solear corium was dressed with a gauze swab soaked in saline and 2% povidone-iodine. The foot was reshod with a plastic pad covering the sole. No further antibiotic treatment was advised because the resection had resolved the infection. The horse was not lame the next day.

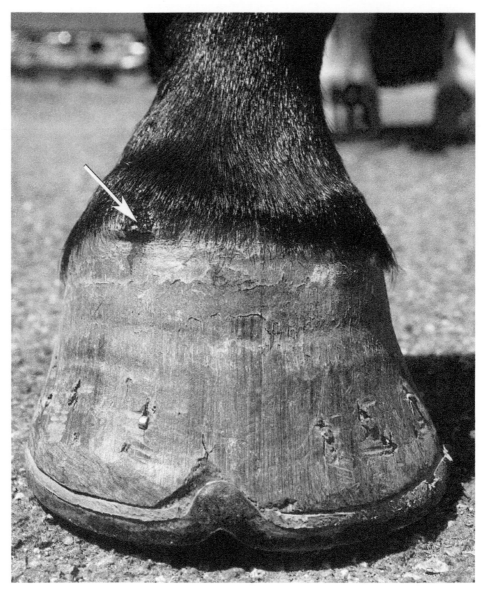

● Figure 20.6 Infected nail hole with coronary band abscess in the foot of an endurance horse. As predicted, an abscess (arrow) formed at the hairline of the coronet, directly aligned with the hoof wall tubules leading to the infected nail hole. The precise location of discharges from the coronet is an important diagnostic point. Sole infections tracking up the hoof wall lamellae to the coronet always discharge at the hairline between the periople and the skin. Note the protective plastic pad between the hoof and the shoe.

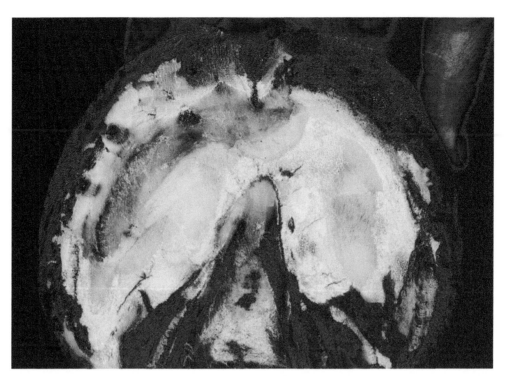

• **Figure 20.7** Infected nail hole with coronary band abscess in the foot of an endurance horse. When examined seven days after the sole resection, the horse was no longer lame. The exposed solear dermis was well covered with a layer of yellow, keratinized epidermis, which was beginning to harden. The horse made an uncomplicated recovery and returned to training three weeks after the resection shod with a protective pad covering the sole. The abscess in the coronary band left a small horizontal defect in the hoof wall, which gradually grew out.

CASE HISTORY 2: INFECTED NAIL HOLE IN THE FOOT OF A COMPETITION HORSE

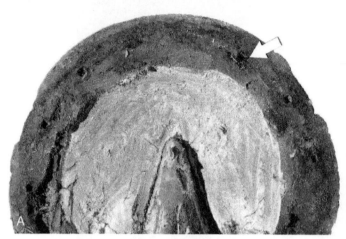
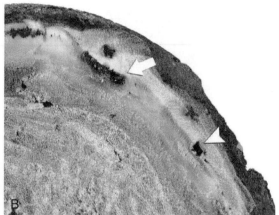

• **Figure 20.8** Infected nail hole in the foot of a competition horse. Two days after routine shoeing with steel competition shoes, this eventing horse became acutely (⅘) lame in the left forefoot. The professional farrier had been shoeing this and other horses for the owner for many years. Nevertheless, the horse reacted to hoof tester pressure over the medial toe and, upon nail and shoe removal (**A**), the medial toe nail hole (arrow) discharged black pus. The sole and the bearing border of the hoof wall (**B**) were pared with a sharp hoof knife, and all the nail holes except the infected one were correctly positioned in the unpigmented inner hoof wall (arrowhead). The infected nail hole was in the terminal horn of the "white line" (arrow) and had likely punctured terminal or sole papillae.

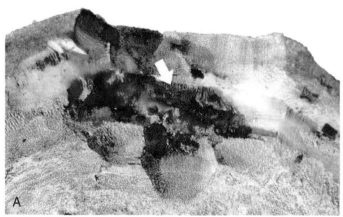
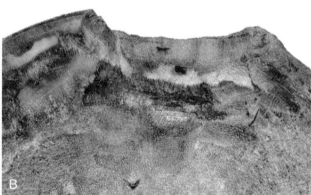

• **Figure 20.9** Infected nail hole in the foot of a competition horse. The hoof wall and sole surrounding the infected nail hole were resected with half round nippers to expose the full extent of the infection (**A**). Necrosis was confined to the lamellae (arrowhead) on either side of the nail hole, and extended up the hoof wall a distance of 15 mm. The sole was not underrun by the infection. The resected area was packed with a povidone-iodine poultice and the foot was wrapped with elastic adhesive tape. The horse was stabled, and received tetanus antiserum and twice daily intramuscular injections of procaine penicillin for five days. The foot dressing and poultice was reapplied every second day, and there was no lameness at the walk. Two weeks after the initial resection, the area was dry and free of discharge (**B**). The foot was reshod a week after that, enabling the horse to return to full work.

Index

261

Printed and bound by CPI Group (UK) Ltd, Croydon, CR0 4YY

08/05/2025

01864668-0001